Quality and Safety in Nursing

A Competency Approach to Improving Outcomes

Second Edition

Edited by

Gwen Sherwood, PhD, RN, FAAN, ANEF
Professor and Associate Dean for Practice and Global Initiatives
School of Nursing
University of North Carolina at Chapel Hill
Chapel Hill, NC

Jane Barnsteiner, PhD, RN, FAAN
Professor Emerita
School of Nursing
University of Pennsylvania
Philadelphia, PA
Editor, Translational Research and QI, American Journal of Nursing

WILEY Blackwell

For general information on our other products and services or for technical support, please contact our Customer Care Department within the United States at (800) 762-2974, outside the United States at (317) 572-3993, or fax (317) 572-4002.

Wiley also publishes its books in a variety of electronic formats. Some content that appears in print may not be available in electronic formats. For more information about Wiley products, visit our Website at www.wiley.com.

Library of Congress Cataloging-in-Publication data applied for:

9781119151678 [paperback]

Cover image: Ralf Hiemisch/Gettyimages
Cover design: Wiley

Set in 10/12pt Warnock by SPi Global, Pondicherry, India

Printed in the United States of America by Sheridan

10 9 8 7 6 5 4 3

To faculty, students, and clinicians who are successfully pioneering the work of QSEN. On a daily basis their work demonstrates their commitment that the highest quality, safest care can only be achieved when all clinicians are delivering *person-and-family-centered care* as members of an *interprofessional team*, emphasizing *evidence-based practice, safety, quality improvement approaches*, and *informatics*.

Contents

Contributors

Editors

Gwen Sherwood, PhD, RN, FAAN, ANEF
Professor and Associate Dean for Practice and
Global Initiatives
School of Nursing
University of North Carolina at Chapel Hill
Chapel Hill, NC

Jane Barnsteiner, PhD, RN, FAAN
Professor Emerita
School of Nursing
University of Pennsylvania
Philadelphia, PA
Editor, Translational Research and QI,
American Journal of Nursing

Contributors

Kathryn R. Alden, EdD, MSN, RN, IBCLC
Associate Professor
School of Nursing
University of North Carolina at Chapel Hill
Chapel Hill, NC

Elizabeth Cerbie Brown, MSN, RN
Director of Nursing Education
Indiana University Health
Indianapolis, IN

Thomas R. Clancy, MBA, PhD, RN, FAAN
Clinical Professor and Associate Dean
Faculty Practice, Partnerships and
Professional Development

School of Nursing
The University of Minnesota
Minneapolis, MN

Linda R. Cronenwett, PhD, RN, FAAN
Dean Emerita and Professor
UNC-Chapel Hill, School of Nursing
Chapel Hill, NC
and
Co-Director, RWJF Executive Nurse Fellows
Program

Lisa Day, PhD, RN, CNE
Associate Professor
Josiah Macy Jr Foundation Faculty Scholar
Duke University School of Nursing
Chapel Hill, NC

Joanne Disch, PhD, RN, FAAN
Professor ad Honorem
University of Minnesota School of Nursing
Minneapolis, MN

Mary A. Dolansky, PhD, RN, FAAN
Associate Professor
Director, QSEN Institute
Frances Payne Bolton School of Nursing
Case Western Reserve University
Cleveland, OH

Carol F. Durham, EdD, RN, ANEF, FAAN
Professor
School of Nursing
University of North Carolina at Chapel Hill
Chapel Hill, NC

Pamela M. Ironside, PhD, RN, FAAN, ANEF
Prairie du Sac, WI

Jean Johnson, PhD, RN, FAAN
Professor, Founding Dean (retired) and
Executive Coach
School of Nursing
George Washington University
Washington, DC

Ellen Luebbers, MD
VA Quality Scholars Fellow
Louis Stokes Cleveland VA Medical Center
Case Western Reserve University School of
Medicine
Cleveland, OH

Shirley M. Moore, PhD, RN, FAAN
Edward J. and Louise Mellen Professor of
Nursing
Frances Payne Bolton School of Nursing
Case Western Reserve University
Cleveland, OH

Mary Jean Schumann, DNP, MBA, RN, CPNP, FAAN
Associate Professor of Nursing and
Senior Associate Dean for Academic Affairs
George Washington University School of
Nursing
Washington, DC

Mamta K. Singh, MD, MS
Associate Professor of Medicine
Case Western Reserve University School of
Medicine
Louis Stokes Cleveland Veterans Affairs
Medical Center
Cleveland, OH

Nancy Spector, PhD, RN, FAAN
Director of Regulatory Innovations
National Council of State Boards of Nursing
Chicago, IL

Mary Fran Tracy, PhD, RN, APRN, CNS, FAAN
Associate Professor/Nurse Scientist
University of Minnesota School of Nursing
University of Minnesota Medical Center
Minneapolis, MN

Beth T. Ulrich, EdD, RN, FACHE, FAAN
Professor, University of Texas Health Science
Center at Houston School of Nursing
Editor, *Nephrology Nursing Journal*
Pearland, TX

Mary K. Walton, MSN, MBE, RN
Director, Patient and Family Centered Care;
Nurse Ethicist
Hospital of the University of Pennsylvania
Adjunct Assistant Professor of Medical Ethics
and Health Policy
Perelman School of Medicine
University of Pennsylvania
Philadelphia, PA

Judith J. Warren, PhD, RN, BC, FAAN, FACMI
Consultant, Warren Associates, LLC
Plattsmouth, NE

Amy Hagedorn Wonder, PhD, RN
Assistant Professor
Indiana University School of Nursing
Bloomington, IN

Foreword

The Carnegie Foundation for the Advancement of Teaching's Preparation for the Professions Program called out important changes needed in the preparation for professional work in medicine, nursing, law, engineering, and the clergy. Professor Patricia Benner led the team for nursing (Benner *et al.*, 2010). They began by noting that profound changes were occurring in the practice of the nursing professional that were arising from science, technology, patient activism, market-driven financing of health care service, and in the settings where these forces come together and where nurses now practice. They noted a practice-to-education gap characterized by the need to match learning with the realities of the work that nursing professionals face. This book begins to address that gap by opening the knowledge and skills needed to understand and improve these new practice settings of nursing.

All professions earn societal recognition as a "profession" by the ongoing improvement of their own work (Houle, 1980). But as Benner and colleagues (2010) note, improving health care service now isn't easy or simple. Health care service for patients and populations today occurs in complex, interdependent systems (Batalden, Ogrinc, and Batalden, 2006). Designing and testing changes for improvement in those systems requires new knowledge and skill. This book is about developing those competencies essential for a sense of professional mastery.

"Doing quality improvement" is not necessarily the same as "improving the quality of what we do"–the profession-enabling work. This is not the work of a small department of zealots who staff offices to meet regulations; it is part of the work of every person who claims designation today as a health care professional.

Improving the quality, safety, and value of health care service invites the use of multiple knowledge disciplines (Batalden *et al.*, 2011). Diverse knowledge-building traditions from biological, social, and physical sciences and the humanities come together to contribute to the development of the knowledge and science of improvement. This book is about those knowledge domains and invites attention to the scholarly and applied work of educators and researchers who develop and foster critical thinking about improving health care.

At the core of professional work in service of improving health for a patient is a series of interactions that can be represented by the simple logic formula:

Generalizable science X Particular patient → Measured improvement.

Each element of this logic comes together millions of times every day as clinical health professionals do their work.

We can use a similar logic representation for improving health care service:

(Individual, population goal + Generalizable science) X Particular context → Measured performance improvement.

Each phrase or symbol of this simple logic formula is informed by knowledge that is developed and tested in customized ways. Because all health care service is co-produced by two parties, the person we know as a "patient" and the person we know as a "health care professional," the process begins by creating a shared aim (Batalden *et al.* 2015). The shared aim comes from knowledge of the goal sought by the patient and identification of the contribution that the professional's generalizable knowledge can offer. They work together. Good professional knowledge about "generalizable science" is developed by carefully controlling and minimizing "context" as a variable. In contrast, particular context knowledge comes from obsessing about context, that is, the systems, processes, traditions, patterns, and so forth, that characterize and give "particular" identity to contexts. Measuring performance improvement means measuring over time–not just at two points in time–and it means using balanced measures to understand the multidimensional aspects of quality, safety, and value of process and outcome of health care service. Even the symbols represent knowledge domains. The "+" sign signifies knowing how to match the contribution that the professional's science can make to the realization of the patient's goal. The "X" signifies the important role that context plays in the results of the shared work. The "→" represents the knowledge of actually executing change–making it happen. Each part and symbol of the formula invites a different way of knowing, and they must all come together to make change for the improvement of health care service. (Batalden and Davidoff, 2007).

Benner and her colleagues (2010) also note that nurses have very diverse entries, pathways, curricula, and time frames to become a nurse. This book invites attention to that diversity by focusing on the content of what must be mastered–the competencies themselves. As health professions engage in competency-based learning, it will be important to avoid reducing all the content that is signaled by the competencies into mechanical packages that fail to invite the whole person to the learning and its application in relationship to another person in need.

What is important in health care service is reducing the burden of illness for individuals and populations. The people, and what they are struggling to do together, is what is real in health care. Together they form some relationship and engage in some activity. This relationship and activity are connected by knowledge, skill, and habit. The intervention for improving health care service quality, safety, and value is a social change that is learned experientially (Batalden *et al.*, 2011). Improvement theories, methods, tools, and techniques are all potentially helpful, but we must never confuse them with the work of improving health care service, lest we make an error similar to the one of confusing a map for the territory it represents.

Creating work environments that sustain the generative, refreshing work of improving health care service involves the inextricable linkage of three aims and invites the work of everyone, illustrated in Figure F.1 (Batalden and Foster, 2012). Health care professionals have an opportunity to help design and weave these together.

It is often noted by practicing nurses and other clinicians that their job is to protect the patient from the system of health care service in which the patient and clinician meet. This frames responsibility for the design of the system and its ongoing improvement as external to the working professional on the front lines of health care service. I prefer a different view of professional work, one that accepts the professional responsibility for health care service system quality, safety, and value. This book can help nurses and other clinicians who are not content to work in alien systems.

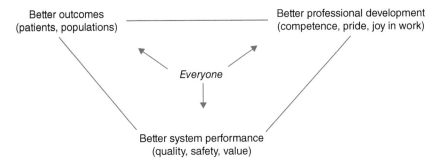

Figure F.1 Creating work environments for improving health care service.

A nurse who was a member of a class I was teaching many years ago said it very succinctly: "We actually have two jobs–to do our work and to improve it."

This book invites the work of improving health care, the work that helps make health care workers professionals. Enjoy it.

Paul Batalden, M.D.
Emeritus Professor, The Dartmouth Institute for
Health Policy and Clinical Practice
Dartmouth Medical School
Lebanon, New Hampshire
USA

References

Batalden, M., Batalden, P. Margolis, P., Seid, M., Armstrong, G., Opipari-Arrigan, L., and Hartung H. (2015) Coproduction of healthcare service. *BMJ Quality & Safety,* Published Online First [15 September 2015] doi:10.1136/bmjqs 2015 004315.

Batalden, P., Bate, P., Webb, D., and McLoughlin, V. (2011) Planning and leading a multidisciplinary colloquium to explore the epistemology of improvement. *BMJ Quality & Safety,* 20, i1–i4.

Batalden, P., and Davidoff, F. (2007) What is quality improvement and how can it transform healthcare? *Quality & Safety in Health Care,* 16, 2–3.

Batalden, P., Davidoff, F., Marshall, M., Bibby, J., and Pink, C. (2011) So what? Now what? Exploring, understanding and using the epistemologies that inform the improvement of health care. *BMJ Quality & Safety,* 20, i99–i105.

Batalden, P. and Foster, T. (eds.) (2012) Sustainably Improving Health Care: Creatively Linking Care Outcomes, System Performance, and Professional Development. London: Radcliffe.

Batalden, P., Ogrinc, G., and Batalden, M. (2006) From one to many. *Journal of Interprofessional Care,* 20, 549–551.

Benner, P., Sutphen, M., Leonard, V., and Day L. (2010) Educating nurses: A call for radical transformation. San Francisco: Jossey-Bass.

Houle, C.O. (1980) Continuing learning in the professions. San Francisco: Jossey-Bass.

Preface

The synergy inspired by the Quality and Safety Education for Nursing (QSEN) project over the past decade is leading the transformation of nursing education and practice to improve quality and safety of health care (Cronenwett *et al.*, 2007; Cronenwett *et al.*, 2009). Through a series of grants from the Robert Wood Johnson Foundation between 2005 and 2012, the QSEN project was led by a steering team, a national expert panel, and an advisory board who identified the knowledge, skills, and attitudes (KSA) for the six competencies first identified by the Institute of Medicine (IOM) think tank (2003): patient-centered care, teamwork and collaboration, evidence-based practice, quality improvement, safety, and informatics. With the second edition of this seminal text, we celebrate the continuing journey to improve our health care systems launched 11 years ago by a group of pioneers who helped identify and lead early adopters through four phases of QSEN.

The original two dozen pioneers who launched QSEN expanded to 40 champions who became QSEN facilitators (www.qsen.org) and then to hundreds of educators, clinicians, and administrators who led the Pilot Schools Learning Collaborative, the American Association of Colleges of Nursing (AACN)/QSEN Faculty Development Institutes, and countless projects. Although transformation has been swift and pervasive in many settings, many gaps remain. The six quality and safety competencies from the QSEN project are firmly embedded in nursing education essential competencies in both the National League for Nurses and the AACN documents and are spreading globally across education and clinical settings. A train-the-trainer approach helped spread educational approaches, preparing thousands of nursing faculty to integrate the new KSAs for the six core competencies. The passion to improve health care has transformed into new education models and teaching strategies, clinical initiatives and applications, evidence-based practices, and safety cultures.

Faculty and clinicians are embracing a new way of thinking about quality and safety; new partnerships are evolving across professions and among academic and service agencies creating a bold new vision for health professions, education, and practice. Consumers and health care professionals both recognize that health care in America remains far from ideal, but believing joint efforts among educators and clinicians across multiple professions can together make it better.

Quality and safety are universal values in health care; nurses in both education and practice settings have the *will* through a common value system if they are helped to develop the *ideas* for leading change, and are provided the tools to *execute* the change needed and in fact are inspired by the opportunity to work in systems focused on safe quality care.

Education is indeed the bridge to quality (IOM, 2003), and progress comes with each generation of nurses prepared with the competencies to work in and lead health care systems focused on safety: patient-centered care, teamwork and collaboration, quality improvement, safety, evidence-based practice, and informatics. Have we reached a tipping point? Nurse leaders have long recognized the imperative to improve patient care outcomes and have been a part of early quality improvement work within nursing. Safety and patient-centered care have been recognized as cornerstones of effective nursing practice, but with new evidence, a science of safety and quality improvement provide a sharper focus to quality and safety initiatives.

The expanded version of this book seeks to address the needs of faculty, practicing nurses, administrators, and nursing students at all educational levels. Each chapter tells a part of the story and collectively offers a roadmap to improve quality and safety. Updated information in each chapter provides a current view of application of quality and safety; consumer efforts driving change are found in Chapter 2; and Chapter 3 presents the first person account from Dr. Cronenwett of how QSEN began as well as the continuing story of this award-winning project to become the QSEN Institute at Case Western Reserve University School of Nursing. Section 2 includes an in-depth current view of each of the six competencies. The chapters provide a resource for faculty, graduate students, practicing nurses, and other leaders including teaching strategies, resources, and current references. Section 3 has redesigned chapters on implementing quality and safety across settings. A revised chapter is provided on the mirror of education and practice to better understand teaching approaches for redesigning teaching approaches. Other instructional approaches include narrative pedagogy, integrating the competencies in simulation, a new chapter to explore application in clinical learning, the critical nature of interprofessional teamwork to improve quality and safety, and developing personal leadership to lead change in organizations focused on improving quality and safety. The last chapter examines global applications of quality and safety, and outlines the need for sharing strategies related to education, research, and practice changes around the world. Three appendices provide additional resources with the knowledge, skills, and attitudes tables for each of the prelicensure and graduate competencies, the results of a Delphi study to assist educators with placing the 162 KSAs for beginner, middle, and advanced placement in nursing programs and staff development, and an extensive glossary.

Each contributor is a leader in quality and safety and offers his or her work to stimulate all nurses and health care professionals to share and disseminate their work around the globe. Together, we hope to rebuild health care as a high-reliability system focused on safety and quality. It is our hope that the shared and expanding story of QSEN provides motivation and *will*, that the expansive tool kit within these pages stimulates *ideas*, and that the continuing efforts for faculty and leader development translate to *execution* as we move toward new generations of nurses fully prepared to lead and work in health care systems based on cultures of quality and safety.

Gwen Sherwood, PhD, RN, FAAN, ANEF
Jane Barnsteiner, PhD, RN, FAAN
Coeditors

Section 1

Quality and Safety

An Overview

Driving Forces for Quality and Safety

Changing Mindsets to Improve Health Care

Gwen Sherwood, PhD, RN, FAAN, ANEF

Julia stashed her umbrella and looked at the overflowing waiting room of the Emergency Department (ED) where she had worked weekends for the past five years. It was summer and staffing was short even for a Sunday evening in August; several staff were on vacation and one called in sick. A storm had pounded the area, and there was a power outage. The hospital was on the emergency generators, and that meant the electronic chart was slow in response because of the overload. Staff were taking shortcuts due to time pressures. She thought about these breakdowns and remembered the workshop she recently attended on quality improvement. The focus had been on identifying problems and applying quality improvement tools to collect data on the problem, analyze results, and design solutions to close the gap between actual and desired practice. She noted that Ms. Masraf was in the waiting area; she had diabetes, and wounds were difficult to heal. Infection was a constant threat so she had been to the emergency department on several occasions. Julia turned at the sound of a crash and saw that one of the nurse aids had fallen where water had collected from wet umbrellas. Falls were common in the ED as a result of the population served. Patients may be unstable due to their disease condition or influence of alcohol or drug use. She wondered if she could initiate a quality improvement study on any of these continuing problems she saw every time she came to work. Other staff seemed to think this was just a part of how the emergency room functioned.

In 1999, the Institute of Medicine (IOM), a not-for-profit organization sponsored by the United States National Academy of Sciences, released *To Err Is Human* (2000), which estimated there were between 44,000 and 98,000 deaths each year as a result of medical harm. Makary and Daniel (2016) declare this number is both limited and out of date. Their projection released in 2016 cites the deaths due to medical error is more likely 251,454, making this the third leading cause of death in the United States. Since the IOM series of reports focused attention on the issues in health care quality and safety, responses have included regulatory changes, new roles and responsibilities for health care professionals, and calls for a new educational paradigm. Still, health care safety remains a major threat (Balik and Dopkiss, 2010; Cronenwett, 2012; Leape and Berwick, 2005; Wachter, 2004; Wachter, 2010).

The original 1999 report was the first evidence of the gap between the status of health care delivered and the quality of health care that the IOM panel believed Americans were entitled to receive. A number of reports have heralded ways to improve the system of care. The 2001 *Crossing the Quality Chasm: A New Health System for the 21st Century* issued recommendations for sweeping changes in

Quality and Safety in Nursing: A Competency Approach to Improving Outcomes, Second Edition.
Edited by Gwen Sherwood and Jane Barnsteiner.
© 2017 John Wiley & Sons, Inc. Published 2017 by John Wiley & Sons, Inc.

our systems. This was followed by the 2003 IOM report, *Health Professions Education: A Bridge to Quality*, which called for a radical redesign of health professions education to achieve six core competencies described as essential to improve twenty-first century health care: patient-centered care, teamwork and collaboration, evidence-based practice, quality improvement, safety, and informatics. The attention from the series of IOM reports over the past 15 years demonstrates that quality and safety are the leading contemporary issues in health care, contributing to costs and poor outcomes. Current health care reform in the United States is based on improving quality outcomes; health care mistakes cost the system between $17 billion and 29 billion each year and costs patients and families economically but also emotionally and physically. Providers who work in flawed systems and deal with inadequate resources experience dissatisfaction and low morale. For all, there is an erosion of trust from the pitfalls experienced.

Health professions education continues to undergo transformation to include preparation in the knowledge, skills, and attitudes (KSA) needed to improve our systems of care (Batalden, Leach, and Ogrinc, 2009; Cronenwett *et al.*, 2007). In 2011, representatives of the major health professions worked together to reach consensus on four domains of interprofessional education competencies that crosswalk these competencies for improving quality and safety: roles and responsibilities, teamwork, communication, and ethics and values (Interprofessional Education Collaborative [IPEC], 2011).

The same questions from 15 years ago continue to need solutions. What are issues in redesigning our systems of care? How do we prepare health professionals with what they need to know and do? How can organizations develop cultures of quality and safety? This chapter will examine the impact of the driving forces for the changes needed, application of quality and safety science to reframe organizational cultures for quality improvement and safety, and a fresh look at how these reframe the education needs for nurses. In a safety culture, the paradigm shifts from individual performance to system initiatives and redesigns to monitor outcomes of care, and situates the patient as a full partner in care.

The Compelling Case for Quality and Safety

When the initial data revealed in the IOM Quality Chasm series of reports became public it, sent shock waves throughout the industry and grabbed the attention of consumers (Textbox 1.1). The evidence reported in this series identified the imperative for changing mindsets to include quality and safety as part of the everyday work of nurses and other health professionals. Prior to release of the first report in 1999, the issues were wrapped in silence; without a reporting system, there was not an evidence base to establish the scope or depth of system issues that contributed to poor quality and safety. There was no national tracking system and little pressure to improve quality and safety outcomes from regulators, health care purchasers, or third-party payers. And, without just culture emphasis, there was little transparency or accountability in sharing information with patients and families who experienced harm.

The 2001 IOM report, *Bridging the Quality Chasm*, identified the STEEEP model to improve health care quality and safety. STEEEP outlines performance measures to assure care is safe, timely, effective, efficient, equitable, and patient centered. These aims provide the measures of quality and accountability that continue to elude health care. Although the United States spends more than any other country on health care, the system has significant shortcomings, particularly in efficiency, quality, access, safety, and affordability (Davis, Schoen, and Stremikis, 2010). The fragmentation and decentralization of the health care system is a barrier to quality and safety; for example, patients may see multiple providers who may not be able to share critical patient information due to a lack of technology infrastructure or have a feeling of ownership that precludes sharing and consultation.

Although most data are based on acute care in patient settings, errors can occur in physician offices, outpatient settings, nursing homes, patient homes, and so forth. An annotation of the reports with their recommendations is provided in Textbox 1.1.

Textbox 1.1 Summary: The Institute of Medicine Quality Chasm Series (www.iom.edu)

- *To Err Is Human: Building a Safer Health System* (2000)
  This first IOM report presented the first aggregate data on the depth and breadth of quality and safety issues in US hospitals. Analysis of outcomes from hospitals in Colorado and Utah concluded that 44,000 people die each year as a result of medical errors and that in New York hospitals, the number is 98,000. Even using the lower number, more people die annually from medical error than from motor vehicle accidents, breast cancer, or AIDS. Medical errors are the leading cause of unexpected deaths in health care settings. Communication is the root cause of 65% of sentinel events. The report presents a strategy for reducing preventable medical errors with a goal of a 50% reduction over five years.
- *Crossing the Quality Chasm: A New Health System for the 21st Century* (2001)
  The IOM issued a call for sweeping reform of the American health care system. A set of performance expectations for twenty-first century health care seeks to assure that patient care is STEEEP. These aims provide the measures of quality to align incentives for payment and accountability based on quality improvements. The report includes causes of quality gaps and barriers to improve care. Health care organizations are analyzed as complex systems with recommendations for how system approaches can help implement change.
- *Health Professions Education: A Bridge to Quality* (2003)
  Education is declared as the bridge to quality based on five competencies identified as essential for health professionals of the twenty-first century: patient-centered care, teamwork and collaboration, evidence-based practice, quality improvement (and safety), and informatics. Recommendations include developing a common language to use across disciplines, integrating learning experiences, developing evidence-based curricula and teaching approaches, initiating faculty development to model the core competencies, and implementing plans to monitor continued proficiency in the competencies.
- *Keeping Patients Safe: Transforming the Work Environment of Nurses* (2004)
  The 2004 IOM report links nurses and their work environment with patient safety and quality of care. The findings of this report have helped shape the role of nurses in patient care quality and safety efforts. Key recommendations are creating a satisfying and rewarding work environment for nurses, providing adequate nurse staffing, focusing on patient safety at the level of organizational governing boards, incorporating evidence-based management in the management of nursing services, building trust between nurses and organizational leaders, giving nurses a voice in patient care delivery through effective nursing leadership and participation in executive decision-making, providing organizational support to promote learning for both new and experienced nurses, promoting interdisciplinary collaboration, and designing work environments and culture that promote patient safety.
- *Identifying and Preventing Medication Errors* (2006)
  Medication errors make up the largest category of error with as many as 3–4% of patients experiencing a serious medical error while hospitalized. This report presents a national agenda for reducing medication errors and the huge costs associated with medication errors. Changes across the health care industry require collaboration from doctors, nurses, pharmacists, the Food and Drug Administration and other government agencies, hospitals and other health care organizations, and patients.

The data are startling, particularly related to medication errors, one of the most common according to *Identifying and Preventing Medication Errors* (Aspen *et al.*, 2007). Medication errors particularly impact nurses. Nurses have the primary responsibility for medication administration with patients in a complex environment. Medication errors account for over 7,000 deaths annually. On average, inpatients may experience at least one medication error per day. At least 1.5 million preventable adverse drug events occur each year. Almost 2% of admissions experience a preventable adverse drug event, which increases hospital costs by $4,700 per admission or about $2.8 million annually for a 700-bed hospital; multiplied, this would account for $2 billion nationally.

The costs associated with quality and safety are complex; accounting includes lost income, health care costs, and other expenses. The national cost for preventable adverse events ranges between $17 billion and $29 billion; additional health care accounts for more than half of these totals because tests and treatments may have to be repeated or others added, and patients may need to extend their hospital stay. In addition to these costs, there are intangible, immeasurable costs, such as patients may suffer or be inconvenienced, have lower satisfaction with care, and lose trust in the system. Most of what is known about the financial and other burdens are hospital related. Data are just beginning to emerge on costs associated with quality and safety across the continuum of care, including ambulatory, home health care, and skilled care.

Health care workers are also affected by the quality of care in the systems in which they work. They may experience loss of morale and lower satisfaction when they are not able to provide the best care possible. *Keeping Patients Safe: Transforming the Work Environment of Nurses* (Page, 2004) is a comprehensive analysis of the factors influencing nurses' work. Health care is value based; as professionals we pledge, first, to do no harm. Quality is an essential value. Professionals take pride in doing the right thing, but quality is more than *will*; it is a mindset of inquiry and the capacity to use appropriate tools to improve systems in which we work. Quality improvement intersects all areas of health care from economic issues to the moral basis undergirding quality for doing our best. It builds on the shared values and moral commitment common to all health professionals. Health professionals have the motivation and ability to *improve* systems if they have the necessary education and training and work in organizations where quality improvement is integrated as part of daily work.

Consumers have helped motivate changes in health care. Patients and families who experienced adverse events have called for reform in how health care systems identify, investigate, report, and share information related to errors. Patients and families who experience health care mistakes leverage their influence to prevent similar events happening to others. National organizations such as the National Patient Safety Foundation (NPSF) (www.npsf.org) serve both consumers and health professionals. Numerous nonprofit organizations created in response to adverse events focus attention on particular care delivery issues as well as broader issues, establishing patient advocacy with an increasing influence in health care. Many patients or their family members now serve on hospital boards or consumer panels, share their stories in learning situations, and bring growing pressures to have systematic participation in all areas of health care.

The health care industry is applying lessons from other industries, particularly those known as high-reliability organizations (www.ahrq.gov). A key difference is that most other industries that have had dramatic improvements in quality and safety were supported by a designated agency that sets and communicates goals, brings visibility, and systematically collects and analyzes error reports for root cause analysis; however, health care lacks a single designated agency, as responsibilities are spread among various groups. Although numerous agencies have emerged to promote the safety and quality agenda, none have the purpose of collecting safety or quality data for systematic analysis with broad dissemination to assure that best practice and safety alerts are implemented across all settings. Schumann (2017) offers a summary of these federal, regulatory, professional, and consumer agencies and organizations.

With lack of information on which errors occur and how they occur, and systematic dissemination of the information we do have, health care has lagged behind other high-risk industries in establishing a safety focus. Aviation has focused on safety for more than 50 years with significant reduction in fatalities. Health care has adopted and adapted principles and approaches from aviation as well as other high-reliability organizations that have similar characteristics, such as intermittent, intense tasks that demand exacting responses. By systematically collecting data on sentinel events for review through standardized processes, these industries have been able to monitor and improve safety in their systems.

Health care delivery organizations have a significant role in safety. Systems are a set of interdependent components that interact to achieve a common goal. For example, a hospital is a system composed of service lines, nursing care units, ancillary care departments, outpatient care clinics, and so forth. The way in which these separate but united system components interact and work together is a significant factor in delivering high-quality, safe care. Organizational leadership helps align quality and safety goals with mission and vision so that it is practiced consistently throughout all areas and levels of the system (Triolo, 2012). High-reliability organizations focus on safety; it is pervasive in their culture to be mindful of where the next error may occur to increase vigilance, establish check lists, or implement other preventions (Barnsteiner, 2012).

Examining Familiar Terms: The Science of Quality and Safety

Quality and safety are intertwined, complex concepts with multiple dimensions. Lack of a comprehensive understanding of the full scope of these terms is but one barrier for implementing quality and safety strategies. It is difficult to reshape the mental model of these broad terms held by health care workers and change attitudes about the necessity of focusing on safety. Overcoming these historic views and overuse of the terms are part of the application of the new KSAs associated with the science of quality and safety.

Though interrelated, quality and safety comprise different concepts. Quality improvement uses data to monitor outcomes of care processes that help guide improvement methods to design and test changes in the system to continuously improve outcomes (Compas, Hopkins, and Townsley, 2008; Johnson, 2017). The goal of quality is to reach for the best practice, and the goal is determined by measuring the reality of the care delivered compared with benchmarks or the ideal outcome. Continuous quality monitoring is the mechanism by which the health care system can be transformed through the collaboration of health care professionals, patients and their families, researchers, payers, planners, and educators. All are working toward a triangle of improvements that lead to better patient outcomes (health), better system performance (care), and better professional development (education) (Bataldan and Davidoff, 2007). All health professionals must know how to assess the scientific evidence to determine what constitutes good care, identify gaps between good care and care delivered in their setting, and implement actions to close gaps (Sherwood and Jones, 2011).

Safety science embraces an organizational framework to minimize risk of harm to patients and providers through both system effectiveness and individual performance by applying human factors as discussed more fully by Barnsteiner in another chapter (2017) and Sammer and colleagues (2010). Safety science builds on Reason's human error trajectory, which uses the model of lining up a stick through the holes of Swiss cheese; sometimes redundancies in the system fail, and all the holes line up (2000).

Error is the failure of a planned action to be completed as intended or the use of an incorrect plan to achieve an aim. Reason identified two kinds of failure that constitute error:

1) Error of execution in which the correct action does not proceed as intended
2) Error of planning in which the original intended action is not correct

An adverse event is the injury that results from care delivered or from care management, not from the underlying patient condition or the reason the patient was seeking care. Preventable adverse events are those attributed to error. There are also various types of errors. Diagnostic errors delay diagnosis, prevent use of appropriate tests, or result in failure to act. Treatment errors can occur while administering treatment, include errors in administering medication, lead to avoidable delay in treatment or response to treatment, or contribute to inappropriate care. Other examples are failure to provide prophylactic treatment, inadequate monitoring or follow-up, failure to communicate, equipment malfunction, or other system failure.

Errors can be defined in multiple ways with varied components. It is a challenge to develop a unified reporting system that can be used across settings or nationally, in the same way that the aviation industry aggregates reports of airline events. Inconsistent nomenclature of a long list of terms adds to the difficulty of consistently reporting similar events in a central system. Organizations with a culture of safety have implemented processes through risk management to collect error reports for root cause analysis, often classifying them using a tiered system of potential for harm. Carefully detailing all steps and decisions leading to an error or near miss can formulate a system redesign of processes that lessens the chance of future occurrence. The focus is on improving the system to prevent future errors rather than merely blaming individuals. Exploring what happened acknowledges the influence of complex systems and human factors that influence safety. In a just culture, the focus is to determine what went wrong rather than identifying exactly who committed the error to establish blame and punishment. Just culture establishes an environment in which errors and near misses are acknowledged, reported, and analyzed for ways to improve the system. Accountability remains a critical aspect of a culture of safety; recognizing and acknowledging one's actions is a trademark of professional behavior.

Nurses are in the forefront of examining the work environment to identify quality and safety issues and the influence of human factors, the interrelationship between people, technology, and the environment in which they work (Page, 2004). Human factors consider the ability or inability to perform exacting tasks while attending to multiple tasks at once. For system improvements, organizational leadership must give attention to human factors such as managing workload fluctuations, seeking strategies to minimize interruptions in work, and attending to communication and care coordination across disciplines. Nurses manage care coordination and employ checklists and other strategies to assure safe hand-offs between providers and settings. Nurses are challenged by other human factors that impact quality and safety, such as multitasking, distractions, fatigue, task fixation that limits environmental scanning, and hierarchy and authority gradients. Staffing, interpersonal relationships, and the lack of education on quality and safety are among the multiple human factors that impact quality and safety.

Assuring quality and safety involves more than individual accountability; poorly designed protocols and system designs also contribute to quality and safety outcomes (Hughes, 2008). The best way to reduce health care harm is by preventing errors before they happen. Focusing on safety helps eliminate discrepancies in care that result from provider actions in delivering care. Safety huddles or safety briefings are becoming a part of daily routine in many hospitals to identify and focus on high risk situations.

Quality improvement is a critical component of safety—it requires assessing safety issues for prevalence, making comparisons across units or departments, and using benchmark data to help clinicians improve their own practice as well as that of the system. When principles and strategies from quality improvement are applied, the rate of medication errors occurring in a given setting can be measured and compared with a peer unit or industry benchmark. Root cause analysis can determine reasons for errors in medication administration to change the system to prevent or lessen the possibility of errors occurring.

National Organizations for Quality and Safety

Many of the improvements in our health care systems are the result of regulatory mandates from groups such as the Joint Commission (www.jointcommission.org), which grants institutional accreditation and opens the possibility of different aspects of federal funding (Wachter, 2004; Wachter, 2010). The Joint Commission also established the National Patient Safety Goals that are updated annually. The goals provide guidance in key areas of high vulnerability and share evidence for solutions by emphasizing a systematic process for quality improvement, patient safety, and monitoring outcomes. The Joint Commission also established regulations to eliminate disruptive behavior among health care professionals and required organizations to have a code of conduct to define acceptable and inappropriate behavior as well as a process for managing such behaviors.

The Institute for Healthcare Improvement (IHI) (www.ihi.org) is a strong advocate for quality and safety innovations, bringing collaboration among all professions. The IHI's 100,000 and 5 Million Lives campaigns are just two examples of focused collective efforts for improving outcomes. IHI describes the goals of health care reform in the US as the Triple Aim: improve population health, reduce costs, and improve the quality of care (Berwick, Nolan, and Whittington, 2014). These goals align with the STEEEP model from the IOM (2001) and also place new demands on health care professions education programs to prepare a workforce capable of changing the system (Reeves *et al.*, 2013). New skills for interprofessional care, quality and process improvement, and population health management-meaning educational institutions must align with practices, health systems and the communities they serve (Brandt *et al.*, 2014). The work of the Affordable Care Act seeks reform and redesign of the systems of care to provide better care, align cost and value, and improve outcomes. Professional nursing organizations have responded to the imperative to improve quality and safety in health care systems (Earnest and Brandt, 2014).

Schumann (2017) provides a comprehensive description of national groups and their goals of quality and safety. The American Nurses Association, following a long history of promoting quality assurance, and the International Council of Nurses (2002) developed a new framework on quality improvement distributed nationally and globally (Doran, 2010). The Magnet recognition program based standards on continuous quality improvement to recognize nursing leadership and organizational quality in nursing care delivery (Triolo, 2012). The standards reinforce conditions in the organization and practice environment that support and facilitate nursing excellence. Recognition is linked to improvement in nurse recruitment, retention, quality outcomes, and patient satisfaction scores. The American Nurses Association also established the National Database of Nursing Quality Indicators in 1998, which maintains data on sustained improvement in a designated nursing-sensitive indicator such as staffing, hospital-acquired pressure ulcers, falls and prevention of injury from falls, staff satisfaction, and pediatric and psychiatric mental health data (Montalvo and Dunton, 2007; Schumann, 2017).

Federal programs in Medicare and Medicaid have helped define nurses' roles and revised the payment structure for health care. Medicare and Medicaid subsequently developed programs to reduce hospital-acquired conditions, or those conditions that were not present at the time of a patient's hospital admission (Bodrock and Mion, 2008; Centers for Medicare and Medicaid Services, 2008). Hospitals are no longer reimbursed for 10 preventable hospital-acquired conditions, many of which were part of nursing care interventions (Hines and Yu, 2009). Other third-party payers and large employers have "pay for performance" plans in which health systems receive additional economic incentives when specific quality targets are met, many of which are nurse driven.

Comparing Progress to Improve Quality and Safety

The IOM (2001) issued four recommendations to change the system:

- Create a national focus through leadership, research, tool kits, and protocols to enhance knowledge about safety.
- Identify and learn from errors by establishing a vigorous error reporting system to assure a safer health care system.
- Increase standards and expectations for safety improvements through oversight groups, professional organizations, and health care purchasers.
- Improve the safety system within health care organizations to assure care improves.

Improvements to quality and safety have been slow and uneven. Two progress reports 5 years and 10 years after the release of *To Err Is Human* (IOM, 2000) examine progress based on these goals. Longo *et al.* (2005) used a 91-item survey to assess changes over time between two survey points in 2002 ($N = 126$) and 2004 ($N = 128$) in hospitals in Missouri and Utah that had collaborated on a patient safety project funded by the Agency for Healthcare Research and Quality (AHRQ). Assessment included seven variables: computerized physician order entry systems and test results, and assessments of safety procedures; specific safety policies; use of data in patient safety programs; drug handling procedures; manner of handling adverse events reporting; prevention policies; and root cause analysis. Five years after the initial report, hospitals were still not satisfactorily meeting the IOM recommendations. Progress is slow, and technology applications that could improve safety lag.

Another study (Wachter, 2004) measured five areas of patient safety five years after the initial release of the IOM data and also reported slow progress in addressing safety and quality goals. Robust regulations had an initial impact on early improvements, but that impact slowed quickly because regulations alone do not result in lasting change. Progress was noted in information technology applications and workforce organization and training. Still, there was little demonstrable impact from early error reporting systems and only small improvement in accountability. At five years after the initial galvanizing report, Wachter concluded, "we are at the end of the beginning," meaning much work remains.

In 2010 Wachter assessed10-year progress following publication of *To Err Is Human* (2000). Using a report card grading system from A (highest) to D (lowest), he assessed 10 key patient safety domains based on 1999–2004 and 2004–2009. Overall, Wachter graded the progress in safety as a B–, a modest improvement from a C+ based on data in the 2004 report. Leadership engagement from provider organizations and reporting systems were gauged as having made the most progress. There is a stronger business case for hospitals to concentrate on their safety efforts due to stronger accreditation standards and error reporting requirements. Interventions across national and international organizations receive the highest grade, including major campaigns from groups such as IHI, AHRQ, the Joint Commission, the National Quality Forum, and the World Health Organization. Few hospitals have moved to fully implement information technology applications. More systems are implementing a safety culture that balances no blame with accountability. Research is advancing in spite of inadequate funding. Progress in workforce and training is limited as few organizations have robust teamwork or culture change, but some impact has been felt from reducing residents' duty hours and easing of the nursing shortage. Patient engagement and involvement remains small, with more progress related to disclosure policies and procedures, also addressed by Balik and Dopkiss (2010). Payment system intervention is uncertain, as pay for performance is only beginning. Wachter concludes that our limited ability to measure safety outcomes is a major barrier to progress.

Measuring the impact of quality and safety efforts is challenging, particularly patient deaths due to preventable harm because of its hidden nature; it sometimes depends on providers being willing to share exactly what happened, varying definitions of what is reportable, and fear of punishment. Since the 1999 IOM report, several studies have issued projections of patient deaths due to preventable harm from a health care encounter.

Inpatient deaths between 2000 and 2002 based on AHRQ Patient Safety Indicators in a Medicare population estimated 575,000 deaths extrapolated to 175,000 per year (Health Grades, 2004). A 2008 report from the Inspector General reported 180,000 deaths annually among Medicare inpatients (Department of Health and Human Services [HHS], 2008). Classen *et al.* (2008) projected roughly 400,000 deaths per year; Landrigan *et al.* (2010) studied North Carolina inpatients over six years and estimated 134,581 deaths; James (2013) projected a range of 250,000 to 400,000 per year, and, as noted earlier, Makary and Daniel (2016) estimated 251,454. These reports demonstrate the challenges in accurate numbers because of reporting issues, and as Makary and Daniel note, there is no diagnosis for death from medical error on death certificates, which they used for their report. Regardless of the exact number, these reports, like the report cards above, indicate change is coming slowly in trying to reduce patient harm due to error. Still, with any number above zero, work remains to be done.

Other indicators show promise. A focused effort implemented by The Joint Commission (2014) reduced patient falls by 35% in seven hospitals. Between 2010 and 2013, there was a 17% decline in hospital-acquired conditions, and 50,000 fewer patients died, saving $12 billion in health care costs.

Many nursing organizations have identified and developed programs to improve quality and safety. For example, the American Association of Critical-Care Nurses (2010) developed multiple approaches including a program on healthy work environments focused on teamwork and collaboration. Competencies were developed for prelicensure and graduate nurses by the Quality and Safety Education for Nurses (QSEN) project (Cronenwett, 2012). The Nursing Alliance for Quality Care (Schumann, 2017) was formed to bring one organized nursing voice to ensure that (a) patients receive the right care at the right time by the right professional; (b) nurses actively advocate and are accountable for consumer-centered, high-quality health care; and (c) policymakers recognize the contributions of nurses in advancing consumer-centered, high-quality health care.

A Systems Approach to Improve Quality and Safety Outcomes: High Reliability Organizations

High-reliability organizations (HRO) have effectively applied a systems approach toward quality and safety. Error prevention shifts from the individual to a shared accountability across the system, which assures errors are analyzed through root cause analyses. Understanding how the adverse event trajectory occurred allows the system to reconsider protocols, procedures, or other actions that will reduce the possibility of a repeat error. The National Patient Safety Foundation (NPSF, 2014) has defined health care errors as unintended health care outcomes caused by a defect in care delivery to a patient, therefore a shared system accountability for patient harm. To prevent harm to patients, organizations adopt operational systems and processes that minimize risk and focus on maximizing interception of errors before harm occurs. Safe care, in fact, is preventing harm to patients during the care that is intended to help them; preventable harm involves errors that could have been avoided through reasonable actions and decisions (Sherwood and Armstrong, 2016).

HROs emphasize just culture as a feature of a safety culture (Oster and Braaten). A non-punitive approach to patient harm is built on the engagement and commitment of everyone from the board room to all staff to accountability, honesty, integrity, and mutual respect in a just culture. Accountability is a critical aspect of a culture of safety; recognizing and acknowledging one's actions is a trademark of professional behavior. All staff are trained and empowered to participate in an error-reporting system without fear of punitive action. Near misses are treated as opportunities to improve by examining gaps and correcting design flaws. Safety principles to eliminate hazards guide job design, management of equipment, and working conditions.

Simplifying and standardizing processes are key components of high reliability organizations so that results are predictable, thus improving reliability. Reliability is expecting to get the same result each time an action occurs; therefore, a reliable system seeks to have defect-free operations in spite of a high risk environment. Health care delivery has intersecting units or microsystems. How these systems function together impacts quality and safety outcomes. For instance, the way patients are assigned beds from the ED to one of the inpatient units, or how the lab responds in urgent situations to the need for blood draws, or how patients are discharged to a skilled nursing facility are opportunities for standardized operational procedures to improve effective outcomes. Five principles guide HROs: sensitivity to operations, preoccupation with failure, reluctance to simplify, deference to expertise, and commitment to resilience. Reliability has economic consequences. Hospital reimbursement is increasingly tied to quality and safety outcomes (Schumann, 2017). Hospitals may not be reimbursed for patient harms such as hospital-acquired infections, therefore reliable procedures are needed to insure adherence to hand-washing procedures, evidence-based catheter insertion and care guidelines, and other evidence-based best practices.

Nurses on the Frontlines: Changing Mindsets, Improving Quality and Safety

Although quality and safety improvements are goals for practitioners in all levels and areas of health care, nurses have particular roles. The IOM website has the following quote from the 2010 report *The Future of Nursing: Leading Change, Advancing Health*:

> Overcoming challenges in nursing is essential to overcoming the challenges in the health care system as a whole. Nurses are the largest segment of the health care workforce, and their skills and availability can directly affect quality, safety, and efficiency. Most nurses work in hospitals or other acute settings, where they are patients' primary, professional caregivers and the individuals most likely to intercept medical errors. However, because hospital systems and acute care settings are often complex and chaotic, many nurses spend unnecessary time hunting for supplies, filling out paperwork, and coordinating staff time and patient care, reducing the time they are able to spend with patients and delivering care.

Considering the scope of the recommendations and the limited progress, what are ways that nurses can help lead innovations to achieve the goals of the IOM Quality Chasm series? Wachter's (2010) review of progress to achieve the IOM recommendations cites moderate progress in addressing workforce and training issues, reporting systems, and research. What does it mean for nursing? Three primary goals can guide nurses in leading change. First, all nurses must develop a mindset of questioning to constantly improve their work and increase their capacity to recognize and acknowledge quality and safety issues in their own work and in the systems in which they work. Second, educational programs must be transformed to address quality and safety competencies to help learners with changes in KSAs. Third, advancing scholarship to determine best practices in education, practice, and systems applications will establish an evidence base to implement effective approaches to transform health care.

Changing Mindset: Inquiry Leading Change

Increasing nurses' awareness of quality and safety developed within new science applications will help nurses recognize quality and safety concerns in their practice and in their settings. Many remain largely unaware of the scope of the problems and have not been taught how to identify, report, and systematically analyze a near-miss or sentinel event or lead a quality improvement team (Chenot and Daniel, 2010). Learning the concepts of new safety science refocuses how errors are reported. Rather than using incident reports to establish blame on an individual provider, organizations committed to quality and safety create a culture in which nurses and other professionals are empowered to disclose near misses and mistakes through a reporting system, and to identify areas in which outcomes do not match benchmarks.

A mindset of inquiry, of asking questions is the first step in change for leading improvements in the system. We must be open and receptive to feedback and be able to see the consequences of our actions and be willing to change. Reflective practice is a change process using systematic questions to examine experiences in the context of what one knows and values, other perspectives, and situational context (Horton-Deutsch and Sherwood, 2008). Asking questions opens the way to innovative approaches, application of evidence-based practice standards, and various methods of quality improvement.

It is a challenge, however, to build the awareness that empowers nurses to make the first step and acknowledge a near miss or mistake. Nurses then need to know what to report, and how, as well as how to follow the steps in the organization's safety plan. In a just culture, there is a shift from establishing blame and punishing someone for a mistake to a systematic analysis for the purpose of learning and change. All providers who had any part in the event come together, led by trained professionals, to establish the chain of actions, decisions, and circumstances that may have contributed to an error so there is the opportunity to learn and develop system changes to prevent future occurrences. Patients and their families should be informed and included in the process to achieve transparency in the system, to have full disclosure of the event. Quality improvement teams can collect information to monitor occurrences of the problem in other parts of the system, compare data, and initiate strategies to eliminate variances.

Asking questions can be used in another way. Conducting an annual safety culture survey identifies areas for workplace improvement and determines priorities for improving quality. Scorecards, dashboards, or report cards are strategies to collect and monitor data about services and care provided to track key areas. In academic settings, educators establish a culture of safety and quality for their own educational processes such as a reporting system of learner near misses and errors to assess processes and increase safety awareness.

Transform Education to Integrate Competencies

The second focus area is transforming nursing education to integrate the competencies based on the KSAs developed from the QSEN project (Cronenwett, 2012). The project goal for the QSEN project in the United States (www.qsen.org) is to (a) change the mindset of nurses to a practice based on inquiry in which questions focus on how to continuously improve care, (b) develop and use evidence-based standards and interventions, (c) investigate outcomes and critical incidents from a system perspective, and (d) work in intra- and interprofessional delivery teams(Cronenwett et al., 2007; Cronenwett et al., 2009; Sherwood, 2012). The IOM (Greiner and Knebel, 2003) identified the following competencies as essential for all health professionals if we are to improve health care: patient-centered care, teamwork and collaboration, evidence-based practice, quality improvement, safety, and informatics. In the initial report, quality and safety were combined competencies, but subsequent definitions recognize the separate knowledge base for each and have made them distinct competencies, so there is a set of six.

The six competencies are not isolated concepts but are interrelated and apply across all health disciplines. The goal of the competencies is to enable health professionals to deliver patient-centered care, work as part of interdisciplinary teams, practice evidence-based health care, implement quality improvement measures and strategies, and use information technology (Cronenwett *et al.*, 2007; Cronenwett *et al.*, 2009; Finkelman and Kenner, 2009; Greiner and Knebel, 2003). Brief descriptions of the competencies are provided in Textbox 1.2, complete definitions and the KSAs can be found in Appendices A and B, and each competency is discussed in separate chapters in Section 2 of this book.

Textbox 1.2 Descriptions of Six Competencies to Improve Quality and Safety*

- Patient-centered care

  In patient-centered care, patients and their families are treated with respect and honor, engaged as partners in their care, treated as safety allies, and participate in shared decisions that are made based on knowledge of patient values, beliefs, and preferences (Walton and Barnsteiner, 2017). Sharing knowledge and information with patients and families enable their participation in the team and agreement on their treatment plan. Helping patients and their families know what to report can help prevent errors.

- Teamwork and collaboration

  The degree of how well health care professionals work together accounts for as much as 70% of health care errors (Institute of Medicine, 2000; TJC, 2016), yet nurses and physicians have few educational experiences together. Coordinating complex care requires cross-disciplinary communication, knowing scope of responsibility, and organizational support for speaking up when safety is compromised (IPEC, 2011). Nurses need skills in problem solving, conflict resolution, and negotiation to be able to coordinate care across interprofessional teams (Dolansky, Luebber, and Singh, 2017). Developing emotional intelligence can help health professionals use their strengths to contribute to effective team functioning. Flexible leadership, effective communication, mutual support, and environmental scanning are effective team behaviors (Disch, 2017).

- Evidence-based practice

  Evidence-based practice standards guide patient care, not tradition or trial and error (Tracey and Barnsteiner, 2017). A spirit of inquiry identifies clinical questions that seek best practices. Reflective practice develops a spirit of inquiry by asking questions about the care that was delivered. Skills in informatics are a part of evidence-based practice to seek current evidence to determine best practices and clarify care decisions. Patient-centered care considers patient preferences, values, and beliefs within an evidence-based approach. Nurses use evidence-based standards and quality improvement tools to measure how care in their own setting compares with benchmark data to determine areas to improve.

- Quality improvement

  A practice attitude of continuously improving care every day with every patient reflects a spirit of inquiry. Quality improvement measures variance in ideal and actual care and implements strategies to close the gap (Johnson, 2017). Nurses use quality improvement tools and informatics to seek evidence and measure care outcomes as well as benchmark data to assess current practice. The ethical responsibility of quality improvement is revealed through the commitment to provide the best practices as well as the ethical conduct of the process itself.

- Safety

  Safety is the effort to minimize the risk of harm to patients and providers through both system effectiveness and individual performance (Barnsteiner, 2017). Competency in safety is based on constantly asking how actions affect patient risk, where the next error is likely to occur, and what actions can prevent near misses. Safety science redirects the examination of errors from the person approach, which blames the individual for forgetfulness, lack of attention, or moral weakness, to one that examines the system in which the error occurred. A systems approach examines the conditions in the environment that may have contributed to the error and designs defenses to prevent errors or mitigate effects.

- Informatics
  Informatics is a thread through all the competencies to help manage care through documentation in electronic health records, decision support tools, and safety alerts (Clancy and Warren, 2017). Providers apply skills in informatics to retrieve information, search for the latest evidence, manage quality improvement data and strategies, and share information across the interprofessional team. Nurses also use informatics knowledge, skills, and attitudes to help guide development of informatics applications, purchases, and ways to use it on the unit.

*Appendices A and B have definitions with the 162 knowledge, skill, and attitude objective statements.

Education transformation cannot happen in isolation. The IOM recommendations demand interprofessional learning experiences for both academic and clinical learning situations. Nursing education most often occurs in silos, or independent departments, with few shared learning opportunities among the many health disciplines with which nurses are expected to work. Knowing what each discipline contributes is crucial to high performance and flexible team leadership that works through authority gradients so all team members have equal opportunity to share information in establishing patient care goals (Disch, 2017). Education transformation applies to all settings—academic and clinical, and all educational entry programs—to prepare nurses in practice as well as those in academic programs.

Resources are available to assist educators in making the transition. The American Association of Colleges of Nursing (AACN) presented a series of QSEN faculty development workshops, and maintains a list of resources on the Association's web site. The QSEN institute continues to present an annual national forum in which participants share outcomes and strategies for integrating the QSEN competencies in academic and clinical settings. The QSEN web site offers teaching strategies, annotated bibliographies, demonstration projects, videos, learning modules, and a facilitator panel to assist with educator development. Educators and organizations responsible for accreditation, licensing, and certification of health professionals have embedded the competencies into nursing education standards to help lead transformation of how we prepare students and nurses to be proficient in these competencies that are essential to quality and safety (Sherwood, 2012).

Advancing Scholarship

A third area of focus is advancing scholarship in all areas of quality and safety. Research can help develop the scientific evidence of quality and safety issues to know how and to what extent patients are harmed as well as ways to mitigate. We need evidence-based educational strategies to determine best practices for teaching and implementing quality and safety concepts in practice. Traditional education methods relying on lecture have not demonstrated the capacity to achieve the KSAs needed to redesign health care across multiple settings (Benner *et al.*, 2010; Day and Sherwood, 2017a; Day and Sherwood, 2017b; Ironside and Cerbie, 2012). To integrate the competencies, educators need evidence-based curricula and teaching strategies for innovative educational interventions, whether as part of their formal education or as staff in clinical settings (www.qsen.org).

- Hobgood *et al.* (2010) compared four pedagogical approaches including high and low fidelity to measure changes in knowledge and attitude of nursing and medical students from an educational intervention for interdisciplinary teamwork.
- Welsh, Flanagan, and Ebright (2010) compared two methods of end-of-shift handoffs to examine communication and potential for adverse events.
- Hayden *et al.* (2015) led a national study on the use of simulation in nursing education. Findings indicated learners could achieve the same learning objectives by substituting up to 50% of the usual hours spent in clinical learning assignments with high fidelity simulation.
- Moughrabi and Wallace (2015) tested the effectiveness of simulation accelerated nursing students in achieving the quality and safety competencies, particularly teamwork and collaboration. Simulation provides a safe place for learners to practice, receive feedback, and apply what they have learned.
- Riley and Yearwood (2012) used a mixed-method approach to investigate students' experiences with infusion of QSEN competencies and their intention to address quality care indicators.

These few examples illustrate opportunities to develop evidence-based approaches to achieving the IOM recommendations. We have an unparalleled opportunity for nursing leadership and scholarship to help improve our health systems. We need to determine the effectiveness of what we are teaching about quality and safety, measure the long-term behavior change, and assess the skills needed in the workplace that will drive curricular changes. Benner *et al.* (2010) call for nurses to claim this opportunity for radical redesign of nursing education that can match the radical changes needed in health care delivery. Scholarly investigation can determine effective pedagogies, outcomes of care interventions, strategies for reporting and investigating errors, system malfunctions that lead to work-arounds, and communication that promotes interprofessional teamwork.

Summary

More than 15 years after the release of *To Err is Human*, patient safety and quality of care remain major health concerns. Various organizations, including professional and consumer groups, have developed regulations, educational programs, and initiatives for leading change. There is progress in establishing a culture conducive to pursuing health care quality and reporting; clinicians are replacing the fear of a punitive response and cover-up with a focus on accountability and reporting events so that through analysis the organization can implement improvements and prevention strategies. Nurses have new roles and responsibilities in continuous quality improvement that encourage a culture of inquiry and asking questions, and investigate outcomes and critical incidents from a system perspective. The QSEN institute continues to lead integration of quality and safety competencies in all levels of nursing education. Progress in evidence-based education approaches and pedagogies will help determine ways to prepare clinicians with new mindsets and lasting changes in behavior based on the six quality and safety competencies.

References

Agency for Healthcare Research and Quality. (2008) Becoming a high reliability organization: Operational advice for hospital leaders. Rockville, MD: U.S Department of Health and Human Services. Last retrieved July 4, 2015: http://www.ahrq.gov/qual/hroadvice/hroadvice.pdf.

American Association of Critical-Care Nurses. (2010) *Clinical practice resources: Healthy work environment.* Retrieved July 10, 2011, from http://www.aacn.org/.

Aspen, P., Walcott, J., Bootman, L., and Cronenwett, L. (Eds.) and the Committee on Identifying and Preventing Medication Errors. (2007) *Identifying and preventing medication errors.* Washington, DC: National Academies Press.

Balik, B., and Dopkiss, F. (2010) 10 years after *To Err Is Human*: Are we listening to patients and families yet? *Focus on patient safety, newsletter of the national patient safety foundation, 13*(1), 1–3. Retrieved June 29, 2010, from http://www.npsf.org/paf/npsfp/fo/pdf/Focus_vol_13_1_2010.pdf.

Barnsteiner, J. (2017) Safety. In G. Sherwood and J. Barnsteiner (Eds.), *Quality and safety in nursing: A competency approach to improving outcomes.* 2nd Ed. Hoboken, NJ: Wiley-Blackwell.

Batalden, P. B., and Davidoff, F. (2007) What is "quality improvement" and how can it transform healthcare? *Quality & Safety in Health Care, 16*(1), 2–3.

Batalden, P. B., Leach, D., and Ogrinc, G. (2009) Knowing is not enough: Executives and educators must act to address challenges and reshape healthcare. *Healthcare Executive, 24*(2), 68–70.

Benner, P., Sutphen, M., Leonard, V., and Day, L. (2010) *Educating nurses: A call for radical transformation.* San Francisco, CA: Jossey-Bass.

Berwick, D., Nolan, T., and Whittington, J. (2014) The Triple Aim: Care, health, and cost. *Health Affairs, 27*(3), 759–769.

Bodrock, J. A., and Mion, L.C. (2008) Pay for performance in hospitals: Implications for nurses and nursing care. *Quality Management in Health Care, 17*(2), 102–111.

Brandt, B., Lutfiyya, M. N., King, J., and Chioreso, C. (2014) A scoping review of interprofessional collaborative practice and education using the lens of the Triple Aim. *Journal of Interprofessional Care. 28*(5): 393–399. doi: 10.3109/13561820.2014.906391.

Centers for Medicare and Medicaid Services. (2008) *Roadmap for implementing value driven healthcare in the traditional medicare fee-for-service* program. Retrieved July 14, 2010, from https://www.cms.gov/QualityInitiativesGenInfo/downloads/VBPRoadmap_OEA_1–16_508.pdf.

Classen, D., Resar, R., Griffin, F., *et al.* (2011) Global "trigger tool" shows that adverse events in hospitals may be ten times greater than previously measured. *Health Aff* 2011;*30*:581–9 doi:10.1377/hlthaff.2011.0190.

Clancy, T., and Warren, J. (2017) Informatics. In G. Sherwood and J. Barnsteiner (Eds.), *Quality and safety in nursing: A competency approach to improving outcomes,* (2nd ed.). Hoboken, NJ: Wiley-Blackwell.

Compas, C., Hopkins, K., and Townsley, E. (2008) Best practices in implementing and sustaining quality of care: A review of the quality of improvement literature. *Research in Gerontological Nursing, 1*(3), 209–215.

Cronenwett, L. (2012) A national initiative: quality and safety education for nurses (QSEN). In G. Sherwood and J. Barnsteiner (Eds.), *Quality and safety in nursing: A competency approach to improving outcomes.* Hoboken, NJ: Wiley-Blackwell.

Cronenwett, L., Sherwood, G., Barnsteiner, J., Disch, J., Johnson, J., Mitchell, P., *et al.* (2007) Quality and safety education for nurses. *Nursing Outlook, 55*(3), 122–131.

Cronenwett, L., Sherwood, G., and Gelmon, S. (2009) Improving quality and safety education: The QSEN learning collaborative. *Nursing Outlook, 57*(6), 304–312.

Cronenwett, L., Sherwood, G., Pohl, J., Barnsteiner, J., Moore, S., Sullivan, D. T., *et al.* (2009) Quality and safety education for advanced practice nursing practice. *Nursing Outlook, 57*(6), 338–348.

Davis, K., Schoen, C., and Stremikis, K. (2010) *Mirror, mirror on the wall: How the performance of the U.S. health care system compares internationally, 2010 Update.* Retrieved July 14, 2010, from http://www.commonwealthfund.org/~/media/Files/Publications/Fund%20Report/2010/Jun/1400_Davis_Mirror_Mirror_on_the_wall_2010.pdf.

Day, L., and Sherwood, G. (2017a) Quality and safety in clinical learning environments. In G. Sherwood and J. Barnsteiner (Eds.), *Quality and safety in nursing: A competency approach to improving out-comes*. 2nd Ed. Hoboken, NJ: Wiley-Blackwell.

Day, L., and Sherwood, G. (2017b) Transforming education to transform practice: integrating quality and safety in unfolding case studies. In G. Sherwood and J. Barnsteiner (Eds.), *Quality and safety in nursing: A competency approach to improving out-comes*. 2nd Ed. Hoboken, NJ: Wiley-Blackwell.

Day, L., and Smith, E.L. (2007) Integrating quality and safety content into clinical teaching in the acute care setting. *Nursing Outlook, 5More 5*(3), 138–143.

Disch, J. (2017) Leadership to create change. In G. Sherwood and J. Barnsteiner (Eds.), *Quality and safety in nursing: A competency approach to improving out-comes*, 2nd Ed. Hoboken, NJ: Wiley-Blackwell.

Disch, J. (2017) Teamwork and collaboration. In G. Sherwood and J. Barnsteiner (Eds.), *Quality and safety in nursing: A competency approach to improving out-comes*. 2nd Ed. Hoboken, NJ: Wiley-Blackwell.

Doran, D.M. (2010) *Nursing outcomes: The state of the science*. 2nd Ed. Sudbury, MA: Jones and Bartlett Learning.

Greiner, A.C. Knebel, E. (2003) Institute of Medicine Committee on the Health Professions Education Summit. *Health Professions Education: A Bridge to Quality*. Washington, DC: National Academies Press.

Department of Health and Human Services. (2010) Adverse events in hospitals: national incidence among Medicare beneficiaries. http://oig.hhs.gov/oei/reports/oei-06-09-00090.pdf.

Earnest, M., and Brandt, B. (2014) Aligning practice redesign and interprofessional education to advance triple aim outcomes. *Journal of Interprofessional Education*. Early Online: 1–4. doi: 10.3109/13561820.2014.933650.

Hayden, J.K., Smiley, R.A., Alexander, M., Kardong-Edgren, S., and Jeffries, P.R. (2014) The NCSBN national simulation study: A longitudinal, randomized, controlled study replacing clinical hours with simulation in prelicensure nursing education. *Journal of Nursing Regulation, 5*(2), S3–S64.

HealthGrades quality study: patient safety in American hospitals. (2004) http://www.providersedge.com/ehdocs/ehr_articles/Patient_Safety_in_American_Hospitals-2004.pdf.

Hines, P. A. and Yu, K.M. (2009) The changing reimbursement landscape: Nurses' role in quality and operational excellence. *Nursing Economic, 27*(1), 345–352.

Hobgood, C., Sherwood, G., Frush, K., Hollar, D., Maynard, L., Foster, B., *et al.*, on behalf of the Interprofessional Patient Safety Education Collaborative. (2010) Teamwork training with nursing and medical students: Does the method matter? Results of an interinstitutional interdidsciplinary collaboration. *Quality and Safety in Health Care, 19*, 1–6.

Horton-Deutsch, S., and Sherwood, G. (2008) Reflection: An educational strategy to develop emotionally competent nurse leaders. *Journal of Nursing Management, 16*(8), 946–954.

Hughes, R.G. (2008) Tools and strategies for quality improvement and patient safety. In Hughes, R. G. (Ed.), *Patient safety and quality: An evidence-based handbook for nurses, 3*, 313–340. Rockville, MD: Agency for Healthcare Research and Quality. Also retrieved from http://www.ahrq.gov/qual/nurseshdbk.

Institute of Medicine. (2000) *To err is human: Building a safer health system*. Washington, DC: National Academies Press.

Institute of Medicine. (2001) *Crossing the quality chasm: A new health system for the 21st century*. Washington, DC: National Academies Press.

Institute of Medicine. (2010) *The future of nursing: Leading change, advancing health*. Institute of Medicine and the Robert Wood Johnson Foundation. Washington, DC: National Academies Press. Retrieved from http://www.iom.edu/Reports/2010/A-Summary-of-the-October-2009-Forum-on-the-Future-of-Nursing-Acute-Care.aspx.

International Council of Nurses. (2002) *Position statement on patient safety*. Retrieved July 14, 2010, from http://www.icn.ch/images/stories/documents/publications/position_statements/D05_Patient_Safety.pdf.

Interprofessional Education Collaborative Expert Panel. (2011) *Core competencies for interprofessional collaborative practice: Report of an expert panel* Washington, DC: Interprofessional Education Collaborative.

Ironside, P., and Cerbie, E. (2017) Narrative teaching strategies to foster quality and safety. In G. Sherwood and J. Barnsteiner (Eds.), *Quality and safety in nursing: A competency approach to improving outcomes*. Hoboken, NJ: Wiley-Blackwell.

James, J.T.A. (2013). A new, evidence-based estimate of patient harms associated with hospital care. *J Patient Saf*; 9:122–128. doi: 10.1097/PTS.0b013e3182948a69 pmid:23860193.

Johnson, J. (2017) Quality improvement. In G. Sherwood and J. Barnsteiner (Eds.), *Quality and safety in nursing: A competency approach to improving outcomes*. Hoboken, NJ: Wiley-Blackwell.

Joint Commission. (2015) Sentinel event data: Root causes by event type. Retrieved May 20, 2016 from http://www.jointcommission.org/assets/1/18/Root_Causes_by_Event_Type_2004-2015.pdf.

Landrigan, C.P., Parry, G.J., Bones, C.B., Hackbarth, A.D., Goldmann, D.A., and Sharek, P.J. (2010) Temporal trends in rates of patient harm resulting from medical care. N Engl J Med;363:2124–34. doi:10.1056/NEJMsa1004404 pmid:21105794.

Leape, L.L., and Berwick, D.M. (2005) Five years after *To Err Is Human*: What Have We Learned? *Journal of the American Medical Association*, *293*, 2384–2390.

Longo, D.R., Hewett, J.E., Ge, B., and Schubert, S. (2005) The long road to patient safety: A status report on patient safety systems. *Journal of the American Medical Association*, *294*(22), 2858–2865.

Makary, M.A., and Daniel, M. (2016) Medical error – the third leading cause of death in the US. *British Medical Journal*. May 3; 353:i2139. doi: 10.1136/bmj.i2139.

Montalvo, I. and Dunton, N. (2007). *Transforming nursing data into quality care: Profiles of quality improvement in U.S. healthcare facilities*. Silver Spring, MD: American Nurses Association.

Moore, S., Dolansky, M., and Singh, M. (2012) Interprofessional approaches to quality and safety education. In G. Sherwood and J. Barnsteiner (Eds.), *Quality and safety in nursing: A competency approach to improving outcomes*. Hoboken, NJ: Wiley-Blackwell.

Oster, C., and Braaten, J. (2016) High reliability organizations: A healthcare handbook for patient safety and quality. Indianapolis: Sigma Theta Tau Press.

Page, A. (2004) *Keeping patients safe: Transforming the work environment of nurses*. Committee on the Work Environment for Nurses and Patient Safety, Board on Health Care Services. Washington, DC: National Academies Press.

Reason, J. (2000) Human error: Models and management. *British Medical Journal*, *320*(7237):768–770.

Reeves, S., Perrier, L., Goldman, J., Freeth, D., and Zwarenstein, M. (2013) Interprofessional education: Effects on professional practice and health care outcomes.(update). Cochrane Database of Systematic Reviews, 3, CD002213.

Riley, J.B., and Yearwood, E.L. (2012) The effect of a pedagogy of curriculum infusion on nursing student well-being and intent to improve the quality of nursing care. *Archives of Psychiatric Nursing*. 26(5):364–73. doi: 10.1016/j.apnu.2012.06.004.

Sammer, C.E., Lykens, K., Singh, K.P., Mains, D.A., and Lackan, N.A. (2010) What is patient safety culture? A review of the literature. *Journal of Nursing Scholarship*, *42*(2), 156–165.

Schumann, M.J. (2012) Policy implications driving national quality and safety initiatives. In G. Sherwood and J. Barnsteiner (Eds.), *Quality and safety in nursing: A competency approach to improving outcomes*. Hoboken, NJ: Wiley-Blackwell.

Sherwood, G. (2017) The imperative to transform education to transform practice. In G. Sherwood and J. Barnsteiner (Eds.), *Quality and safety in nursing: A competency approach to improving outcomes*. Hoboken, NJ: Wiley-Blackwell.

Sherwood, G., and Armstrong, G. (2016) Current Patient Safety Drivers. In C. Oster and J. Braaden (Eds), *Achieving High Reliability through Patient Safety and Quality – A Practical Handbook*. Indianapolis: Sigma Theta Tau Press, 25–48.

Tracey, M.F., and Barnsteiner, J. (2017). Evidence-based practice. In G. Sherwood and J. Barnsteiner (Eds.), *Quality and safety in nursing: A competency approach to improving outcomes*. Hoboken, NJ: Wiley-Blackwell.

Triolo, P. (2012) Creating cultures of excellence: Transforming organizations. In G. Sherwood and J. Barnsteiner (Eds.), *Quality and safety in nursing: A competency approach to improving outcomes*. Hoboken, NJ: Wiley-Blackwell.

Wachter, R.M. (2004) The end of the beginning: Patient safety five years after "To Err Is Human." *Health Affairs*, W4–534–W4–545.

Wachter, R.M. (2010) Patient safety at ten: Unmistakable progress, troubling gaps. *Health Affairs*, 29(1), 165–173.

Walton, M.K., and Barnsteiner, J. (2017). Patient-centered care. In G. Sherwood and J. Barnsteiner (Eds.), *Quality and safety in nursing: A competency approach to improving outcomes*. 2nd Ed. Hoboken, NJ: Wiley-Blackwell.

Welsh, C.A., Flanagan, M.E., and Ebright, P. (2010) Barriers and facilitators to nursing handoffs: Recommendations for redesign. *Nursing Outlook*, 58(3), 148–154.

Resources

Agency for Healthcare Research and Quality: www.ahrq.gov

American Association of Colleges of Nursing: www.aacn.nche.edu

American Association of Critical-Care Nurses, Clinical Practice Resources: www.aacn.org/DM/MainPages/PracticeHome.aspx?lastmenu=divheader_clinical_practice

American Nurses Association. The National Center for Nursing Quality Indicators: www.nursingquality.org

American Organization of Nurse Executives: www.aone.org

Center for Studying Health System Change: www.hschange.org

Commonwealth Fund: www.commonwealthfund.org

Consumers Advancing Patient Safety: www.patientsafety.org

Empowered Patient Care Coalition: www.empoweredpatientcoalition.org

Institute for Healthcare Improvement: www.ihi.org

Institute of Medicine: www.iom.edu

Institute for Safe Medication Practices: www.ismp.org

International Council of Nurses. www.icn.ch

Joint Commission: www.jointcommission.org

Nursing Alliance for Quality Care: http://www.gwumc.edu/healthsci/departments/nursing/naqc/

National League for Nursing: www.nln.org

National Quality Forum: www.qualityforum.org

National Patient Safety Foundation: www.npsf.org

Quality and Safety Education for Nurses: www.qsen.org

Robert Wood Johnson Foundation: www.rwjf.org

Robert Wood Johnson Foundation (2008) *Transforming care at the bedside toolkit*. Retrieved July 10, 2015, from http://www.rwjf.org/pr/product.jsp?id=30051

2

Policy Implications Driving National Quality and Safety Initiatives

Mary Jean Schumann, DNP, MBA, RN, CPNP, FAAN

Even though individual providers and clinicians of every discipline can elect to improve their own practice, strive to provide higher quality care, and reduce errors in their own work environments, much of the effort to reach higher levels of quality and safety must also occur through high-level policy setting. Without policies that focus prioritization of resources on quality health care as a goal, individual efforts will be subsumed by other challenges such as stressful working conditions, short staffing and limited access, and demands for cost containment. This chapter addresses the policy strategies and initiatives that have emerged since 1990, from coalition building, to standard setting, to rule making and regulation, to the development of new incentives, and even legislation. Nurses' roles in these efforts will also be described, as well as opportunities to influence policy, priorities, outcomes, and implementation today and in the decade that follows. Although quality and safety are distinct, the inclusion of safety is considered in any discussion of health care quality. Because so many measures of health care quality seem rooted in the absence of negative outcomes, such as falls, development of infections, pressure ulcers, and harm as a result of medication errors, safety has become synonymous with quality improvement in many discussions.

Policy in the Context of Health Care Quality and Safety

From the outset, this chapter is based on the premise that policy encompasses many strategies and certainly is not limited to or even best achieved in most instances by legislation. Simon (1966) defines policy as "a set of processes, including at least 1) setting the agenda, 2) specifying alternatives from which to choose, 3) an authoritative choice among those specified alternatives, as in a legislative vote or a presidential decision, and 4) implementing the decision." Although Kingdon (2003) ascribes multiple definitions to the term *agenda setting*, one is most applicable in the arena of health care quality. He includes as a definition of agenda setting "a coherent set of proposals, each related to the others and forming a series of enactments its proponents would prefer." There is considerable evidence in this chapter to support the value of that definition.

For purposes of this chapter's discussion, policy encompasses alternatives that include not only legislative action but also rule making, statements of positions, establishment of standards, the adoption of guidelines or principles of best practice, and national consensus strategies. While policy is not confined to federal or national actions, the policy initiatives and opportunities discussed here will be largely at that level, given the scope and nature of the quality issues.

Quality and Safety in Nursing: A Competency Approach to Improving Outcomes, Second Edition.
Edited by Gwen Sherwood and Jane Barnsteiner.
© 2017 John Wiley & Sons, Inc. Published 2017 by John Wiley & Sons, Inc.

Another important concept espoused by Kingdon (2003), useful to understanding not only policy formation but also nursing's role in shaping it, is that multiple process streams exist. Kingdon describes these as streams of problems, policies, and politics. Indeed, accurate formulation of problems is often a crucial first step to figuring out how to move toward solutions that derive from useful policy. Unless the problem is correctly identified, one can chase many alternative solutions without getting to any that might lead to resolution of the real problem. Kingdon concludes that the greatest policy changes grow out of that coupling of problems, policy proposals, and politics. If we think more broadly about passage of still-controversial health care reform legislation, the Affordable Care Act, policy emerged where there was a convergence of health care delivery challenges, support of stakeholder groups and alliances around policy proposals to improve care, and the political will to enact legislation, modify funding streams, and adjust priorities.

The Landscape of Formal Stakeholders in the Ongoing Quality Dialogue

Many collective efforts have been initiated over the last 25 years to drive quality and safety improvement through policy channels. This chapter will describe formalized efforts that grew out of a need to address health delivery challenges, using organizational structures or alliances whose missions were substantially focused on quality. The list is necessarily broad and incorporates federal agencies as well as others. Certainly this list is not exhaustive; the intent has been to include those efforts in which nursing has or needs to have a voice in the formal agenda, solutions, and policy formulations. In addition, this chapter will touch on some of the additional opportunities for policy input through regulation and rule making that inevitably emerge from massive policy enactment.

This chapter will begin with a discussion of the result of two decades of effort—the passage and early efforts to implement the Affordable Care Act (ACA) and the many provisions within it that support health care quality and safety. However, the subsequent discussion centers around understanding that other policy efforts have also been required to achieve convergence, successful legislation, and full-scale implementation.

Affordable Care Act Emerged Where Efforts Converged

In March 2010, the US Congress passed and the president signed into law the ACA. Although the provisions were many and even six years later remain controversial, from the perspective of driving improvements in quality, several key provisions of the law, as they have been phased in, have provided significant opportunity to reshape the future delivery of care. Nurses played a critical role in designing and supporting passage of these provisions and have since had significant opportunity to influence, recommend, and in some cases design innovations in care delivery that are consistent with these provisions and with implementation of various aspects of the law focused on the improvement of quality. The following are some of the key provisions specific to quality and safety.

Improving Health Care Quality and Efficiency

The law established a new Center for Medicare and Medicaid Innovation that conducts pilot demonstrations to test new ways of delivering care to patients. In addition, this center continues to search for existing and promising innovative programs that can be replicated or scaled up to improve the quality and safety of health care delivered, while also reducing the rate of growth in health care spending for Medicare, Medicaid, and the Children's Health Insurance Program. Included in this provision, the HHS was required to submit a National Strategy for Quality Improvement in Health Care that would include these programs in addition to those of third-party payers. This National Strategy, a strategic plan for improving the delivery of health care services, achieving better patient outcomes, and improving the health of the US population, continues to be updated yearly. The ACA called for the establishment of an Interagency Working Group on Health Care Quality, composed of senior officials representing 24 federal agencies with major responsibility for health care quality and quality improvement. The working group's function is to provide a platform for collaboration, cooperation, and consultation among relevant agencies regarding quality initiatives as a means to ensure alignment and coordination across federal efforts and with the private sector. It continues to meet annually to provide guidance and oversight to the collective quality efforts.

Linking Payment to Quality Outcomes

ACA established a Hospital Value-Based Purchasing program for traditional Medicare participants. No longer do hospitals receive reimbursement for care based exclusively on the quantity of services delivered. This program offers financial incentives to hospitals to improve the quality of care provided to Medicare patients. This method of payment rewards institutions based on how closely they adhere to best clinical practice, as well as on their improvement of the patients' experiences of care during hospitalization. In keeping with the intent of transparency and accountability, hospital performance is publicly reported using a star rating system in Hospital Compare. Reporting is based on measures relating to events like heart attacks, heart failure, pneumonia, surgical care, health care-associated infections, and patients' perception of care. Early in the development of this process stakeholders and quality alliances, including nursing, submitted public comments regarding the proposed rules that would implement the value-based purchasing provision.

The work of developing and endorsing performance measures that meet the intent of this provision are the result of work in which various entities, alliances, and individual stakeholder organizations engage. Measure development remains some of the more important and most challenging work in policy related to ACA. Measures, if appropriately defined, can quantify the quality of the care delivered for payments, and they also focus attention on issues that are major factors in whether patients survive medical or surgical interventions and hospitalizations. Measure development is challenging because although electronic systems are more efficient methods of data monitoring and capture than manual (paper) documentation that can track institutions' progress and success, few measures are electronically available in many of these domains, particularly as they might pertain to items that fall most directly into the realm of nurses and nursing care. Equally challenging is the expensive pilot testing and subsequent endorsement process to demonstrate the adequacy and accuracy of such measures for reporting to the public, and for payment. Nurses have great opportunities for influence in the development and adoption of measures that reflect the outcomes and patient experiences of nursing care.

Encouraging Integrated Health Systems

ACA provides incentives for physicians and other providers to join together to form Accountable Care Organizations (ACO), which allow physicians and other providers to better coordinate patient care and improve health care quality, help prevent disease and illness, and reduce unnecessary hospital admissions. When an ACO provides high quality care while reducing costs to the health care system, rules allow the ACO to keep some of the money saved. Key stakeholder groups, including nursing, engaged in public comments in response to controversial ACO rules proposed by the Centers for Medicare and Medicaid Services (CMS) prior to the establishment of most of the ACOs currently in existence. Although ACOs clearly would benefit from the services of RNs, advanced practice registered nurses (APRN), and other clinicians, certain exclusions in the rules could have negative impact in recognizing their contributions or sharing cost savings.

Paying Providers Based on Value, Not Volume

Provisions in the ACA tie provider payments to the quality of care they provide. Providers are expected to see their payments modified so that those who provide higher value care will receive higher payments than those who provide lower quality care. This provision is taking place in progressive stages. In fiscal years 2013 to 2015, hospitals have become accountable in both reporting and in receipt of payment for specific domains of care that expand to include an additional domain each year. These domains include the following: the clinical process of care domain measures such as venous thromboembolism prophylaxis, appropriate surgical use of postoperative antibiotics, and urinary catheter removal postoperatively; the patient experience of care domain such as nurse communication, doctor communication, hospital staff responsiveness, pain management, medicine communication, and discharge information; the outcome domain measures such as acute myocardial infarction (AMI) 30-day mortality rate, heart failure (HF) 30-day mortality rate, pneumonia (PN) 30-day mortality rate, central line-associated blood stream infection (CLABSI); and in 2015 the efficiency domain, which focuses on Medicare spending per beneficiary. CMS assesses each hospital's performance by comparing its scores on achievement and improvement related to each measure of performance (Department Of Health And Human Services Centers for Medicare and Medicaid Services, Hospital Value-Based Purchasing Program Fact Sheet, accessed at https://www.cms.gov/Outreach-and-Education/Medicare-Learning-Network-MLN/MLNProducts/downloads/Hospital_VBPurchasing_Fact_Sheet_ICN907664.pdf).

Partnership for Patients

Partnership for Patients was a national partnership initiated in April 2011 by HHS that projected to save 60,000 lives by preventing injuries and complications in patient care over three years. HHS stated upon its inception that the Partnership for Patients also had the potential to save up to $35 billion in health care costs, including up to $10 billion for Medicare. Over the next 10 years, the Partnership for Patients could reduce costs to Medicare by $50 billion and save billions more in Medicaid. More than 3,500 hospitals, physician and nurse groups, consumer groups, and employers pledged their commitment to the Partnership for Patients. Oversight for this program has been under CMS's Center for Medicare and Medicaid Innovations.

This public-private partnership was invested in reforms that help achieve two shared goals:

- ***Keeping hospital patients from getting injured or sicker:*** By the end of 2013, preventable hospital-acquired conditions were expected to decrease by 40% compared to 2010. Achieving this goal meant approximately 1.8 million fewer injuries to patients, with more than 60,000 lives saved over the next three years.
- ***Helping patients heal without complication:*** By the end of 2013, preventable complications during a transition from one care setting to another were expected to decrease so that all hospital readmissions would be reduced by 20 compared with those of 2010. Achieving this goal would mean that more than 1.6 million patients will recover from illness without suffering a preventable complication requiring re-hospitalization within 30 days of discharge.
- The partnership asks hospitals to focus on nine types of medical errors and complications where the potential for dramatic reductions in harm rates has been demonstrated by pioneering hospitals

and systems across the country. Examples included preventing adverse drug reactions, pressure ulcers, childbirth complications, and surgical site infections. The CMS Innovation Center had pledged to help hospitals adapt effective, evidence-based care improvements to target preventable patient injuries on a local level, developing innovative approaches to spreading and sharing strategies among public and private partners in all states. Members of the partnership were to identify specific steps they will take to reduce preventable injuries and complications in patient care.

- How has the Partnership for Patients done so far in meeting these goals? As reported by Blumenthal in May 2015, 30-day readmission rates for Medicare enrollees declined nationally from more than 19% to less than 18.5% in 2012 and to 17.5% in 2013; this is equivalent to 150,000 fewer readmissions between January 2012 and December 2013. The first ever decline in hospital composite rates of hospital-acquired conditions (HAC) nationally decreased from 2010 to 2013. It is estimated that this prevented roughly 50,000 deaths and saved $12 billion. The overall 9% in the decline in the incidence of hospital acquired conditions from 2010–2012 includes 560,000 fewer HACs in just two years, with the prevention of 15,000 deaths due to reductions in adverse events, falls, and infections, and a savings of $3.2 billion in 2012 alone. In addition, through the end of 2013, falls and trauma decreased by nearly 15%, pressure ulcers decreased by 25%, ventilator associated pneumonias decreased by over 50%, and venous blood clotting complications decreased by 13% (Blumenthal, Abrams, and Nuzum, 2015).

National Quality Strategy Is the Future

In compliance with ACA, the National Quality Strategy was released via a report to Congress in March 2011. Consistent with the initiatives of the National Quality Forum and the National Priorities Partners Goals and Priorities, the National Quality Strategy pursued three broad aims—similar to those referenced by the Institute for Health Care Improvement as the Triple Aims—to guide and assess local, state, and national efforts to improve the quality of health care. The aims included the following:

- *Better Care:* Improve the overall quality by making health care more patient centered, reliable, accessible, and safe.
- *Healthy People/Healthy Communities:* Improve the health of the US population by supporting proven interventions to address behavioral, social, and environmental determinants of health in addition to delivering higher quality care.
- *Affordable Care:* Reduce the cost of quality health care for individuals, families, employers, and government.

The National Quality Strategy was based on recognition that in the end, all health care is local, and its intent has been to help assure that these local efforts remain consistent with shared national aims and priorities. The Secretary of HHS developed this initial strategy and plan through a participatory, transparent, and collaborative process that reached out to more than 300 groups, organizations, and individuals who provided comments. The AHRQ was tasked with supporting and coordinating the implementation plan and further development and updating of the strategy, which it has continued to do.

At the federal level, the National Quality Strategy has guided the development of HHS programs, regulations, and strategic plans for new initiatives, in addition to serving as a mechanism for evaluating the full range of federal health efforts. The first year strategy did not include HHS-specific plans, goals, benchmarks, and standardized quality metrics, but AHRQ developed these through collaboration of the participating agencies and private sector consultations. The 2015 Strategy speaks to the following six evolving priorities that inform the advancement of efforts to keep patients safe:

- Making care safer by reducing harm caused in the delivery of care
- Ensuring that each person and family members are engaged as partners in their care
- Promoting effective communication and coordination of care
- Promoting the most effective prevention and treatment practices for the leading causes of mortality, starting with cardiovascular disease
- Working with communities to promote wide use of best practices to enable healthy living
- Making quality care more affordable for individuals, families, employers, and governments by developing and spreading new health care delivery models (reference AHRQ, Working for Quality web site accessed at http://www.ahrq.gov/workingforquality/nqs/overview.htm

Starting in 2015 annual reports on the progress on the aims and priorities of the National Quality Strategy will be based upon AHRQ's National Healthcare Quality and Disparities Reports. These reports will include updated measurement data regarding the Nation's progress on each priority. Current measurement data can be found on the National Health Care Quality and Disparities web site at http://www.ahrq.gov/research/findings/nhqrdr/index.html.

Building the Momentum for Quality

The inclusion of such far-reaching provisions related to quality and safety in the ACA was made possible largely because of efforts over two decades of health care industry stakeholders to identify the challenges and build multiple supportive allegiances, leading to addressing the issues through policies at every level. As by-products, professionals in the health care industry became educated about quality principles, and consumer awareness of the complexities of health care systems was raised. The following pages describe how powerful such efforts would be.

National Quality Forum: A Strategic Model

In 2000, following the IOM reports on medical errors and the quality chasm, the National Quality Forum (NQF), a new private not-for-profit entity, became central to the establishment of standards and policy relative to health care quality. NQF grew out of the Presidential Advisory Commission on Consumer Protection and Quality in Health Care Industry convened in 1996. The advisory commission was one of many ways that entities concerned about the eroding quality of care began to consider how they might drive improvement. Ultimately, the commission recommended the creation of a private sector entity, which then became the NQF. The expanding role of NQF over the next decade is an instructive example of the collective efforts of many entities, whether professions, consumers, insurers or others, working to shape and implement national policy, including the National Quality Strategy.

NQF's overall purpose is to provide key leadership for a national health care quality measurement and reporting system. Its mission is focused on three themes: 1) build consensus on priorities and goals for health care quality; 2) play a major role in the endorsement of national consensus standards; and 3) use its collective membership to promote attainment of these standards in the delivery of care to consumers. From inception, the CMS, the Office of Personnel Management, and the AHRQ have been part of NQF. In addition, standard setting bodies like the Joint Commission, the National Commission for Quality Assurance, the IOM, the National Institutes of Health, and Physician

Consortium for Performance Improvement (PCPI)-American Medical Association (AMA) have had key liaison roles as well. Today, there are nearly 450 NQF organizational members.

The development and expansion of NQF has included input from nurses with representation from organizational membership in NQF from its inception and at the 23-member board by nursing experts. The American Nurses Association (ANA) was the first NQF nursing organization member, with others following suit over the next decade. As many as 23 entities representing nursing have been NQF members, and nursing continues to hold a seat on the NQF Executive Board.

The NQF employs three strategies to collectively move quality as a national priority as well in driving performance improvement. These three strategies have been used by other coalitions and individual professions as well: 1) convening experts across the industry to define quality by developing standards and measures; 2) gathering information from measurement of performance through data reporting and analysis; and 3) identifying gaps that are provided back to providers, institutions, and others about performance to initiate performance improvement and public reporting. In addition, NQF, as do other collective efforts, places ongoing focus on dissemination of tools and educational activities that promote health care improvement in the United States.

The expansiveness of the NQF structure has provided many touch points for nursing to influence its direction. Calls for endorsement of standards or measures require formal comment and ballot-type voting. Calls for nominations to work groups based on content expertise or representation allows for formally nominating nursing leaders who can speak on behalf of quality through a nursing lens. Nursing leaders have had opportunities to serve in leadership roles within committees and work groups, to react to the work of colleagues from other disciplines, and to inform, persuade, or dissent as needed, in the shaping of policy.

Measure Applications Partnership Driving Selection of Measures

The NQF has been named as a consensus endorsement agency, as required by Section 3014 of the ACA. In the habit of convening multi-stakeholder groups, it is expected to provide input to the US Secretary of Health and Human Services through federal government appointment, on the selection of performance measures for public reporting and performance-based payment programs. An NQF board work group met in early 2010 to consider the charge and structure for a potential new partnership to serve this purpose, called the Measure Applications Partnership (MAP). MAP has been designed as a two-tiered structure that includes a standing multi-stakeholder coordinating committee to provide direction to and synchronize with the second tier of advisory work groups. The coordinating committee establishes the strategy for the partnership. The work groups advise on measures needed for specific uses. NQF through the coordinating committee recommends measures for use in public reporting, performance-based payment, and other programs to HHS. At least one nursing organization, the ANA, is a member of the coordinating committee, and several nursing organizations have representatives, and individual nursing leaders and content experts have been appointed through a nominations process to the various work groups.

National Database of Nursing Quality Indicators: Capturing the Data

Even before the release of *To Err is Human* (Institute of Medicine, 2000) and *Crossing the Quality Chasm* (Institute of Medicine, 2001), the nursing profession had begun to speak up about the eroding of the quality of care patients received. Not surprisingly, this concern surfaced early at the national nursing policy level. In 1994, the ANA House of Delegates at its annual meeting approved a house resolution that urged ANA leadership to address the problem of declining patient care quality experienced in many institutions, perceived by nurses to be due in part to reductions in staffing levels implemented following declining revenue. ANA, when addressing this problem with its interdisciplinary colleagues, was repeatedly asked to show the evidence that reduced nursing staffing led to such declines in quality care. Nurse leaders determined that not only was there a need for education about principles of quality, but that in fact, data were required that would put to rest the criticisms of those claiming that the value of nursing could not be substantiated.

In the mid-1990s, ANA began a national effort to educate nurses about the value of data and quality through regional conferences. ANA simultaneously convened nurse experts Dr. Norma Lang, Dr. Marilyn Chow, and others to identify structural, process, and outcome measures that would support the relationship between staffing levels, skill mix, and the quality of nursing care. Those initial measure definitions became the basis for the NQF-endorsed nursing sensitive measures. As a result of recommendations from this group of experts, ANA funded a contract to develop a national database with Dr. Nancy Dunton as principal investigator, that could receive and aggregate data collected via these measures. In 1998, ANA awarded grants to seven state nurses associations to encourage hospitals in those states to collect and submit data to this new database, National Database of Nursing Quality Indicators (NDNQI), a proprietary database of the ANA (Montalvo and Dunton, 2007). Since 1998, the number of acute and specialty hospitals that submit quarterly nursing-related quality data has grown to more than 2,000, more than one-third of all US acute care facilities.

The impact of NDNQI on policy conversations at the institutional, state, or national level has been far reaching. Studies published at the national level utilizing the aggregated data support the impact of the quantity and skill mix on the quality of nursing care, the link between nursing satisfaction and improved satisfaction of patients with their care, and the impact of levels of nursing education with the outcomes of care. It has provided comparisons of similar institutions and unit types, both within the state and across the country, to assist chief nursing officers and nurse managers to defend the appropriate levels and skill mix of nurse staffing in their institutions, describe the impact of decreased levels on patient outcomes, and drive performance improvements at unit and institutional levels. NDNQI data reports provided back to the institutions point to opportunities for deeper examination of the processes of care and the need for evidence that supports care decisions.

Data from NDNQI has been used at the state level for public reporting, driving state initiatives, and supporting staffing legislation that defends the hospital and the nursing unit-level leaderships' rights to make decisions about safe staffing levels based on the evidence, rather than on state-mandated ratios. Major insurers provide higher ratings to those institutions that participate in NDNQI, based on their conviction that institutions that care about nursing care quality are more likely to have positive outcomes.

In 2014 ANA made a decision to divest itself of NDNQI and arranged for its purchase by Press Ganey, an established for-profit business that supports data collection and reporting on the patient experience of care. ANA retains stewardship of certain NDNQI measures and retains an advisory role in the further development of NDNQI.

Institute for Healthcare Improvement Focused on System Improvement

Founded in 1991, IHI has been a major driver of quality care and health care change based on the philosophy that almost any product or service, including health care, can be improved. The IHI encouraged systems thinking with improvement of a systems idea; if one can change the way things are done, one can get better results. IHI aims to improve the lives of patients, the health of communities, and the joy of the health care workforce by focusing on the IOM's six improvement aims for the health care system: safety, effectiveness, patient-centeredness, timeliness, efficiency, and equity (Institute of Medicine, 2001). IHI may be best known for its campaigns to Save 100,000 Lives, later to Save Five Million Lives, and currently the Triple Aim initiatives of better care, better health, at lower cost. IHI provides a variety of services and educational programs and tools to assist hospitals and other stakeholders to achieve these aims. IHI's structure and campaigns have enabled institutions and individual providers of care, including nurses, to share their "near misses" and successes in instructive ways. Nursing organizations have participated in IHI to contribute to discussions and to influence actions that have global and national consequences.

Informatics, Electronic Health Records, and Impact of Technology on Quality and Policy

While also helping align the health care industry with quality expectations in other industries, dialogue about the use of technology, nursing terminologies, and consistent specifications for data capture, including physician order entry, diagnoses, interventions, and decision support, became part of the quality discussion. Harnessing complex technology for quality improvement and reporting purposes has become crucial. Although NDNQI has been able to function successfully in a manual data capture environment to accommodate institutions with insufficient progress toward electronic health records, driving policy changes that impact future quality requires the ability to capture that data electronically according to widely agreed upon specifications. Unless data for measures are able to be gathered as well as submitted electronically, the ability of nurse leaders to drive progress in the policy world of quality will erode.

Data collection burdens, the accuracy of electronic data extractions, the timeliness of the data reporting and analysis, the ability to have timely comparisons to benchmarks, all impact not only the performance improvement process but also the ability to ensure that patients are receiving the care they deserve within a safety culture. The challenge of many electronic systems, as may have already been mentioned, is that while much data go into the system, particularly in the delivery of nursing care, it can be nearly impossible to extract it for reporting and analysis. Further, decision supports based on data that identifies a patient with a stage two pressure ulcer, for instance, must also incorporate in a timely way from the patient perspective, an evidence-based appropriate plan of action to both prevent further skin breakdown and begin healing. From a public reporting perspective, is it enough to know a patient is at risk of experiencing a pressure sore while hospitalized? Engaged consumers and insurers will want to know what the data show about not only the prevention of decubiti but also the appropriateness of treatment, the speediness of recovery, lost work days, and impact on the quality of life. Policy makers are interested in lengths of stay and other factors that drive up the cost of such hospital-acquired conditions.

Nursing continues to drive forward in the development of electronic measures (eMeasures), particularly data collection on the incidence of pressure ulcers. As of yet, no pressure ulcer eMeasure has been endorsed by NQF, nor is there national level public reporting of any nursing measures.

Nursing informatics and the use of nursing terminologies are central to capturing key data elements in a consistent way. Adherence to consensus-based terminologies, both for the collection of data around the nursing sensitive measures, but also the processes of care, are necessary to articulate the actual contributions of nurses, their importance in keeping patients safe, and improving the quality of care, as identified in both the IOM reports and the QSEN competencies (Cronenwett *et al.*, 2007; Cronenwett *et al.*, 2009).

A major contributor to this agenda is the Technology Informatics Guiding Education Reform (TIGER Initiative), launched as a result of a 2006 conference convened to create a vision for the future of nursing, bridging the quality chasm with information technology, enabling nurses to use informatics in practice and education to provide safer, high-quality patient care (Warren, 2012). Laying the groundwork for an interdisciplinary collaborative, TIGER is implementing Phase 3 to integrate TIGER recommendations for a virtual learning network on health information technology, for the nursing community as well as the larger interdisciplinary health care community. While at first this may seem to be about education and practice, the implications for policy are clear. As national initiatives improve electronic interoperability and the development and implementation of health records, the collection of meaningful data that can be used to influence improvements in care has the potential to revolutionize nurses' care delivery. At the same time, issues of privacy and confidentiality of data confront every nurse practicing or teaching in such environments, necessitating policies that address these issues and electronic patient data for research and quality improvement.

National Priorities Partnership and Implementation of the National Quality Strategy

The National Priorities Partnership is another national collaborative effort, initially including 28 national health care organizations, convened in 2008 as an initiative of the NQF. Its role is to join stakeholders from both public and private sectors to influence policy encompassing every aspect of the health care system. Stakeholder groups currently include consumer groups, employers, government, health plans, health care organizations, health care professions, scientists, accrediting and certifying bodies, and quality alliances. Since 2008, the number of organizations has expanded to more than 40 stakeholder groups. Nursing was represented only by ANA in the initial stakeholder group, but the newly formed Nursing Alliance for Quality Care (NAQC) was added as the group expanded. The partnership took the early step of identifying a set of national priorities and goals to coalesce efforts toward achieving performance improvement by stakeholders on high-leverage areas with the potential to make the most substantial contributions in the near term to the health care delivery systems of the nation and ultimately to consumers. In 2011 the National Priorities Partnership expanded its focus. Significantly, the full list of priorities and goals, consistent with the QSEN competencies identified earlier, had substantial impact on the final recommendations of the National Quality Strategy. The list included:

- Engaging patients and families in managing their health and making decisions about their care
- Improving the health of the population
- Improving the safety and reliability of America's health care system
- Ensuring patients receive well-coordinated care within and across all health care organizations, settings, and levels of care
- Guaranteeing appropriate and compassionate care for patients with life-limiting illnesses
- Eliminating overuse while ensuring the delivery of appropriate care
- Improving access
- Improving the health care infrastructure

As a second step, the partnership agreed to align the drivers of change and the performance measures around goals for each priority. Each goal reflects those aspects that will most likely lead to achievement of the priority, along with a road map consisting of examples of successful actions and targets for describing success. Taking an important step, the partnership agreed to commit its leadership to support the drivers (below) in order to effect change at the federal, state, and local levels:

- Performance measurement
- Public reporting
- Payment systems
- Research and knowledge dissemination
- Professional development: education and certification
- System capacity

In 2009, the ANA and NQF nursing member organizations, supported by NQF and the Robert Wood Johnson Foundation (RWJF), hosted the Invitational Conference on Nursing and the National Priorities Partnership Goals: Next Steps. Its purpose was to examine each of the priorities, goals, and drivers to 1) identify priorities for nursing quality measurement to align nursing measures with current national quality initiatives, 2) develop specific strategies to fast-forward achievement of these priorities, and 3) envision new frameworks that would advance performance measurement to improve health and well-being. As a result of that conference, two American Academy of Nursing (AAN) scholars summarized the proceedings, detailing the nursing opportunities and action plans for each of the priority areas.

Quality Alliances Influence Policy Actions Through a Professional Lens

Various professions have followed a model similar to that of NQF while determining their own efforts to influence the measurement of quality, support quality improvements, and take action at a national policy level. From a positive perspective, these alliances create a pipeline for their profession's or specialty's representation at national stakeholder tables, for grooming nominees with the expertise to inform measure development and policy setting, and for providing national leadership for the overall quality agenda. Each faces similar challenges, including that of determining membership and governance structures and dues for long-term financial sustainability. Each needs to coordinate with other stakeholders and standard setters among its own discipline in order to lead with one voice. Externally, each alliance forms a coherent, coordinated, and consistent approach to quality and measurement that moves the health care system forward as a whole, without becoming counterproductive. Most alliances have some combination of stakeholders among their membership or board that reflects other disciplines, as well as federal agencies such as AHRQ, CMS, or NQF, to provide some level of transparency, consistency, and connectedness. Financial support of each alliance varies, but for most, ongoing sustainability becomes a challenge to the mission of the stakeholders in each alliance.

Nursing Alliance for Quality Care

Nursing through the NAQC has created its own alliance of national nursing stakeholder organizations in partnership with patient care advocacy organizations representing consumers. NAQC's membership continues to grow and to find that space where nursing can collectively make the largest contribution to the quality arena. Although formed only in early 2010 from an earlier RWJF-funded planning grant, NAQC is committed to advancing the highest quality, safety, and value of consumer-centered health care for patients, their families, and their communities. Governed by an independent board of directors, NAQC first sought long-range expected outcomes that include the following:

- Patients receiving the right care at the right time by the right professional
- Nurses actively advocating and being accountable for consumer-centered, high-quality health care
- Policymakers recognizing the contributions of nurses in advancing consumer-centered, high-quality health care

NAQC focused on four goals to accomplish these three outcomes: 1) support consumer-centered health care quality and safety goals to achieve care that is safe, effective, patient-centered, timely, efficient, and equitable; 2) performance measurement and public reporting that strengthens the role of nursing in transparency and accountability activities; 3) advocacy, by serving as a resource to partners and stimulating policy reform that reflects evidence-based nursing practice and advances consumer-centered, high-quality health care; and 4) building nursing's capacity to serve in leadership roles that advance consumer-centered, high-quality health care. NAQC provided national level conferences that supported important policy changes, including nurse-led medical homes, nurses' roles in accountable care organizations, and nurses' roles in fostering patient and family engagement.

In 2013, NAQC determined that its long-term strategy for sustainability as an alliance required a more permanent home within one of the existing member organizations. It now resides within ANA, maintaining memberships from among the leading national nursing associations. NAQC still retains a seat as an alliance at various national tables.

Other similar alliances are included here to provide a perspective on the interdisciplinary reach and nursing's inclusion in those efforts to improve quality.

The Hospital Quality Alliance

In 2002, the Hospital Quality Alliance (HQA) was formed from organizations representing America's hospitals, consumer representatives, physician and nursing organizations, employers and payers, oversight organizations, and governmental agencies. It was a national public-private collaboration committed to making meaningful, relevant, and easily understood information about hospital performance accessible to the public and to informing and encouraging efforts to improve quality. HQA was effective in initiating changes in national policy, perhaps most visibly in terms of quality reporting.

HQA facilitated continuous improvement in patient care through implementation of measures that portray the quality, cost, and value of hospital care; the development and use of measurement reporting in the nation's hospitals; and sharing of useful hospital performance information with the public through Hospital Compare. Hospital Compare (www.hospitalcompare.hhs.gov) contains performance information about more than 4,000 hospitals, and data are updated quarterly. Hospital Compare is a voluntary national report card of the performance among hospitals, evolved with the support and strong encouragement from HQA, while retaining the right to suppress data it deems not appropriate to share. HQA dissolved as the National Priorities Partnership flourished and the National Quality Strategy took center stage in shaping the quality measures environment.

The Ambulatory Care Quality Alliance

Shortly after the formation of HQA, the American Academy of Family Physicians, the American College of Physicians, America's Health Insurance Plans, and AHRQ joined together in 2004 to initiate efforts to improve performance measurement, data aggregation, and reporting in the ambulatory care setting. Since then, the mission and membership have grown to a broad-based collaborative of over 100 organizations, and include all areas of physician practice as well as a variety of other stakeholders, now known simply as the Ambulatory Care Quality Alliance (AQA). To distinguish itself from the HQA, this collaborative focused initial efforts on physician or other clinician performance. AQA's most recent strategic plan focuses on being a convener to promote and facilitate alignment among the public and private sector efforts, on promoting best practice quality improvement strategies that address the gap between measurement and improvement, and on advising HHS as it implements health care reform initiatives. While ANA has sent representatives to monitor this alliance's activities, no nursing organizations are listed among its current membership. Of late, AQA has been actively focused on measure development and on public reporting of outcomes.

Pharmacy Quality Alliance

The Pharmacy Quality Alliance, in place since 2006, focuses on its intersection with the health care system. Its stated mission is to improve the quality of medication use across health care settings through a collaborative process in which key stakeholders agree on a strategy for measuring and reporting performance information related to medications. This alliance, like many of its counterparts, includes representatives from CMS and NQF among its board, as well as at least one consumer representative. Once again, nursing organizations are not listed among its members, yet it has issued an invitation to NAQC to learn more about its structure and work efforts, with the potential for future collaboration.

Alliance for Pediatric Quality

Four national organizations formed the Alliance for Pediatric Quality (APQ) to establish a unified voice for improving the quality of pediatric health care. These organizations are the American Academy of Pediatrics, the American Board of Pediatrics, the Child Health Corporation of America, and the National Association of Children's Hospitals and Related Institutions (NACHRI). The focus is to improve the quality of care for children by promoting effective, systematic efforts to improve children's health care and to ensure that health information technology works for children by developing standards that incorporate pediatric requirements and advocating for health information technology that enables systematic improvement. Both NACHRI and the Child Health Corporation of America include nursing in their purview, but neither organization focuses primarily on nursing. There is, however, collaboration on measures that reflect nursing in pediatric quality care, such as pediatric falls and skin breakdown. ANA and NACHRI have worked together to align specifications for pediatric measures and to strengthen opportunities to measure improvements in nursing care for children. The APQ web site states its interest is in recognizing systematic, well-designed and well-run improvement initiatives. APQ is currently active in supporting ImproveCareNow as one of its four *Improve First* projects focused on improved outcomes.

Long-Term Quality Alliance

The Long-Term Quality Alliance was established in 2010 to respond to increasing demands for long-term services and support and for expanding the field of providers delivering that care in the United States. It is governed through a broad-based board of 30 of the nation's leading experts on long-term care and related care issues including consumers, family caregivers, health care providers, private and public purchasers, federal agencies, and others. The web site for this alliance states it is focused on facilitating dialogue and partnerships among all provider organizations that serve people needing long-term services and supports to help break down the provider silos in which quality initiatives have occurred, on bringing consumers and family caregivers together with long-term care (LTC) providers and government agencies to agree on goals and associated measures of greatest concern, on making stronger links between quality measurement goals and evidence-based practices to achieve them, and on collaborating with other quality improvement organizations on common priorities and goals. Nursing is well represented and has been a key player in the formation of this alliance.

Kidney Care Quality Alliance

Active since 2006, this alliance was formed by persons committed to kidney care and the health care community at large to involve patients and their advocates, care professionals, providers, suppliers, and purchasers in developing performance measures focused on institutions and physicians. The intent was to also focus on developing data collection and aggregation strategies while promoting transparency by reporting performance measures. The broad membership included two specialty nursing organizations serving that patient population and nurses specializing in nephrology care. Current information reflects four quality measures for managing End Stage Renal Disease (ESRD), which resides on the AHRQ web site but no other Alliance activity. These measures evaluate whether facilities' and physicians' patients have had documented discussions of alternate renal replacement therapies during their ESRD management, whether patients receiving dialysis have functional arteriovenous (AV) fistulas, grafts, or cannulas, and whether patients receiving dialysis are appropriately offered or receive influenza vaccine.

Quality Alliance Steering Committee

The Quality Alliance Steering Committee (QASC) was formed in 2006 through a collaboration of HQA and AQA to better coordinate the promotion of quality measurement, transparency, and improvement in care. This alliance included close relationships with CMS and AHRQ, already members of both AQA and HQA. The new steering committee was expected to expand several ongoing pilot projects focused on combining public and private information to measure and report on performance in new ways to enhance the goals of transparency and meaningful information. Nursing organizations and the NAQC have been members of this alliance. No current information is available on QASC's activities.

Institute of Pediatric Nursing

Gaining status as a private not-for-profit entity in early 2011, the Institute of Pediatric Nursing was an alliance of diverse pediatric nursing organizations and major children's hospitals, acting collaboratively to maximize pediatric nursing's contribution to child and youth health through unified leadership, knowledge, and expertise. Its goals were to influence 1) nursing education, 2) health care access, 3) child and youth advocacy, 4) care coordination, and 5) safe, quality evidence-based care. Governed by an independent board that reflects the various major settings of care for children and youth, this alliance served as a catalyst and collaborative voice in addressing key issues in pediatric health care and the pediatric nursing specialty. Early efforts focused on ensuring that Medicaid provisions are actually resulting in high-quality care by meeting the medical needs of children. The group also helped create new partnerships to support the quality of transitions from acute to school-based care for many chronically ill children.

Alliance for Home Health Quality Innovation

The Alliance for Home Health Quality Innovation is dedicated to improving the nation's health care system by supporting research and education to demonstrate the value of home-based care. Nursing is engaged in this alliance, both through the Visiting Nurse Association of America and the Visiting Nurses Association of New York.

Federal Agencies Engage with Alliances

It becomes clear from studying the configuration of most of the alliances that allegiance and partnerships with federal agencies such as AHRQ and CMS are critical to any strategy driving health care system change that is focused on higher quality. CMS, at the behest of Congress, controls decisions determining reimbursement for services, how to reward for higher quality care, and in making deductions in reimbursement due to preventable negative outcomes of care. NQF has been made the arbiter of measure endorsement and of which measures' data, gathered by institutions and providers, point to the outcomes that either get rewarded or penalized. And AHRQ plays a major role from a federal perspective in the creation and validation of standards, guidelines for best practice, and research related to quality, safety, and best practice. Any professional alliance looking to develop measures or to suggest that given measures are or are not appropriate for considerations of payment would do well to bring these entities along to the discussion, keep them informed of challenges and lessons learned, and either heed or shape the future they want to see. Some of the alliances that have developed and achieved endorsement of their measures from NQF ensured their measures continued through AHRQ representation.

Centers for Medicare and Medicaid Services

CMS is a federal agency that administers Medicare, Medicaid, and the Children's Health Insurance Program. CMS reports to HHS. Even though Medicaid services are provided by each state, CMS provides guidance for administering services and can audit services provided to Medicare recipients. CMS has several newly created offices as a result of the ACA, including the Center for Medicare and Medicaid Innovation and the Center for Dual Eligibles. In recent years, CMS has created a Nursing Steering Committee that includes several CMS officials willing to address concerns that arise from external nursing organizations about Medicare and Medicaid reimbursement and service issues for Medicare or Medicaid recipients. This steering committee includes a number of nursing organizations and continues to meet quarterly by conference call.

As policy efforts have shifted from passage of the ACA to defining the rules and regulations that impact implementation of its many provisions, the CMS Nursing Steering Committee has been extremely valuable in identifying opportunities for the profession to weigh in with public comment on proposed rules, and in calling to attention and advocating for changes to language that would disadvantage nursing practice or reduce nursing's ability to keep patients safe. It continues to serve as a venue for getting timely information about CMS initiatives that potentially affect the profession and consumers.

Agency for Healthcare Research and Quality

AHRQ is the lead federal agency charged with improving the quality, safety, efficiency, and effectiveness of health care for all Americans. AHRQ is one of 12 agencies within the HHS. AHRQ supports research that helps people make more informed decisions and improves the quality of health care services. AHRQ is committed to improving care safety and quality and does this through successful partnerships and the development of knowledge and tools needed for long-term improvement. AHRQ's research goals include measurable improvements in health care, with a focus on improved quality of life, improved patient safety and outcomes, and high-value care for each dollar spent.

Standard Setting by Nonfederal Agencies

Accreditation bodies such as the Joint Commission, the National Commission on Quality Assurance, the Utilization Review Accreditation Commission, and others impact how quality is recognized in practice settings. They drive quality through formal policy mechanisms of setting, monitoring, and evaluating accreditation standards and recognition criteria. Although accreditation is voluntary and paid for by the institution seeking it, accreditation processes wield a great deal of power in shaping expectations of quality and safety. To ensure the reasonableness of standards and evaluation criteria, professional organizations and alliances participate in the development and revision of accreditation and recognition criteria and measures. ANA and others seek to ensure that nurses provide board representation, public comments, or advocacy efforts as a check and balance on the rigor of the accreditation standards and recognition criteria these entities use as the yardstick by which performance is evaluated.

The Joint Commission

The Joint Commission is a 105-year-old independent, not-for-profit organization that accredits and certifies more than 19,000 health care organizations and programs in the United States, including acute care and long-term care facilities, ambulatory care services, hospice and home care programs, behavioral health programs, managed care entities, and health care staffing services. The Joint Commission states that these activities are undertaken to continuously improve the safety and quality of care provided to the public. The Joint Commission uses Professional-Technical Advisory Committees to establish or modify existing standards and determine patient safety goals. Nursing input into these activities occurs through multiple professional nursing organizations with representation on the various advisory committees, through ongoing dialogues and via a separately established Nursing Advisory Council that meets periodically to consider nursing issues where the Joint Commission standards play a role in shaping policy. The Joint Commission has at least one board seat held by a nurse.

The National Committee for Quality Assurance

Founded in 1990, the National Committee for Quality Assurance (NCQA) is a private, not-for-profit organization dedicated to improving health care quality and elevating health care quality to the top of the national agenda. NCQA is governed by an independent board composed of multiple stakeholder groups. NCQA develops quality standards and performance measures for a broad range of health care entities. These standards and measure are the tools that organizations and individuals can use to identify opportunities for improvement. Annual reporting of performance against such measures provides direction for improvement. NCQA collects Healthcare Effectiveness Data and Information Set data known as HEDIS (Health Plan Employer Data and Information Set Measures) from more than 700 health plans; conducts accreditation, certification, and state plan surveys; and develops and conducts formal recognition programs including the Primary Care Medical Home Recognition Program. No nursing organizations are included in the governance of NCQA, although nurses have been in key positions at one time or another. However, nursing organizations have actively engaged with NCQA to urge acceptance of APRNs as leaders of medical homes, so that several nurse-led medical homes are now recognized by NCQA's programs. Nurse faculty and others have worked with NCQA to mine relevant data regarding APRN practice and the outcomes of patients receiving care by APRNs in practice settings.

Utilization Review Accreditation Commission

The Utilization Review Accreditation Commission (URAC), initiated in 1990, is a not-for-profit organization promoting health care quality by accrediting health care organizations, developing measurement, and providing education. URAC's mission is to protect and empower the consumer. URAC's first mission was to improve the quality and accountability of utilization review programs. Its spectrum of services has grown to include a larger range of service functions, including the accreditation of integrated health plans. URAC is governed by a board with representatives from multiple constituencies including consumers, providers, employers, regulators, and industry experts. Nursing has a long well-established presence on URAC's Board.

"Stand for Quality in Health Care"-focused Health Reform Efforts

A driving force for the inclusion of vital principles for quality in health reform legislation emerged from the various quality alliances. This joint effort, formed in 2008 and known as Stand for Quality in Health Care, included more than 200 health care organizations, including nursing organizations. It achieved consensus around the most important features of quality as the health care reform initiatives took shape—consensus that was so strong it evoked bipartisan support. Stand for Quality established recommendations for building a foundation for high-quality affordable health care that linked performance measurement to health reform. In addition, it linked the investment in health information technology to the improvement of the quality of care and helped drive a quality agenda during the framing of the ACA. It outlined the case for supporting performance measurement, reporting, and improvement through the articulation of Core Principles Linking Performance Measurement, Improvement, and Health Reform; through identification of the Key Functions of the Performance Measurement, Reporting, and Improvement Enterprise; and through the development of deliverables. The key functions included the following:

- Function 1. Set national priorities and provide coordination.
- Function 2. Endorse and maintain national standard measures.
- Function 3. Develop measures to fill gaps in priority areas.
- Function 4. Use effective consultative processes so stakeholders can inform policymakers on use of measures.
- Function 5. Collect, analyze, and make performance information available and actionable.
- Function 6. Support a sustainable infrastructure for quality improvement.

Based on the final provisions of ACA, the above functions are driving the creation of the various commissions and strategies for quality.

Today Stand for Quality states it is engaged in a long-term strategy to 1) extend current funding for measure endorsement and 2) to secure major funding for further measure development. Specifically, funding will support ongoing endorsement of measures for high-priority conditions, endorse measures that cross settings and conditions, support new areas of measurement such as value-based purchasing and registries, and work to facilitate the transition to eMeasures.

Common Strategies Run Through Formalized Initiatives

There are common strategies each collective effort employs to gain political will for change. The various alliances and other collaborative initiatives have several strategies in common, which in and of themselves contribute to a set of tactics around quality that may be applied to other policy discussions. Strategic themes among these initiatives include the following, which are critical when considering quality and safety:

- Most formal entities include consumers on their governing bodies or among the stakeholder groups they convene to ensure that the needs of the recipients of the care are heard and addressed.
- The inclusion of a broad base of stakeholders is almost universally applied, acknowledging the complexity of the challenges facing health care.
- The inclusion of multiple disciplines in most formal collaboratives reinforces that developing policy solutions is a team sport, with no discipline having the political clout to dictate or finalize solutions independently.
- Most formal collective efforts include one or more federal agencies among its board members in some capacity to ensure federal efforts and other entities are moving in concert.
- Professional organizations and other stakeholder groups participate in multiple efforts, maximizing their opportunities to influence policy.
- Participants on the various alliances, agencies, and accrediting bodies often participate with multiple groups. Questions remain whether this is more expeditious or not.
- Consensus building is the preferred approach to derive proposed solutions.
- Convergence on proposed solutions occurs among stakeholders and alliances, with the result that while the details might look a bit different, the same conceptual underpinnings run similarly across many collaborative efforts.

Challenges All Collective Efforts Face in Improving the Quality of Care

With approximately 200 national entities, including professional organizations, consumer groups, and thousands of hospitals and other institutions and agencies engaged in the effort to improve quality, there has been substantial investment of financial and other resources, including manpower, over the last 25 years. The timing of many of these efforts in the early 1990s suggests that long before the publication of *To Err is Human* and *Crossing the Quality Chasm*, leaders in the health care industry understood that the lack of quality was a significant problem. Nurses were early adopters in hospital efforts to identify opportunities for continuous quality improvement. Many engaged in dialogue with individual physicians who were being challenged by state performance review boards and utilization review committees. Then the focus was primarily on local quality improvement and policy initiatives rather than state or national efforts. Global quality leaders (Deming, 1986; Juran, 1998) stated that 85% of errors in complex organizations were due to system design rather than to inadequate individual job performance. But even their discussions were addressed in departmental, corporate, or institutional policy terms. Twenty-five years later in 2015, the magnitude of the current efforts to transform the health care system into a high quality system dwarfs all previous efforts. Why has this exploded to such mammoth proportions?

Prior to the implementation of the ACA, looking at any acute care facility, large or small, the number of outpatient procedures and the revenue generated from them had kept pace or overtaken the revenue from acute care services. Numbers of providers in even the smallest facility have increased, including increases in specialists, whether providing virtual or face-to-face medicine.

The enormity and complexity of the system needing improvement did not differ all that much, whether one considered the problems of the critical access hospital or the largest multihospital system. The technology needs of the solo practitioner bore an alarming resemblance to technological capabilities needed by larger health service plans to which many providers belong. At the same time, fewer and fewer patients saw their own primary provider once they entered an acute care facility, regardless of the size of the institution. The hospitalist providing their care may have never seen them previously and would have no connection to their care once they were discharged. Home care and hospice programs were beginning to use technology to replace the face-to-face time that nurses and others have traditionally relied upon with homebound patients to determine their unspoken needs and vulnerabilities, including electronic profiles on patient caseloads and communication about patients only via electronic records.

The challenges of ensuring effective care transitions, care coordination, and engagement of patients are difficult without effective communication systems. But alas, one electronic system in a hospital department is still often unable to share information with another department, in a timely manner, or more frequently with someone outside the institution. Faxes and phone calls may seem antiquated by comparison to today's technology, but they did work. Electronic records and communications are expected to have filled the gap, but they have not. Patients suffer from the lack of effective communication with and among professional staff. The situation is magnified when ineffective communication couples with the payment system and reimbursement that rewards undesired outcomes of care, such as continued disease rather than wellness or health, or complications of hospitalization rather than speedy recovery and discharge. One begins to see how local policies and regulations have little effect. As the interconnectedness has grown, so have the problems and the solutions required to correct them.

Part of the anticipated effectiveness of ACA was the inclusion of millions of previously uninsured US citizens under Medicaid expansion. The unevenness of implementation across states has impacted services, costs, and meeting chronic health needs, particularly for underserved and minority populations (Long *et al.*, 2014) In addition, despite many efforts to harness the costs of caring for high needs patients and dual eligibles (those whose services are covered by both Medicare and Medicaid), this is a challenge not yet well managed. These are challenges faced by the various collaboratives striving to improve upon the policies, regulations, and incentives incorporated in every community hoping to improve the quality of care. The challenge resembles the analogy of the global epidemic, which nonetheless requires "immunity in every community" (American Nurses Association, 2011) to bring order out of the chaos.

What Can Every Nurse Do to Influence Policy That Improves Quality?

The QSEN project is an example of nurses taking the responsibility for improving quality and safety outcomes (Cronenwett *et al.*, 2007; Cronenwett *et al.*, 2009). Nurses prepared with the six competencies (patient-centered care, teamwork and collaboration, evidence-based practice, quality improvement, safety, and informatics) have the tools and resources to impact policy at the local, state, and national levels (Textbox 2.1; also see Appendices A and B; Sherwood, 2011). Improving quality and safety requires the dedicated work of all, and with the work of the QSEN project, nurses will be able to participate in all levels of policy making.

To impact **institutional** policy, every nurse, regardless of setting or specialty, has expertise to contribute to the discussions focused on health care improvement. Nurses can:

- Take the opportunity to question practices that lack a base of evidence, or seek literature that informs practice questions.
- Collect data and utilize National Database of Nursing Quality Indicators to inform and lead better practices that will improve fall assessments or reduce falls, or improve one's own assessment skills regarding stages of decubiti.
- Devise local studies with the assistance of more senior experts, to explore or establish the evidence that either supports or disproves care practices.
- Teach colleagues what has been learned and review institutional or specialty policies about ineffective practices employed.
- Publish findings, experiential learning, and literature reviews to influence policy changes in others.
- Engage with others in the institution to review proposed rules and regulations that impact them and offer public comment on professional organizations' position statements, local or state proposed rules, or CMS-proposed rules. Proposed rules are published along with the timeline for comment in the Federal Register.

To **impact local or community** policies, nurses can:

- Assess community needs or practices that perpetuate risks for falls, whether due to poor sidewalks, potholes in grocery parking lots, or cluttered hallways and aisles in stores, schools, or churches.
- Advocate for community consensus on policies or regulations to reduce danger to children and elderly pedestrians.
- Provide education about reducing falls, improving medication adherence, or increasing patient engagement in making care decisions or choices about end-of-life care.
- Volunteer to serve on local YMCA boards, hospital boards, or other local service organizations that may be able to effect changes in services, provide access to better nutrition, or offer safer alternatives for exercise.

To impact **state** policy nurses can:

- Demand greater clarity and compliance with CMS guidance regarding Medicaid services for children who are not receiving the supplies they need for their chronic illness, or who lack the services to keep them safe in schools or after school.
- Engage with local or state chapters of professional nursing associations to coordinate advocacy for change, for modifications to practice acts, or improved services for at-risk populations.
- Actively engage in political campaigns around platforms on health care, agree to serve on state licensing boards, or attend state legislative hearings and meetings.

To impact **national** policy nurses must:

- First keep themselves and their colleagues informed of the issues.
- Develop skills and expertise at representing their specialty.
- Engage in leadership roles within their preferred professional national nursing association.
- Take action to contact congressmen or senators regarding passage of bills that affect their state and community.
- Share stories with their representatives that highlight the need for changes in health care.
- Work with their institutions to invite a congressman or senator to walk a day in the shoes of a nurse, in order to better understand the challenges of short staffing, limited resources, or other needs of the community.

Summary

The improvement of nursing and health care quality is the responsibility of every nurse. It can and needs to occur at every level, from the direct one-on-one interaction with a patient or family to the advocacy for changes in rules or regulations at every level of government, within an institution or in the local community. It takes many forms, but at its most basic level, it requires being unwilling to accept the status quo, and taking the risk to challenge practice behavior. It requires moral courage to stand up to nursing peers or physician colleagues and dissent when something begins to occur that violates basic principles of quality and safety. Even though many are working on the national level to effect policy change, at the end of the day, all health care is local. It comes back to the individual nurse providing care and living in a community, to articulate when a policy is being crafted, and how its implementation will improve or hinder quality of care or the safety of patients. It comes back to each nurse understanding the intent of that policy and implementing it on behalf of patients. Only then, when every patient is provided the same care we would want for our parent, or sister, or best friend, or child, will high-quality health care be achieved.

References

American Nurses Association. (2011) ANA Immunize: Bringing immunity to every community. Retrieved July 8, 2011, from http://www.anaimmunize.org.

Blumenthal, D., Abrams, M., and Nuzum, R. (2015) *N Engl J Med* May 8, 372:2451–2458.

Cronenwett, L., Sherwood, G., Barnsteiner, J., Disch, J., Johnson, J., Mitchell, P., *et al.* (2007) Quality and safety education for nurses. *Nursing Outlook, 55*(3), 122–131.

Cronenwett, L., Sherwood, G., Pohl, J., Barnsteiner, J., Moore, S., Taylor Sullivan, D., *et al.* (2009) Quality and safety education for advanced practice nursing practice. *Nursing Outlook, 57*(6), 338–348.

Deming, W.E. (1986) *Out of crisis.* Cambridge, MA: MIT Press.

Institute of Medicine (2000) *To err is human: Building a safer health system.* Washington, DC: National Academy Press.

Institute of Medicine. (2001) *Crossing the quality chasm: A new health system for the 21st century.* Washington, DC: National Academy Press.

Juran, J.M. (1998) *Juran's quality handbook.* New York: McGraw-Hill.

Kingdon, J.W. (2003) *Agendas, alternatives and public policies.* 2nd Ed. New York: Addison-Wesley.

Long, S., Karpman, M., Shartzer, A., *et al.* (2014) *Taking Stock: Health insurance coverage under the Affordable Care Act as of September 2014.* Washington, DC: Urban Institute.

Montalvo, I., and Dunton, N. (2007) *Transforming nursing data into quality care: Profiles of quality Improvement in US healthcare facilities.* Silver Spring, MD: Nursebooks.org.

Sherwood, G. (2011) Integrating quality and safety science in nursing education and practice. *Journal of Research in Nursing, 16*(3), 226–240.

Simon H. (1966) Political research: the decision-making framework. In D. Easton (Ed.), *Varieties of political theory* (p. 19). Englewood Cliffs, NJ: Prentice-Hall.

Warren, J. (2012) Informatics. In G. Sherwood and J. Barnsteiner (Eds.), *Quality and safety in nursing: A competency approach to improving outcomes.* Hoboken, NJ: Wiley-Blackwell.

Resources

Agency for Healthcare Research and Quality (AHRQ) at a Glance. Accessed May 2011. http://www.ahrq.gov/about/ataglance.htm

Agency for Healthcare Research and Quality (AHRQ), Working for Quality. Accessed October 2015 at http://www.ahrq.gov/workingforquality/nqs/overview.htm

Alliance for Home Health Quality Innovation. http://www.ahhqi.org/

Alliance for Pediatric Quality. http://improvecarenow.org/care-providers/our-supporters/31-our-supporters-apq

Ambulatory Care Quality Alliance. http://www.ambulatoryqualityalliance.org/

Centers for Medicare and Medicaid Services. http://www.cms.gov/

Centers for Medicare and Medicaid Services, Hospital Value-Based Purchasing Program Fact Sheet. Accessed October 2015 at https://www.cms.gov/Outreach-and-Education/Medicare-Learning-Network-MLN/MLNProducts/downloads/Hospital_VBPurchasing_Fact_Sheet_ICN907664.pdf

Hospital Quality Alliance. http://www.hospitalqualityalliance.org/

Institute for Healthcare Improvement. http://www.ihi.org/ihi

Institute of Pediatric Nursing. http://www.ipedsnursing.org/ptisite/control/index

Kidney Care Quality Alliance. http://kidneycarepartners.com/kcp_creating.html

Long-Term Quality Alliance. http://www.ltqa.org/

Measure Applications Partnership. http://www.qualityforum.org/setting_priorities/partnership/map_coordinating_committee.aspx

National Committee for Quality Assurance. http://ncqa.org/

National Database of Nursing Quality Indicators. https://www.nursingquality.org/

National Priorities Partnership. http://www.nationalprioritiespartnership.org/aboutnpp.aspx

National Quality Forum. http://www.qualityforum.org/about/

National Quality Strategy. http://www.healthcare.gov/center/reports/quality03212011a.html

Nursing Alliance for Quality Care. http://nursingaqc.org

Partnership for Patients. www.healthcare.gov/center/programs/partnership

Pharmacy Quality Alliance. http://www.pqaalliance.org/

Quality Alliance Steering Committee. http://www.healthqualityalliance.org/about-qasc

Stand For Quality in Health Care. http://www.standforquality.org/sfq_report_3_19_09.pdf

Technology Informatics Guiding Education Reform (TIGER Initiative). http://tigersummit.com/summit.html

The Joint Commission. http://www.jointcommission.org/about_us/about_the_joint_commission_main.aspx

Utilization Review Accreditation Commission. http://www.urac.org/docs/programs/urac_annual_publication_2010.pdf

3

A National Initiative

Quality and Safety Education for Nurses

Linda R. Cronenwett, PhD, RN, FAAN and Jane Barnsteiner, PhD, RN, FAAN

Note: Linda Cronenwett wrote the first part of this chapter for the first edition of this book. Jane Barnsteiner wrote the second part, which begins with the heading QSEN: 2012–2017, for the second edition of this book.

As I was writing this chapter, a colleague sent an e-mail saying, "I've been doing grant reviews for HRSA [U.S. Health Resources and Services Administration], and half or more of the applications cite QSEN competencies or QSEN work as part of their justification." Two textbook authors inquired about permission to reprint QSEN materials. A visiting scholar from Sweden reported that QSEN is being used as the framework for action for nursing in Sweden this year. Medical colleagues set up a conference call to talk about what they could learn from QSEN to apply to a national initiative on interprofessional education. Almost 400 people have registered for the 2011 QSEN National Forum, and the conference is yet a month away. The number of forum paper and poster presentations has doubled since last year.

QSEN is an initiative that has been funded since 2005 by the RWJF. The purpose of this chapter will be to posit answers to the questions often asked of those of us who have been involved in leading QSEN, namely, how did QSEN come to be and what do you think accounts for the extent of its spread and impact? A summary of aims and activities for the first three QSEN grants are provided in Figures 3.1 and 3.2. Further information about QSEN outcomes is reported elsewhere, for example, for QSEN Phase I (Cronenwett *et al.*, 2007; Smith, Cronenwett, and Sherwood, 2007), Phase II (Cronenwett, Sherwood, and Gelmon, 2009; Cronenwett *et al.*, 2009), and initial activities of Phase III (Sherwood, 2011). What follows in this chapter is one person's view of the QSEN story, a story that is not yet over. Future historians will evaluate QSEN's outcomes using data that will emerge during the decade to come.

The title *Quality and Safety Education for Nurses* emerged one summer afternoon in 2005 when I spent many hours on my screened porch generating an endless list of ideas for what to call a grant proposal that was due to the RWJF offices within the month. But of course, QSEN began long before that day.

Quality and Safety in Nursing: A Competency Approach to Improving Outcomes, Second Edition.
Edited by Gwen Sherwood and Jane Barnsteiner.
© 2017 John Wiley & Sons, Inc. Published 2017 by John Wiley & Sons, Inc.

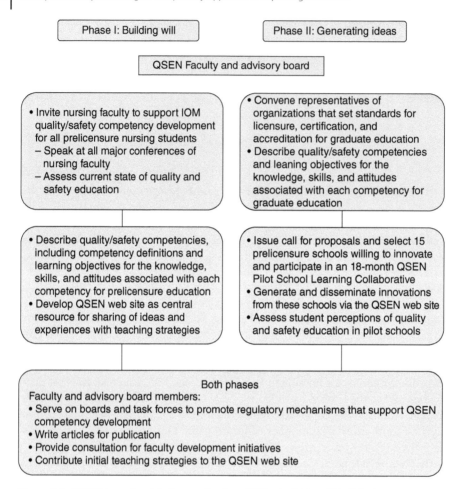

Phase I: Building will

Phase II: Generating ideas

QSEN Faculty and advisory board

- Invite nursing faculty to support IOM quality/safety competency development for all prelicensure nursing students
  – Speak at all major conferences of nursing faculty
  – Assess current state of quality and safety education

- Convene representatives of organizations that set standards for licensure, certification, and accreditation for graduate education
- Describe quality/safety competencies and leaning objectives for the knowledge, skills, and attitudes associated with each competency for graduate education

- Describe quality/safety competencies, including competency definitions and learning objectives for the knowledge, skills, and attitudes associated with each competency for prelicensure education
- Develop QSEN web site as central resource for sharing of ideas and experiences with teaching strategies

- Issue call for proposals and select 15 prelicensure schools willing to innovate and participate in an 18-month QSEN Pilot School Learning Collaborative
- Generate and disseminate innovations from these schools via the QSEN web site
- Assess student perceptions of quality and safety education in pilot schools

Both phases
Faculty and advisory board members:
- Serve on boards and task forces to promote regulatory mechanisms that support QSEN competency development
- Write articles for publication
- Provide consultation for faculty development initiatives
- Contribute initial teaching strategies to the QSEN web site

Figure 3.1   QSEN Phases I and II: Aims and actions (IOM = Institute of Medicine).

QSEN Origins: 2000–2005

Any initiative of the magnitude of QSEN depends on two groups of leaders: thought leaders in the field and thought leaders within a funding organization. Within the professional community, the seeds for what became QSEN were sown in a series of annual summer week-long conferences initiated and led by Paul Batalden, a pediatrician and one of the earliest health care quality thought leaders (Kenny, 2008). Started in 1995, these Dartmouth Summer Symposia (DSS) were invitational meetings for 60 to 70 participants, about 12 to 20 of whom were nurses in any given year. The nurse, physician, and hospital administrator educators who attended DSS described themselves as *an interprofessional community of educators devoted to building knowledge for leading improvement in health care*. Linda Norman, Associate Dean at Vanderbilt, was the first nursing leader who worked with Dr. Batalden to attract nursing deans and faculty members to this work.

I had worked with Dr. Batalden during my years at Dartmouth-Hitchcock Medical Center (1984–1998), participated in Quality Improvement Camp training, attended one summer

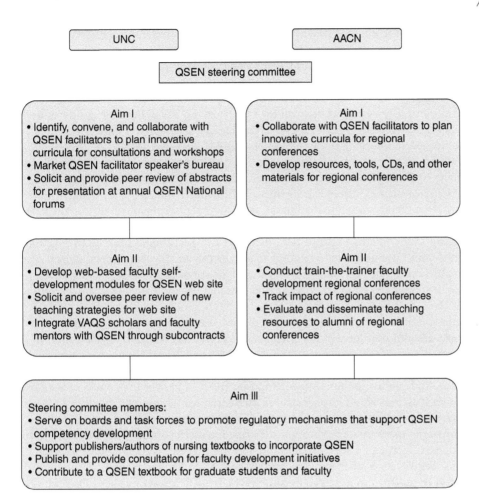

Figure 3.2 QSEN Phase III: Embedding new competencies (UNC = University of North Carolina-Chapel Hill; AACN = American Association of Colleges of Nursing; VAQS = Veterans Administration Quality Scholars Program).

symposium, and worked on a number of quality improvement projects. After I became a faculty member at the University of North Carolina (UNC) at Chapel Hill in 1998, I was invited to DSS regularly and subsequently served as the second representative of nursing in the leadership of the DSS community.

From 1997 to 2002, the DSS topics involved work under way within the physician community to alter educational objectives, curricula, and residency training accreditation and certification standards to include requirements for competency development related to the continuous improvement of health care. Leaders of the professional organizations responsible for these initiatives participated with us as we created and advanced ideas about content and learning opportunities that would, as was the stated DSS goal, "change the world." Many subsequently participated in the IOM conference that resulted in the 2003 IOM publication *Health Professions Education: A Bridge to Quality*, wherein the charge was issued that all health professionals should be educated to deliver *patient-centered care* as members of an *interdisciplinary team*, emphasizing *evidence-based practice, quality improvement approaches*, and *informatics*. It was fascinating and exciting work.

Each summer, Dr. Batalden would ask who was going to lead this work for nursing. We nurses would plot strategies for finding funding to advance this agenda and agreed that if anyone could secure funding, the rest of us would help. Each took away an assignment, and, for a couple of years, we came back empty-handed. I presented proposal ideas to RWJF and one other foundation without results. Yet we persisted.

During this same period, seeds were being sown for QSEN on the RWJF leadership side as well. When I first unsuccessfully proposed the idea for a nursing faculty development initiative in quality and safety education to RWJF's nursing leader, Susan Hassmiller, she was involved in directing the RWJF initiative Transforming Care at the Bedside (TCAB). She had recognized the importance of linking nursing faculty to the TCAB initiative and its quality/safety/cost goals. Beginning in 2002, first I and then Patricia Chiverton, dean of the University of Rochester School of Nursing, initiated attempts to work with the faculty in schools affiliated with the hospitals involved in the initiative. Few successes were achieved, however, primarily because nursing faculty were generally disconnected from the patient safety/quality improvement methods and goals being adopted by hospitals at the time. As Dr. Hassmiller pressed hospital leaders to engage nursing faculty in their projects, she experienced the faculty knowledge gap firsthand, and this evidence of the need for faculty development would eventually provide the strong rationale Dr. Hassmiller used to convince RWJF executive leaders to fund QSEN.

In another development, Rosemary Gibson, a senior program officer for RWJF and coauthor of the book *Wall of Silence: The Untold Story of the Medical Mistakes that Kill and Injure Millions of Americans* (Gibson and Singh, 2003), joined the DSS community in 2003 as a participant who could contribute the patient advocacy perspective to our conversations. She and Dr. Hassmiller were leading efforts that crossed the quality and nursing portfolios at RWJF, and over the course of the next year, we continued in discussions about ideas for an initiative that would improve quality and safety education in nursing.

In 2004, Ms. Gibson and I spent hours during DSS debating the merits of various approaches to an initiative and its proposed products. One consideration was whether this work should be housed in a nursing professional organization, an idea promoted by the AACN. Nurses in the DSS community argued that we needed to reach *all* of nursing education, which by definition included diploma and associate degree schools as well as faculty in collegiate schools that are affiliated with the National League for Nursing. We proposed that the "thought leader" work would be stronger if done by experts in quality and safety rather than appointees of professional organizational task forces who at times are assigned for reasons other than topical expertise. We wanted to involve and share the work with leaders from *all* the organizations that supported nursing licensure, certification, or accreditation of nursing education programs and thought that would more likely occur if the initial grant were housed in a neutral site. In the end, these views prevailed, and we received an official invitation to submit a proposal.

As the RWJF decision-making processes advanced, Ms. Gibson provided guidance about the need to break the initiative into short phases that, if successful, could build on each other. We were charting unknown territory and did not yet have a basis for knowing how open or resistant nursing faculties would be to this paradigm shift. She suggested taking the work one piece at a time so that we could adapt the methods to the needs that emerged. Her experience with other major RWJF initiatives (e.g., palliative care) was invaluable, and the final proposal was a true partnership with a visionary philanthropic leader.

Members of the DSS community responded to proposal drafts and, most importantly, agreed to play key roles as members of the QSEN faculty (Barnsteiner, Disch, Moore, and Mitchell) and advisory board (Batalden and Hall). Ironside's participation in the DSS community began soon thereafter.

At the same time, Dr. Gwen Sherwood became the Associate Dean for Academic Affairs at UNC-Chapel Hill. As someone experienced with patient safety initiatives, she was not only a knowledgeable local colleague but also someone with whom I could share the responsibilities of project management. We invited the participation of people we thought would be the strongest contributors with respect to each competency, area of pedagogical expertise, and the major nursing organizations associated with licensure and accreditation. Amazingly, every person invited to participate said yes.

Building Will: Phase I (October 2005–March 2007)

Funding for Phase I began October 1, 2005, and we held the first faculty/advisory board meeting 30 days later. For 18 months, this group (see Table 3.1) worked intensively to propose competency definitions and learning objectives for the quality and safety domains outlined in the IOM (2003) report on health professions education, assess faculty views about the current state of quality and safety education, and develop a web site through which we could share teaching strategies, annotated bibliographies, and other quality and safety education resources.

Phase I Impact Factors

What Phase I factors contributed to QSEN's eventual influence? First, the underlying issue was a major public concern based on documented quality and safety problems (Kohn, Corrigan, and Donaldson, 2000). The need for changes in health professions education had been made, strongly and clearly, by respected leaders (IOM, 2003), but the knowledge of the implications of this work by health professional faculties was minimal at best. We needed QSEN thought leaders who had the requisite expertise in the competencies (patient-centered care, teamwork and collaboration, evidence-based practice, quality improvement, safety, and informatics) and teaching pedagogies (clinical, classroom, skills/simulation laboratory, and interprofessional education). But we also needed leaders who had bridged the academic and practice worlds through personal commitments and experiences working to improve the health of populations, health care system performance, and professional development. We needed people who could tell stories about the knowledge, skills, and attitudes needed to fundamentally improve health and health care.

QSEN faculty and advisory board members brought these attributes to the work and deepened their learning in dialogue with each other as the work progressed. For starters, QSEN's spread was derived from the importance of the problem and the unique expertise of QSEN leaders whose collective experiences with improving *both* patient care and health professions education provided a strong platform for new ways of thinking about quality and safety education in nursing.

Second, eight faculty and advisory board members were members of the Dartmouth Summer Symposium community, and thus, they were familiar with how to use group processes to generate new ideas. These QSEN leaders had witnessed change in the world of health care improvement and health professions education as a result of DSS community work and were experienced at "thinking big" in attempts to improve health, health care, and health professions education. We were also imbued with the philosophy of community work expressed annually by Dr. Batalden, namely:

- Practice hospitality that invites open sharing. Help keep the space open for exploration.
- Practice your own trustworthiness and enhance the trustworthiness of the commons.
- Share generously, but no stealing. Protect each other's futures.
- Practice listening and dialogue, more than telling and discussion.
- Reflect into the gift of silence when it occurs, rather than rushing to obliterate it with words.

Table 3.1 QSEN faculty, staff, and advisory board members.

Project Team	Faculty-Competency Experts	Faculty-Pedagogy Experts	Advisory Board Members
Project	Jane Barnsteiner[3]	Carol Durham	Paul Batalden[3,4]
Investigators	University of Pennsylvania	UNC-Chapel Hill	IHI, ACGME
Linda Cronenwett[3,4]			
UNC-Chapel Hill		Lisa Day	Geraldine (Polly)
Gwen Sherwood	Joanne Disch[3]	UC-San Francisco	Bednash
UNC-Chapel Hill	University of Minnesota		
		Pamela Ironside[3,4]	AACN Executive Director
Librarian		Indiana University	
Jean Blackwell	Jean Johnson		
	George Washington	Shirley Moore[3]	Karen Drenkard
Project Managers	University	Case Western	AONE
Elaine Smith		Reserve University	
Assistant: C. Meyers	Pamela Mitchell[1,3]		Leslie Hall[3]
Denise Hirst[2]	University of Washington		RWJF ACT
Assistant: D. O'Neal			Initiative;
Web Manager	Dori Taylor Sullivan		IHI Health Professions
Steve Segedy[2]	Sacred Heart		Education
	University, Fairfield,		Collaborative
	CT, and Duke		
	University		Mary (Polly)
			Johnson
	Deborah Ward[2]		NCSBN Vice
	University of		President
	Washington		
	and UC-Davis		Maryjoan Ladden
			Director, RWJF
	Judith Warren		ACT Initiative
	University of Kansas		
			Audrey Nelson
			PI, ANA Safe
			Patient Handling
			Initiative
			Joanne Pohl[2]
			NONPF President
			Elaine Tagliareni
			NLN President
			Elect

[1] Phase I only
[2] Phase II only
[3] Dartmouth Summer Symposium community
[4] IHI board members

Note: UNC = University of North Carolina; IHI = Institute for Health Care Improvement; ACGME = Accreditation Council for Graduate Medical Education; UC = University of California; AACN = American Association of Colleges of Nursing; AONE = Association of Nurse Executives; RWJF = Robert Wood Johnson Foundation; ACT = Achieving Competence Today; NCSBN = National Council of State Boards of Nursing; PI = principal investigator; ANA = American Nurses Association; NONPF = National Organization of Nurse Practitioner Faculties; NLN = National League for Nursing.

QSEN leaders easily adopted DSS values and methods for generating ideas and making decisions. As a result, people from multiple professional organizations were able to take QSEN work, yet unpublished, into organizational deliberations regarding standards for licensure, accreditation, and certification. They invited QSEN faculty to provide special sessions at annual meetings to build will for proposed changes. They provided in-kind support for announcements of QSEN activities and products. They envisioned the parts of the work that could best be done by their own organizations. Beyond anyone's hopes or expectations, the work was spread, as it was envisioned, as a product of the profession itself.

Another impact factor was the QSEN decision to forge a path slightly different from medicine's response to the IOM (2003) report. Physician leaders who had worked to create alignment on descriptions of system-level competencies for undergraduate, graduate, and continuing medical education chose not to outline learning objectives for the competencies, believing that being overly prescriptive would lessen their ability to attract faculty to the goal of improving quality and safety education. With hundreds of community college, diploma, and university-based nursing education programs, and with the need to develop *thousands* of nursing faculty who taught in classroom, clinical, and simulation/skills laboratory teaching roles, QSEN leaders decided we could not assume everyone would be attracted, willing, and able to independently invent their own objectives and teaching strategies. In fact, QSEN's explicit goal was to make it as easy as possible for nursing faculty to envision their roles in supporting quality and safety education.

As we embarked on the iterative work to outline KSA objectives for each of the six QSEN competencies, we completed an initial assessment of undergraduate program leader views of how well nursing was doing currently in each domain. As reported by Smith, Cronenwett, and Sherwood (2007), when QSEN competency definitions were the *sole* reference point, survey respondents from 195 schools reported that they were already teaching to these competencies, albeit with room for some improvement, and that students were generally leaving their programs having developed competencies in patient-centered care, teamwork and collaboration, evidence-based practice, quality improvement, safety, and informatics.

QSEN leaders clearly needed to outline the gap in professional development they knew existed. Collectively, the KSAs provided a template against which schools could identify gaps between current curricular content and the desired future. The intensive group work to define learning objectives, therefore, turned out to be an essential element in the process of building the will to change.

Generating and Sharing Ideas: Phase II (April 2007–October 2008)

Phase I ended with a burst of national presentations, the publication of a special issue of *Nursing Outlook* (2007), and the launch of the QSEN web site, each activity aimed at stimulating the will to change through sharing of initial ideas about competency definitions, learning objectives, and annotated bibliographies. The QSEN faculty/advisory board debated logical next steps and decided the field was not ready for a widespread faculty development initiative. We needed a robust package of teaching ideas to move to a train-the-trainer initiative comparable to the End-of-Life Nursing Education Consortium (Malloy *et al.*, 2008). Phase II objectives, therefore, were to develop, seek feedback, and build consensus for KSAs applicable to *graduate* education and widen the network of QSEN experts and advocates by attracting prelicensure faculty innovators to develop, test, and disseminate teaching strategies for QSEN competency development (see Figure 3.1).

QSEN leaders were familiar with the IHI's use of learning collaboratives to inspire innovation and quality improvement (IHI, 2003) and decided to test the use of that model to accomplish Phase II goals for prelicensure education. Proposals to participate in the QSEN Pilot School Collaborative required

Table 3.2 Participants in April 2007 workshop to generate graduate-level QSEN competencies and associated knowledge, skills, and attitude learning objectives.

Professional organizations	Number of representatives
American Association of Colleges of Nursing[1]	1
American Association of Critical Care Nurses Certification Board	1
American College of Nurse Midwives	1
American Nurses Association	2
American Nurses Credentialing Center	2
American Psychiatric Nurses Association	1
Council on Accreditation of Certified Registered Nurse Anesthetists	1
Commission on Collegiate Nursing Education	2
National Association of Clinical Nurse Specialists	2
National League for Nursing[1]	1
National Organization of Nurse Practitioner Faculties	2
Oncology Nursing Certification Corporation	1
Pediatric Nursing Certification Board	2

[1] Members of QSEN Advisory Board

that applicants describe curricular changes, faculty development strategies, and other activities that they would conduct within their specific nursing education programs. Cross-collaborative learning was an expectation as well, with attendance at two meetings required of all school teams, which comprised clinical, classroom, and simulation lab faculty members plus a clinical partner (Cronenwett, Sherwood, and Gelmon, 2009).

For the work related to education for APRN roles, we added APRN leaders to both the QSEN faculty (Ward) and advisory board (Pohl) and invited the input of multiple organizations involved in setting standards for licensure, certification, or accreditation of APRN education programs. Representatives of 13 organizations (see Table 3.2) participated in the generation and organizational reviews of KSA learning objectives for graduate education (Cronenwett *et al.*, 2009).

Phase II Impact Factors

As in Phase I, linking QSEN with professional organizations potentiated the ideas generated by thought leaders and early innovators. Advisory board members participated fully in both the Pilot School Collaborative and APRN education work and built on this work from the perspectives of their own organizations. For example, the National Council of State Boards of Nursing (2011) began building a *Transition to Practice* model (QSEN link–Jane Barnsteiner) that required attention to QSEN competency development (now in its pilot phase in three states). The American Association of Colleges of Nursing (QSEN links–Polly Bednash and MaryJoan Ladden) created new standards for accreditation of baccalaureate (AACN, 2008) and clinical doctoral education (AACN, 2006) that included quality and safety competencies. The National League for Nursing (2010; QSEN link–Gwen Sherwood and Elaine Tagliareni) developed its education competencies model with a quality and safety thread. The NONPF (QSEN links–Linda Cronenwett and Joanne Pohl) engaged in analyses of core and practice doctorate competencies for evidence of inclusion of the QSEN graduate KSAs (Pohl *et al.*, 2009). The 12 QSEN faculty experts had wide professional networks and were invited to speak at numerous professional conferences, but the efforts of these few alone could not have produced the spread of QSEN-related work throughout the profession. As the major professional organizations associated with licensure and accreditation standards demonstrated the need for and will to change, the momentum for innovation grew.

With that momentum came a need for growing the pool of nursing faculty who could provide consultation among peers in classroom, clinical, and simulation/skills laboratory teaching. A total of 53 schools applied for membership in the QSEN collaborative, and we suspect that the act of applying stimulated attention to improving quality and safety education, even though only 15 schools could be funded. Once again, we used DSS values and methods with 45 expert teachers, and they exceeded our expectations in terms of the breadth and quality of the innovative teaching strategies they developed.

We achieved our goal to end Phase II with at least 40 people who could join the QSEN faculty ranks and provide consultation for associate degree, diploma, and university programs in geographical areas around the country. In addition, a group of collaborative members conducted and published a Delphi study to assist faculties with determining the logical progression of quality and safety competency development across curricula (Barton *et al.*, 2009). We also populated the QSEN web site with teaching strategies that became available for faculty throughout the world to use. QSEN leader Pamela Ironside served as coeditor for a special edition (December 2009) of the *Journal of Nursing Education*, where numerous innovative ideas for developing QSEN competencies (many from collaborative members) were published.

Another influential factor in this phase was our commitment to linking QSEN to practice. Pilot schools were expected to bring clinical partners to the QSEN meetings, and those participants enriched the discussions of both the problem and potential solutions. Many of the teaching innovations required access to root cause analyses, quality improvement project data, methods of error reporting, or electronic health records. Without the common goal of improving quality and safety education for the next generation of nursing graduates, clinical settings often prevented faculty and student access to these learning opportunities. In evaluating their participation in the QSEN Collaborative, faculty participants often commented that a valuable and important outcome had been the extent to which their work on QSEN had strengthened academic-clinical partnerships.

Another potential explanation is that clinical partners helped keep nursing faculty aware of the rationale for the need to change our approaches to nursing professional identity formation. Batalden and Foster (2012) proposed that creating an environment in which people generate never-ending improvement of the quality-safety-value of health care requires a commitment that holds three aims together: 1) better outcomes of care; 2) better system performance; and 3) better professional formation and development. Indeed, QSEN leaders noted that faculty responded with energy and commitment when it was clear how the work we were asking them to do was linked to the needs of patients, families, and communities. Apart from this link, the call for curricular change to accommodate a paradigm shift in thinking about quality and safety may not have found fertile ground.

Embedding New Competencies: Phase III

(November 2008–November 2011 [UNC]; February 2009–February 2012 [AACN])

As Phase II entered its final months, QSEN relationships shifted in preparation for a major faculty development initiative. Program manager Rosemary Gibson resigned her position at RWJF, and we worried about the impact the loss of this long-term partner would have on QSEN work. By some

---

Textbox 3.1 QSEN Phase III: Three Aims

1) Promote continued *innovation* in the development and evaluation of methods to elicit and assess student learning of the knowledge, skills, and attitudes of the six IOM/QSEN competencies and the widespread *sharing* of those innovations.
2) Develop the *faculty expertise* necessary to assist the learning and assessment of achievement of quality and safety competencies in all types of nursing programs.
3) Create *mechanisms to sustain the will to change* among all programs through the content of textbooks, accreditation and certification standards, licensure exams, and continued competence requirements.

---

good fortune, QSEN advisory board member MaryJoan Ladden was hired by RWJF shortly thereafter and was appointed our new program manager and spokesperson within the foundation. Her intimate knowledge and support for the work of QSEN was crucial during the downturn in the economy (and foundation resources) that occurred as Phase III began.

In another shift in relationship, Geraldine (Polly) Bednash, the executive director of the AACN, moved from QSEN advisory board member to principal investigator of the train-the-trainer faculty development initiative portion of Phase III. Three QSEN faculty members (Barnsteiner, Disch, and Johnson) joined Dr. Bednash to develop the resources and lead the teaching of the regional conferences sponsored by the AACN Phase III grant. Three other QSEN faculty members (Ironside, Moore, and Coinvestigator Sherwood) worked with me on UNC-based initiatives. Collectively, we made up the Steering Committee, which oversaw the incredible investment that RWJF made (see Textbox 3.1 and Figure 3.2).

Finally, Paul Batalden and Mark Splaine, another DSS community member and head of the Veterans Administration Quality Scholars (VAQS) program, suggested that we explore the possibility of making VAQS, until then a program for physicians only, into an interprofessional program that would include nursing pre- and postdoctoral scholars. The Veterans Administration (VA) had mechanisms for paying nursing scholars, but since nursing faculties were not employed by the VA in the way medical faculties were, they had no way to pay faculty members for mentoring VAQS nursing scholars. I met with Dr. Hassmiller to explore the possibility of additional RWJF support for this purpose, and she was enthusiastic about the possibility of partnering with the VA to educate the first quality improvement scholars in nursing. Shirley Moore, a QSEN faculty member, proceeded to work with Dr. Splaine to codirect this new interprofessional VAQS program.

Thus began a three-year intensive effort (still under way at the time of writing) to develop faculty expertise for integrating QSEN competency development in curricula throughout the country.

Phase III Impact Factors

One of the Phase III factors that we believe assisted forward progress in faculty development was the following multimodal approach that was taken across two major grants using one steering committee:

- For prospective faculty (pre- and postdoctoral scholars) with an interest in quality improvement science, the VAQS initiative provided a unique opportunity for interprofessional learning and development of scholars in an area of science that was new to nursing.
- Faculty members worldwide could seek their own self-development opportunities on the QSEN web site, through teaching strategies submitted from the field at large and through learning modules developed with expert editorial support from Pamela Ironside.
- For schools that wanted to contract with one or more consultants to conduct faculty development activities with entire faculties on their own campuses, descriptions of QSEN facilitators were accessible through the QSEN web site.

- For schools that wished to send QSEN champions to train-the-trainer opportunities, nine conferences were held in regions across the country (sold out for each one held to date). These early adopters received extensive resources for themselves and for educating colleagues at home.
- For innovator faculty members who were experimenting with new curricula, pedagogies, and clinical and simulation teaching, the opportunity to submit their work for peer review and presentation at QSEN national forums was provided.

In sum, a faculty development opportunity was in reach of anyone, anywhere. Furthermore, the impact of each faculty development method was potentiated by others. Web site learning opportunities were mentioned at conferences, and conferences were advertised on the web site. QSEN facilitators presented and moderated panels at the national forums, thus increasing their visibility and subsequent solicitation as consultants. Through the generosity of RWJF, this multimodal, multi-grant approach was possible. Add to that the 2009 special issues of *Nursing Outlook* and *Journal of Nursing Education*, and QSEN *was* everywhere.

Another important factor was a conscious focus on what would be needed to support the execution phase of improving quality and safety education for faculty, regardless of whether they were innovators, early adopters, or late adopters. Innovators needed to be able to get together and stimulate each other's creativity and motivation to persist in innovating for the field. The QSEN Pilot School Collaborative, QSEN facilitators group, VAQS program, and QSEN National Forums were designed for these purposes.

Early adopters needed faculty development and consultation opportunities that could bring QSEN ideas to them and their schools without requiring everyone to "reinvent the wheel" from KSA learning objectives alone. QSEN web site resources, train-the-trainer regional conferences, and QSEN facilitators, along with this group's publications and presentations, all served to support early adopters.

In spite of the enthusiasm of innovators and early adopters, there remains a large group of faculties who either have never heard of the QSEN competencies (in IOM or QSEN terms) or do not appreciate the fact that accomplishing improvements in this domain requires the knowledgeable support of every faculty member in every school. For those faculty members not innately attracted to or unaware of the work, changing standards for licensure and certification (and continuing competence in both domains) and changing standards for accreditation of nursing education programs are important tools for encouraging continuous improvement.

Another strategy for late adopters was changing the content of the textbooks used in courses. We had expected to have to *push* in this area. Instead we were (and still are) being *pulled* into the processes of change. Textbook authors, working on next editions of more than 20 textbooks, have requested assistance or authorship of sections related to QSEN competency development. Others are undoubtedly making these changes without our knowledge or assistance. One major publisher of nursing textbooks currently requires authors to document the manner in which they are addressing each QSEN competency. Finally, after many calls for a "QSEN Textbook," Drs. Sherwood and Barnsteiner agreed to coedit the book in which this chapter appears.

QSEN and Beyond

In May 2011, our RWJF program manager, MaryJoan Ladden, invited Dr. Bednash and me to submit proposals for one final QSEN phase, so the end of this story and the eventual impact on professional identity formation and continuing competency development of nurses is not yet clear. IPEC, which is sponsored by six professional organizations that represent those who educate allopathic and osteopathic physicians, nurses, pharmacists, dentists, and public health, recently published (2011) a monograph that calls upon the health professions to prepare graduates with interprofessional team and team-based care competencies. The four competencies (values/ethics for interprofessional practice, roles/responsibilities for collaborative practice, interprofessional communicaton, and interprofessional teamwork and team-based care) and their learning objectives overlap significantly with QSEN competency definitions and KSAs. We hope that QSEN has prepared nursing faculty with ideas and resources that will increase the quality of their contributions to this important initiative.

What should we expect to see over time if QSEN's impact, along with other national initiatives, "changes the world"? Initially, curricula have to change so that students develop their professional identity assuming that to be a good nurse means being competent in patient-centered care, teamwork and collaboration, evidence-based practice, quality improvement, safety, and informatics. Using a sample of new nurses who graduated August 2004 to July 2005, Kovner, Brewer, Yingrengreung, and Fairchild (2010) reported analyses of data from a 2008 survey where 39% of the nurses thought they were "poorly" or "very poorly" prepared about or had "never heard of" quality improvement. Fortunately, Drs. Kovner and Brewer, also funded by RWJF, will follow more recent cohorts of newly licensed nurses during their 10-year study, enriching the assessments and analyses of outcomes pertaining to development of quality and safety competencies. We hope that over time we will be able to answer the question posed in Gregory, Guse, Dick, and Russell's (2007) research brief "Patient Safety: Where is Nursing Education?"

In the end, however, returning to Batalden and Foster's (2012) triangle, we will hopefully find health professionals who, as part of their daily work, care for individual patients while simultaneously improving population health, system performance, and professional development. To be successful, we will need to discover ways to support nursing faculty as key contributors to the interprofessional work of continuous quality improvement so that they are role models as well as guides for what it means to be a good nurse. If we succeed in reaching these lofty aims and QSEN has been one of the optimistic catalysts for this magnitude of change, it will be a legacy of which to be proud.

QSEN: 2012–2017

The pioneering work begun in early 2000 has continued at the same fast pace and with broadened dissemination and use in academic and health care organizations, in this country and abroad. What originally began as an initiative to teach faculty the IOM safety competencies has been transformed into an interprofessional, international movement that is bringing passionate advocates together with far-ranging interests to improve quality and safety. This section will describe what has evolved within the nursing education arena. It will also provide a brief overview of where the movement is now heading to improving clinical practice through academic-clinical partnerships, to promoting interprofessional education and practice, and to spreading the word to, and learning from, our international colleagues.

Education

Faculty in schools of nursing continue to integrate the QSEN competencies, with the requisite knowledge, skills and attitudes, into curricula, and share innovative strategies for use in the classroom, simulation laboratories, and clinical settings. As of June 2016, Google scholar indicated that the quality and safety education for nurses publication (Cronenwett *et al.*, 2007) describing the QSEN initiative with the competencies and requisite knowledge, skills and attitudes had been cited in 684 publications. Many of the articles describe how the competencies are being demonstrated in innovative teaching strategies across programs and how outcomes are measured. The first edition of *Quality and Safety in Nursing: A Competency Approach to Improving Outcomes* (Sherwood and Barnsteiner, 2012), received the American Journal of Nursing first place award for Leadership in 2013 and has been translated into Swedish, Korean, and Chinese.

Hundreds of articles and editorials have been written on the competencies and their implementation. Authors who have numerous QSEN publications include Gwen Sherwood, Mary Dolansky, Joanne Disch, Pam Ironside, Gail Armstrong, and Amy Barton. In addition to those previously published, a number of professional nursing journals published special topic issues on quality and safety and the QSEN project, including the following:

- *Archives of Psychiatric Nursing*: October 2012
- *Nursing Clinics of North America*: September/October 2012
- *Journal of Professional Nursing*: March/April 2013

The home of QSEN has successfully transitioned from the University of North Carolina at Chapel Hill to Francis Payne Bolten School of Nursing at Case Western Reserve University. This includes the QSEN Institute, which is the annual meeting that serves as a focal dissemination point for educators, researchers, and increasingly clinicians to present the latest innovations in quality and safety; the QSEN web site; and the consultation service for incorporating the QSEN competencies into nursing curricula.

Expanding Focus

The QSEN work with the leadership of Mary Dolansky, PhD, RN, has expanded from an essentially educational focus to one that seeks to improve the quality and safety of care by promoting stronger academic-practice partnerships. The expanded network includes nurses from academia and practice, other healthcare professionals, nursing professional organizations (American Nurses Association [ANA], Association of Operating Room Nurses [AORN], American Nurses Credentialing Center, National Council of State Boards of Nursing [NCSBN], American Association of Colleges of Nursing [AACN], Association of Nurse Executives [AONE]) and interprofessional organizations (IHI, American Association of Medical Colleges [AAMC], and the Veterans Administration [VA]).

These networks are enabling clinicians to apply the latest evidence and best practices. One example is the QSEN partnership with ANA. A QSEN pre-conference, QSEN Quality Competencies: Connecting Academic and Nursing Practice, was held at the 2016 annual ANA staffing conference and also at the 2015 AONE. Examples of application in clinical settings include the use of the QSEN framework for orientation at the Children's Hospital of Denver, the University of Pennsylvania Health System, the University of Alabama Birmingham hospital, and the ProMedica Health System. The University of Pennsylvania Health System and Denver Children's Hospital are also using the QSEN framework for their clinical advancement program.

Numerous statewide initiatives have been developed. Two examples are 1) the Florida Statewide Initiative Integrating Quality and Safety Education for Nurses (QSEN) Through Academic/Clinical Partnerships to Improve Health Outcomes, and 2) the Michigan Academic Practice Partnership. In Ohio, Dr. Mary Dolansky worked with the Ohio Organization of Nurse Executives to develop a white paper calling for the QSEN framework to be used in all nursing education programs and in the practice arena. In the Michigan example, former Dean Mary Mundt worked with Deans and Chief Nursing Executives to foster academic clinical partnerships based on the QSEN competencies.

The direction is also spreading from a largely nursing focus to an interprofessional one that is influencing how all health professions' students are improving quality and safety together. Successful examples include the collaborative partnership among health professions' schools, titled the Interprofessional Education Collaborative, which was spearheaded by the AACN to offer annual quality and safety workshops to develop interprofessional academic/clinical teams doing safety and quality improvement work. The Veterans Administration Quality Scholars Fellowship Program brings together researchers to work together through interprofessional learning and scholarly inquiry about quality and safety.

The work of QSEN has also moved into the international arena. In addition to numerous international publications, partnerships have been developed between the QSEN Institute and the Swedish Society of Nursing and collaborators in Canada, Japan, and China. QSEN experts have been working with colleagues in Sweden, Saudi Arabia, Spain, United Kingdom, Finland, Japan, France, China, and Thailand. These partnerships are assisting faculty and clinicians in countries other than the United States to learn the competencies and integrate them in nursing education and practice.

Moving forward there is a need to continue to stay focused on QSEN's purpose, that is, ensuring that nurses and other healthcare professionals have the requisite knowledge to provide the highest quality, safest care by delivering *person-and-family-centered care* as members of an *interprofessional team*, emphasizing *evidence-based practice, safety, quality improvement approaches,* and *informatics.*

References

American Association of Colleges of Nursing. (2006) *The essentials of doctoral education for advanced nursing practice.* Retrieved April 21, from http://www.aacn.nche.edu/dnp/pdf/essentials.pdf.

American Association of Colleges of Nursing. (2008) *The essentials of baccalaureate education for professional nursing practice.* Retrieved April 21, 2011, from http://www.aacn.nche.edu/education/bacessn.htm.

Barton, A.J., Armstrong, G., Preheim, G., Gelmon, S.B., and Andrus, L.C. (2009) A national Delphi to determine developmental progression of quality and safety competencies in nursing education. *Nursing Outlook, 57*(6), 313–322.

Batalden, P., and Foster, T.C. (2012) Sustainably improving health care: Creatively linking care outcomes, system performance and professional development. Radcliffe Publishing Ltd., London, UK. ISBN-13: 978-1846195211.

Cronenwett, L., Sherwood, G., Barnsteiner, J., Disch, J., Johnson, J., Mitchell, P., *et al.* (2007) Quality and safety education for nurses. *Nursing Outlook, 55*(3), 122–131.

Cronenwett, L., Sherwood, G., and Gelmon, S.B. (2009) Improving quality and safety education: The QSEN Learning Collaborative. *Nursing Outlook, 57*(6), 304–312.

Cronenwett, L., Sherwood, G., Pohl, J., Barnsteiner, J., Moore, S., Sullivan, D. T., *et al.* (2009) Quality and safety education for advanced nursing practice. *Nursing Outlook, 57*(6), 338–348.

Gibson, R., and Singh, J.P. (2003) *Wall of silence: The untold story of the medical mistakes that kill and injure millions of Americans.* Washington, DC: Lifeline Press.

Gregory, D.M., Guse, L.W., Dick, D.D., and Russell, C.K. (2007) Patient safety: Where is nursing education? *Journal of Nursing Education, 46*(2), 79–82.

Institute for Healthcare Improvement. (2003) *The breakthrough series: IHI's collaborative model for achieving breakthrough improvement.* IHI Innovation Series white paper. Boston: (available on www.IHI.org).

Institute of Medicine. (2003) *Health professions education: A bridge to quality*. Washington, DC: National Academies Press.

Interprofessional Education Collaborative. (2011) *Core competencies for interprofessional collaborative practice: Report of an expert panel*. Retrieved June 24, 2011, http://www.aacn.nche.edu/Education/pdf/IPECReport.pdf.

Kenny, C. (2008) *The best practice: How the new quality movement is transforming medicine*. New York: Public Affairs Perseus Books Group.

Kohn, L.T., Corrigan, J.M., and Donaldson, M.S. (Eds.). (2000) To err is human: Building a safer health system. Washington, DC: National Academies Press.

Kovner, C.T., Brewer, C.S., Yingrengreung, S., and Fairchild, S. (2010) New nurses' views of quality improvement education. *The Joint Commission Journal on Quality and Patient Safety*, 36(1), 29–35.

Malloy, P., Paice, J., Virani, R., Ferrell B.R., and Bednash, G. (2008) End-of-life nursing education consortium: 5 years of educating graduate nursing faculty in excellent palliative care. *Journal of Professional Nursing*, 24(6), 352–357.

National Council of State Boards of Nursing. (2011) *Transition to practice*. Retrieved April 21, 2011, from https://www.ncsbn.org/363.htm.

National League for Nursing (NLN) Nursing education advisory council for competency development. (2010) *The NLN Education Competencies Model*. Retrieved April 21, 2011, from http://www.nln.org/facultydevelopment/competencies/index.htm.

Pohl, J.M., Savrin, C., Fiandt, K., Beauchesne, M., Drayton-Brooks, S., Scheibmeir, *et al.* (2009) Quality and safety in graduate nursing education: Cross-mapping QSEN graduate competencies with NONPF's NP core and practice doctorate competencies. *Nursing Outlook*, 57(6), 349–354.

Sherwood, G. (2011) Integrating quality and safety science in nursing education and practice. *Journal of Research in Nursing*, 16, 226–240.

Smith, E.L., Cronenwett, L., and Sherwood, G. (2007) Current assessments of quality and safety education in nursing. *Nursing Outlook*, 55(3), 132–137.

Section 2

Quality and Safety Competencies

The Quality and Safety Education for Nurses Project

4

Patient-centered Care

Mary K. Walton, MSN, MBE, RN and Jane Barnsteiner, PhD, RN, FAAN

Gus was a tall man; everything about him was big and strong. He was a beloved husband, father, father-in-law, grandfather—the family patriarch. He was diagnosed with pancreatic cancer. He chose to fight. Whipple procedure, chemotherapy…. He got C-difficile. Over months of treatment, he suffered a dramatic weight loss, pain, and GI distress. Picture the downward spiral. We hate to see it as we try to conquer a formidable cancer.

His legal name was Harry, an Americanized version of his name in Greek. He never used it. In fact many members of his large loving family never knew Harry was his legal name. "Call me Gus." Every time he was asked in the hospital, he said, "Call me Gus." The name on his chart and records was Harry. Guess what name we called him by? Harry.

Think about Gus as he lost his health, his ability to be the strong family leader. He lost his physical strength. Did he need to lose his name? This is one of the indignities that his family still remembers several years after his death. It bothered Gus and it bothered his family when we called him Harry.

How do we create systems and structures to help us to call the person by their preferred name?

The relationship between patients and nurses has always revolved around care, but the nature of the relationship has varied greatly, ranging from totally caring *for* patients—and the health care professionals making all health care decisions—to a full partnership *with* the patient and the family if that is the patient's wish, in identifying the problem, developing a plan, and evaluating the plan's success. For reasons of quality, safety, and consumer preference over the past decade, this relationship is shifting toward one of active involvement, even control, by the patient and family, which is requiring cultural and organization change across the health care arena (Disch, 2010). Although this QSEN competency (see Appendices A and B) reads "patient-centered care," the term patient- and family-centered care (PFCC) has emerged as more representative of the concept and acknowledges the significant role that family plays in the health care experience. Here, "family" are those individuals the patient chooses to call family, rather than those defined by providers. Furthermore, the term person-centered care is being increasingly used because the term patient is inadequate for representing recipients of care who are less often hospitalized and receive care in ambulatory care centers, clinics, schools, community centers, pharmacies, and in their own homes (Barnsteiner, Disch and Walton, 2014). Person-centered care reflects the growing recognition that the person receiving care needs to be a partner with health care providers to maximize effectiveness and quality of care.

Patient- and family-centered care is a culture, and as such, demands reflection on deeply held values and meaningful life experiences (Barnsteiner, Disch, and Walton, 2014). Uncovering and exploring

Quality and Safety in Nursing: A Competency Approach to Improving Outcomes, Second Edition.
Edited by Gwen Sherwood and Jane Barnsteiner.

these values and experiences may be uncomfortable or even threatening to learners. Teaching PFCC requires didactic approaches and engagement through exercises that prompt critical thinking, coupled with demonstration of knowledge and skill acquisition. Learners must be prompted to identify what they experienced through guided reflection connecting them to the didactic content and application to practice. Reflections on personal values and beliefs and their influence on practice should enable learners to explore and grasp the culture of PFCC and contrast it with provider-centered approaches to care. As the learner comes to recognize the relationship of personal values to practice and acquire skill in communication and eliciting patient values, the goal of care reflecting the patient's values and beliefs can be achieved.

Recalling the personal experiences with health care, illness, and death that shaped the learner's values may evoke memories of mistreatment, suffering, loss, grief, and unresolved relationship issues. Reflections on both personal and professional experiences may prompt distress, anger, and the uncovering of painful life events. Teachers need to be attentive to the range of emotional responses generated through this work and be prepared to respond (Brien, Legault, and Tremblay, 2008). The full engagement of the "hearts and minds" of care providers through respectful partnerships and a commitment to shared values of PFCC is identified as one of the primary drivers for an exceptional inpatient hospital experience (Balik *et al.*, 2011).

The creation of partnerships in learning, rather than the traditional hierarchy of education, is recognized as essential to meeting the needs of today's student and practicing clinician. This shift is reflected in the needs of patient care where the move from provider-centered care to one of partnership among patients, their loved ones, and nurses is recognized as essential for quality and safety in today's complex arena of health care. These learner-teacher partnerships mirror the partnerships of PFCC, ranging from a focus on an individual's care to that of a health care organization's systems and structures.

Definitions

The Institute of Medicine (IOM), in its landmark book *Crossing the Quality Chasm* (2001), defined patient-centered as "providing care that is respectful of and responsive to individual patient preferences, needs, and values and ensuring that patient values guide all clinical decisions." Thus, the IOM boldly redirected the orientation of the health care industry to one in which full patient engagement is an essential precursor to quality and safety rather than merely an option (Disch, 2010). Patient-centered care is one of the six dimensions of quality (safe, timely, effective, efficient, equitable, and patient-centered) espoused by the IOM (2001).

An important variation of patient-centered care is family-centered care. Henneman and Cardin (2002) suggest that family-centered care is an extension of patient-centered care, "widening the circle of concern to include those persons who are important in a patient's life." They go on to note that family-centered care does not negate the patient's rights to privacy or control but rather recognizes that this is a choice that can be made by the patient. Family-centered care is a philosophy that considers the patient as the unit of attention within the patient's network of relationships. Patient- and family-centered care is a term describing a philosophy and culture that emphasizes partnerships between patients, family members, and health care providers. Several organizations have studied and influenced the shift in culture from provider-centered care to that of patient-centered care over the past several decades. Although they vary slightly, the definitions offered by the Picker Institute, the Institute for Patient- and Family-Centered Care, and Planetree share common elements (Balik *et al.*, 2011) (refer to Textbox 4.1).

Textbox 4.1 Definitions of Patient- and Family-centered Care

Source: Balik B. et al. Achieving an exceptional patient and family experience of inpatient hospital care (IHI Innovation Series white paper), 2011. Cambridge, MA: Institute for Healthcare Improvement (available on www.IHI.org). Reproduced with permission of IHI.

The Picker Institute

Patient- and family-centered care is defined as "improving health care through the eyes of the patient." All patients deserve high-quality health care and patient views and experiences are integral to improvement efforts.
  Patient-centered care includes the following principles:

- Effective treatment delivered by staff you can trust;
- Involvement in decisions and respect for patients' preferences;
- Fast access to reliable health care advice;
- Clear, comprehensive information and support for self-care;
- Physical comfort and a clean, safe environment;
- Empathy and emotional support;
- Involvement of family and friends; and
- Continuity of care and smooth transitions.

Institute for Patient- and Family-centered Care
Patient-and family- centered care has these characteristics:

- People are treated with dignity and respect;
- Health care providers communicate and share complete and unbiased information with patients and families in ways that are affirming and useful;
- Patients and family members build on their strengths by participating in experiences that enhance control and independence; and
- Collaboration among patients, family members, and providers occurs in policy and program development and professional education, as well as in the delivery of care.

Planetree
Patient- and family-centered care includes the following components:

- Human interaction;
- Family, friends, and social support;
- Information and education;
- Nutritional and nurturing aspects of food;
- Architectural and interior design;
- Arts and entertainment;
- Spirituality;
- Human touch;
- Complementary therapies; and
- Healthy communities.

The Joint Commission adopts the definition of PFCC established by the Institute for Patient- and Family-Centered Care, described as "an innovative approach to plan, deliver, and evaluate health care that is grounded in mutually beneficial partnerships among health care providers, patients, and families." Patient- and family-centered care applies to patients of all ages, and it may be practiced in any health care setting" (2010).

Work led by the IHI to improve the health of individuals and populations focuses on five areas, one of which is Person-and Family-Centered Care defined as "putting the patient and the family at the heart of every decision and empowering them to be genuine partners in their care" (http://www.ihi.org/about/Pages/default.aspx).

A recent definition of person- and family-centered care put forth by the NQF (2015) emphasizes the inclusivity of the recipients of health care and their families and caregivers: "an approach to the planning and delivery of care across settings and time that is centered on collaborative partnerships among individuals, their defined family, and providers of care. It supports health and well-being by being consistent with, respectful of, and responsive to an individual's priorities, goals, needs, and values" (http://www.qualityforum.org/Publications/2015/03/Person-_and_Family-Centered_Care_Final_Report_-_Phase_1.aspx).

Establishing partnerships with patients and their families is an essential element of PFCC including partnerships beyond the individual patient level. Patients and family members as advisors involved in all operations of the organization, from task forces to governing boards, can transform the health care organization to one centered on the patient and family experience of care rather than that of the providers. PFCC is *not* conceptually similar to patient-*focused* care. In this form of care, although the patient/family may be involved, the health care provider retains control over decision-making. Patient needs and preferences may or may not be sought and rarely drive care decisions.

The QSEN competencies support the concept of PFCC (Cronenwett *et al.*, 2007, 2009). It is the most inclusive option, underscoring the philosophy that both the patient and family, as defined by the patient, are recipients of care by nurses. This holistic focus on the family unit is a distinguishing characteristic of nursing (Disch, 2010).

Balint (1969) contrasted patient-centered medicine with illness-centered medicine and described positive patient outcomes when physicians understand their patients as a unique human being in addition to their focus on the illness and create space for "their patients to tell them what they want in their own time and in their own way." Over the ensuing years, researchers and clinicians as well as consumers have examined the outcomes of shifting from provider- or illness-focused care to one that engages the patient and provider in a partnership where patient preferences and values direct care. The recent IOM report *The Future of Nursing: Leading Change, Advancing Health* notes the need for patient-centered care to improve quality, access, and value yet recognizes that "practice still is usually organized around what is most convenient for the provider, the payer, or the health care organization and not the patient" (2011).

A growing body of evidence shows that improving the patient experience and developing partnerships with patients are linked to improved health outcomes. For example, evidence shows that patients who are more involved in their care are better able to manage complex chronic conditions, seek appropriate assistance, have reduced anxiety and stress, and have shorter lengths of stay in hospital (Balik *et al.*, 2011).

A business case for hospital redesign reflecting patient-centered principles includes both evidence-based design innovations and experience-based innovations that result in outcomes such as fewer patient falls, reduced adverse drug events, fewer health care-acquired infections, and reduced length of stay (Sadler *et al.*, 2011).

Key Concepts

The IHI works with health systems to improve the care experience through improved coordination and communication and also compassion. The engagement of patients and family members in both the care of the individual as well as in developing new models of care is promoted so that their values and care preferences are central. IHI characterizes their goal as shifting the conversation from "What's the matter?" to "What matters to you?" (http://www.ihi.org/Topics/PFCC/Pages/Overview.aspx). IHI and its partners are starting to demonstrate that engagement and co-design and co-production with individuals and families improves health, quality, and value.

IHI's focus on person- and family-centered care includes:

- Developing care pathways that are co-designed and co-produced with individuals and their families;
- Ensuring that people's care preferences are understood and honored, including at the end of life;
- Collaborating with partners on programs designed to improve engagement, shared decision making, and compassionate, empathic care; and
- Working with partners to ensure that communities are supported to stay healthy and to provide care for their loved ones closer to home" (IHI, http://www.ihi.org/Topics/PFCC/Pages/Overview.aspx).

Patient and family engagement is now recognized as an effective strategy and integral part of improving quality, safety and patient outcomes. It is defined as "patients, families, their representatives, and health professionals working in active partnership at various levels across the health care system—direct care, organizational design and governance, and policy making—to improve health and health care" (Carman *et al.*, 2013). Leaders are now systematically partnering with patient and family members in improvement efforts (Health Research and Educational Trust, 2015; Herrin *et al.*, 2015). "Health care today is a profoundly mutual enterprise" where patients and family caregivers have increased responsibilities to achieve the best possible outcomes (Gruman, 2013).

The Institute for Patient- and Family-Centered Care identifies four core concepts for PFCC: dignity and respect, information sharing, participation, and collaboration (www.ipfcc.org). The foundation for PFCC is the special relationship between the patient/family and the caregivers. "In the therapeutic relationship the needs of the person receiving care are of overriding concern, and the needs of the clinician are intentionally attended to elsewhere. …The purpose of the therapeutic relationship is to promote, guide, and support the healing of another person through knowledgeable and authentic connection" (Koloroutis and Trout, 2012).

Gerteis *et al.* (1993) identified several dimensions of patient-centered care. These include the following:

- *Respect for patients' values, preferences, and expressed needs.* Respect is evident in the sharing of desired information with the patients and families; the active partnering with them to determine care priorities and a plan; tailoring their level of involvement according to their preferences, not those of the care providers; and reformulating the plan as the situation changes.
- *Coordination and integration of care.* As care becomes more complex due to the coexistence of multiple chronic conditions, an increasing number of care providers, numerous care sites, and shorter episodes of care, the need for creating smooth transitions across the episodes of care becomes even more vital.
- *Information, communication, and education.* Some individuals prefer comprehensive explanations, while others prefer none. Some people learn best visually, while others favor the personal experience. Adjusting the message and its delivery according to the individual patient's preferences

is a major challenge yet a cornerstone to patient-centered care. What is common to all situations is that patients want to be able to trust what they are being told, and to receive it in a manner that makes sense to them, at a level they can understand.

- *Physical comfort.* Assuring that patients will be comfortable, and free from pain, is a basic expectation of patient-centered care. However, for a variety of reasons, this is often not adequately addressed and must form the basis for any personalized plan of care.
- *Emotional support.* Similarly, patients and their families may experience anxiety and distress from a number of sources, and the underlying factors need to be identified and dealt with. This is nursing's work and what enables us to make unique contributions to the patient/family experience.
- *Involvement of family and friends.* For more than 40 years, research has indicated that children need their parents nearby. Patient-centered care requires that visiting hours, and engagement of family and friends in all aspects of the process as defined by the family, are structured to meet the patients' needs, regardless of the age of the patient.

Background: What Do Patients and Families Want?

Growing evidence for more than 30 years has examined what patients and families want from the care experience. Churchill, Fanning, and Schenck (2013) sought to answer the fundamental question "What do patients see as the core elements in forming therapeutic relationships with their health care providers?" through extensive interviews with individuals with significant chronic illnesses. Koloroutis and Trout (2012) emphasize that "no matter who the patient is, the purpose of the therapeutic relationship remains the same: to connect with another *as a person* in order to facilitate healing." Earlier authors focused on the needs of patients in specific clinical settings, for example, in the critical care environment (Daley, 1984; Hickey and Leske, 1992; Leske, 1986; Mundy, 2010). The results have been fairly consistent with those identified by Molter (1979) in her classic study of relatives of intensive care unit patients, that is, the need for information, to be near the patient, and for reassurance and support.

Despite this extensive body of evidence, many critical care units continue to struggle with finding ways to implement patient-centered policies (Davidson, 2007). Nurses lack consensus as to what constitutes "appropriate" patient-family involvement. This is witnessed in the disagreements about visiting hours and presence of family members during resuscitation, among other examples. A qualitative study examining the experience of nurse family members of critically ill patients highlights the tension and conflict that can develop when care is not individualized and reflects the values and beliefs of providers over those of the family member (Salmond, 2011). Mounting evidence describes the benefits of family members' presence at the resuscitation of their loved ones (Emergency Nurses Association, 2009; Halm, 2005; Howlett, Alexander, and Tsuchiya, 2010; MacLean *et al.*, 2003; Mangurten *et al.*, 2005) and reflects the increasing inclusion of family throughout the care process. More controversial is the inclusion of family members in the process for disclosing adverse events to patients and, in some organizations, inviting them to participate in root cause analysis of adverse events (Cantor *et al.*, 2005). This form of inclusion requires clear policies, consumer preparation, and close monitoring of the process.

Planetree, established in 1978 as a "non-profit organization that provides education and information in a collaborative community of healthcare organizations, facilitating efforts to create patient centered care in healing environments," is another example of an organization that has whole-heartedly embraced the concept of patient-centered care and become an international leader in promoting it (www.planetree.org/about/html). This is accomplished through conferences, publications, networks, and consultations.

In 2001, the IOM issued its call for patient-centered care and, in 2006, the IOM report *Preventing Medication Errors* outlined patients' expectations. These include "being listened to and respected as a care partner, being told the truth, having care and information sharing coordinated with all members of the team, and partnering with staff who are able to provide both technically and emotionally supportive care" (Spath, 2008). Spath (2008) offers a Patient/Family Engagement Self-Assessment tool assessing whether staff are "personally ready to engage patients and families in improving safety." The *American Journal of Nursing*'s "Putting Patients First" series offers examples of patient-centered approaches to the provision of nursing care developed by the Planetree group (Frampton, 2009; Frampton and Guastello, 2010; Frampton, Wohl, and Cappiello, 2010; Michalak *et al.*, 2010).

Patients and families have been engaged for decades in various activities that have equipped them to be partners in their care. Examples include receiving preoperative and home instructions, learning to take medications and perform treatments, monitoring vital signs, and watching for complications. More recently, however, patients and family members are being invited to actively participate on health system boards, committees, and task forces. For example, hospitals are now including patients and/or families as members of patient safety committees, interview teams, and participants in new employee orientation (Herrin *et al.*, 2015). Likewise, increasingly faculty in schools of nursing include patients in classrooms, such as panels discussing patient-centered care, family involvement in chronic care, or care for the caregiver.

National Standards and Regulations

Over the past few years, the stakes have been raised as more knowledgeable consumers actively select where they will receive care, and patient's evaluation of their experience of care begins to have an effect on payment patterns. National regulatory agencies are weighing in on the issue of PFCC. For example, the Joint Commission, the NCQA, and the CMS are increasingly involved in stipulating expectations and monitoring performance. The federal government uses its Hospital Consumer Assessment of Healthcare Providers and Systems (HCAHPS) survey to measure patients' perceptions of their hospital experience and posts public results (www.hospitalcompare.hhs.gov). It is the first tool to help consumers compare hospitals nationally on key variables that include communication, responsiveness, cleanliness, noise, and pain management. Of particular importance to nursing is that some questions specifically relate to nursing performance, which allows for comparisons across organizations. CMS has designed an incentive program to reward facilities that use the tool and, more importantly, report their data (www.cms.gov).

Another example of a national organization using its influence to promote patient and family involvement is the NQF, a voluntary consensus standards-setting body that has endorsed more than 500 measures of quality and safety. The NQF, through its National Priorities Partnership (2008), identified six priorities with the greatest potential for improving care, reducing disparities, and eliminating waste. One priority is patient and family engagement. The group is working to ensure that all patients:

- will be asked for feedback on their experience of care, which health care organizations and their staff will then use to improve care;
- will have access to tools and support systems that enable them to effectively navigate and manage their care; and
- will have access to information and assistance that enables them to make informed decisions about their treatment options.

In 2014 the NQF convened a multi-stakeholder action team and issued a Patient and Family Engagement Action Pathway toward the goal of anchoring healthcare in patient and family preferences. They offer strategies and exemplars for dialogue, partnership, and change (http://www.qualityforum.org/Publications/2014/07/Patient_and_Family_Engagement_Action_Pathway.aspx).

New accreditation standards and federal regulations for hospitals provide a powerful stimulus toward a culture of patient- and family-centered care. The Joint Commission issued *Advancing Effective Communication, Cultural Competence and Patient- and Family-Centered Care: A Roadmap for Hospitals* (2010) and *Advancing Effective Communication, Cultural Competence, and Patient- and Family-Centered Care for the Lesbian, Gay, Bisexual, and Transgender (LGBT) Community: A Field Guide* (2011) to provide specific methods to improve quality and safety initiatives and implement new accreditation standards. These documents detail many strategies and practices for care improvement with summary checklists focused on points along the care continuum: admission processes, assessment, treatment, end-of-life care, discharge, and transfer, as well as organizational readiness (Joint Commission, 2010). Specific recommendations on assessment and approaches to elicit and understand the patient's values and perspectives are included (Joint Commission, 2010).

The Joint Commission standards now include the patient's right to identify a support person and have access to that person throughout an inpatient admission. Surveyors will examine the process for notifying patients of this right and identifying the support person. This individual, based on the patient's preference, may be involved in patient care rounds, education, and planning for transitions in care. Patients in intensive care units are particularly vulnerable, with complex communication needs. "These patients must have unrestricted access to their chosen support person while in the intensive care unit (ICU) to provide emotional and social support" (Joint Commission, 2010).

A presidential memorandum focused on hospital visitation and specifically noting the issues of lesbian, gay, bisexual, and transgender patients and their families directed CMS to establish federal regulations for patient rights (White House, 2010). Effective in January 2011, CMS issued a new condition of participation standard, requiring hospitals to inform patients of visitation rights and the patient's right to receive visitors whom he or she designates, including a spouse, domestic partner, family member, or friend. Thus, these new Joint Commission and CMS requirements recognize the vulnerability of hospitalized individuals and formally establish the role of a "support person" in the hospital setting (HHS/CMS, 2010). Now patients may choose to have an ally at their bedside to ensure that their preferences, needs, and values are respected and to guide clinical decision-making. And, finally, consistent with the above, the 2015 revisions of the ANA Scope and Standards of Practice recognize the health care consumer as the authority on their own health and embrace the need for partnership to achieve the goals of nursing care (ANA, 2015).

Teaching the Competencies

Recognizing the patient as the source of control and full partner in providing compassionate and coordinated care is a challenge for any health care professional given the hierarchical nature of Western medical care. Furthermore, most practice settings have long been established as provider centered, although some organizations have successfully embedded a philosophy of PFCC and instituted the processes and systems to make this a permanent change (Balik *et al.*, 2011; Frampton, Wohl, and Cappiello, 2010; Herrin *et al.*, 2015; Reid-Ponte *et al.*, 2003; Wasson *et al.*, 2003; Zarubi, Reiley, and McCarter, 2008). Clinical experiences in PFCC organizations offer exposure to a physical environment and a culture of partnership among clinicians, patients, and loved ones in all aspects of operations. Until all care settings reflect PFCC, prelicensure nursing students and practicing nurses alike will need to develop competency in providing patient-centered care without necessarily experiencing it. Education to gain competency in PFCC demands a curriculum and learning experiences that are participatory, active, and experiential. Providing patient-centered care reflects a nurse's values and attitudes, arises from a deep knowledge base, and requires skilled communication to practice. Below are teaching strategies for the classroom, simulation, and clinical settings to engage students and practicing clinicians at all levels in learning the knowledge, skills, and attitudes necessary to engage the patient as a full partner in providing compassionate and coordinated nursing care based on the patient's preferences, values, and needs.

Didactic Strategies

Narrative Pedagogy

The relationship between storytelling, or narrative and health care is vital to clinical practice. Narrative practices can hone clinical skills and promote the trust and relationship building necessary to navigate the complexities of health care (Wahlert, 2014). Narrative thinking is recognized as an approach to help clinicians shift their gaze from a clinical lens to that of the individual seeking care. In clinical ethics where consultants address value-laden concerns, narrative approaches offer effective ways to enter into and understand the experience of patients and families. In 2014, The Hastings Center issued a special report, Narrative Ethics: The Role of Stories in Bioethics in which clinical ethicists illustrate how to think through patient stories (Montello, 2014). Nurse leaders also recognize the contributions of a narrative culture to clinical outcomes (Erickson *et al.*, 2015).

Fictional and autobiographical literature is particularly suited to teaching PFCC. Autobiographical stories told by patients about their experiences of illness rather than about the disease process express the truth of personal experience in the patient's own voice (Sakalys, 2003). Illness narratives have evolved into a major literary genre and are increasingly used as an effective teaching strategy (Brown *et al.*, 2008; Diekelmann, 2005; Ewing and Hayden-Miles, 2011; Gazarian, 2010; Kumagai, 2008; Sakalys, 2002; Sakalys, 2003; Shattell, 2007; Wall and Rossen, 2004).

The depictions of illness, disease, and caring found in fiction, poetry, drama, film, and paintings are far more powerful and sensitive than the explanations contained in textbooks. Engaging students and clinicians in reading/viewing, interpreting, and critiquing promotes reflective thinking and the consideration of alternate perspectives and meanings in situations. Participants change from reading for information, key points, main ideas, or answers and take authority for their own learning by reading reflectively, observing both their own reactions and the questions the work evokes and actively creating meaning. They gain an understanding of the human experiences and the capacity to adopt another's perspective (Sakalys, 2002). Teachers and learners challenge assumptions and interpret situations from multiple perspectives. "Narratives offer an opportunity for discourse that opens up new possibilities for student-centered learning" (Ewing and Hayden-Miles, 2011). Incorporating narrative strategies promotes critical thinking, reasoning, and analytical skills along with introspection and self-reflection to facilitate the participants' shifting their view from their personal and professional lens to the patient's perspective. There are an infinite variety of ways that patient narratives can be used to develop the knowledge, skills, and attitudes for competency in PFCC. Sakalys (2002) offers numerous strategies to engage students and clinicians in careful reading and reflections on illness narratives. Wahlert (2014) also offers a range of approaches including ones suited to clinical practice such as writing with patients and their families, for example asking a patient to write a parallel chart or a family member to write about the patient's illness. Comparing and contrasting narratives offers opportunities to reimagine the experiences and learn from each other. It is the opportunity to be creative and engage learners in identifying published narratives, films, and artwork for class study. Examples of suggested learning strategies are offered below.

Evaluating the Hospital Experience Through the Patient's Eyes

Illness narratives by patients offer the reader the opportunities to see the patient's experience without a clinical lens. Discuss their stories and compare and contrast to the definitions of PFCC. Introduce the HCAHPS tool. Direct the learners to complete the survey based on a published narrative, thus engaging them in reading for context and meaning as well as learning the evaluation process. Participants will vary in how they "see," appreciate, and evaluate the patient narrative. Explore these variations in classroom discussion. Evaluate these narratives for evidence of patient engagement and activation as well as for evidence of clinician support. Jesse Gruman chronicles her cancer journey, illustrating how patients can improve outcomes (Gruman, 2013). Nurse Amy Berman offers her perspective on quality of life while living with terminal cancer (Berman, 2015). Narratives such as these illustrate patient engagement and activation; learners see the concepts in action.

Narratives of health care experiences published in the professional literature provide first-person narratives by nurses and physicians and offer the reader the opportunity to "see" a patient's experience through the dual lens of professional and patient. Read, discuss, and evaluate the specific examples in terms of patient-centered care. Was the patient the source of control? Was the care compassionate and coordinated and reflective of the patient's preferences, values, and needs? How was the experience and narrative shaped by the author's professional perspective? Prompt the identification of both patient-directed and provider-directed aspects of care. Where were the missed opportunities to meet patients' needs? What promoted the PFCC aspects of the care experience? What thwarted it? Was nursing visible in the narrative? Did the nurse support patient engagement?

Art Interpretation

The visual arts offer nonverbal narratives that can prompt reflection on the artist's perspective and help learners develop insight and empathy. Art calls for viewers to listen attentively and think about what is openly expressed or hidden from view and to bring this knowledge to spoken language, providing information about values, conflicts, and beliefs (Ewing and Hayden-Miles, 2011). Because learners differ in their cultural, social, and historical backgrounds, multiple interpretations will be generated through the study of a single image. Many of artist Frida Kahlo's works reflect her life experiences of trauma, surgery, hospitalization, suffering, pain, and loss; one example for study is "Henry Ford Hospital." Viewing, discussing, and journaling about art provides a "refreshing way to enlighten students to gain access to others, make connections, and gain a deeper understanding and appreciation for multiple perspectives and levels of knowledge" (Ewing and Hayden-Miles, 2011). This serves to reinforce the need to recognize the variety of perspectives and to elicit the patient's perspective in the provision of care.

Films

Films tell stories. Film is used successfully in both health professions and ethics education (Alexander, Lenahan, and Pavlov, 2005; Ber and Alroy, 2001; Volandes, 2007). Film provides context and can serve to illustrate the patient's perspective. Selecting and using complete films or short clips is a recognized approach to foster the learner's reflection and improve education in the affective domains (Blasco *et al.*, 2006; Wall and Rossen, 2004). As one example, the HBO movie *Wit*, based on the Pulitzer Prize-winning play, is a first-person, fictional narrative of a woman treated for stage IV ovarian cancer. The patient speaks directly to the viewer when narrating her hospital experience. One theme to explore is how the specialty and organizational values influence the patient's experience of care. Clinical research and physician education goals continually override patient care considerations. Other themes to explore are the nurse's partnership with the patient, value conflicts, and moral distress.

Classroom Forums for Patient/Family Advisors or Student Health Care Narratives

Organizations that embrace the philosophy of PFCC establish formal roles for patient and family advisors. In these organizations, patient/family advisors share their experiences in orientations, grand rounds, and staff development programs. These forums are considered essential to a PFCC organizational culture. Patient and Family Advisors introduced to improvement theory will move beyond simply sharing their perspectives; their health care stories may be used to inform, inspire and serve as a catalyst for change (Health Research and Education Trust [HRET], 2015). Local health care organizations may have advisors interested in classroom presentations. If this is not feasible, an alternate approach would be to engage learners in developing and sharing a first-person account of a health care encounter to illustrate PFCC. Effective strategies to maximize the effectiveness of patient storytelling for improvement are offered in the literature (HRET, 2015) The learner can embrace the principles of PFCC, including roles of advisors, offering the class a range of experiences for reflection and critique.

Value Identification Exercises

Recognition of personal and professional values is a fundamental component to competency in PFCC. Life experiences shape and inform personal values, beliefs, and practice. A variety of personal experiences and values lead each student to select nursing. Published exercises can help; for example, *Toward Culturally Competent Care: A Toolbox for Teaching Communication Strategies* from the Center for the Health Professions, University of California, San Francisco (UCSF) contains exercises to promote introspection and identification of personal as well as professional values and beliefs (Mutha, Allen, and Welch, 2002). This lays the groundwork for approaches to eliciting and understanding the patient's perspective and experience of illness. Two examples follow:

- *Exercise: Family Healing Traditions* (UCSF Toolbox Exercise IB): The purpose is to create an atmosphere where each individual's experiences are valued and to begin to examine cultural differences in healing practices. Participants are asked to write down some of the health beliefs and practices instilled by their families. First in pairs and then in the group, participants share and discuss them. Personal traditions are compared and contrasted with Western biomedical approaches. The use of complementary and alternative medicine approaches and effectiveness in their personal experience can be explored. Learners reflect on how they would feel sharing a personal healing tradition that is not consistent with evidence-based practice with their own provider. How might this healing tradition be received? How could it be incorporated into a treatment plan?
- *Exercise: What Do We Need to Know About Ourselves to Provide Culturally Competent Care?* (UCSF Toolbox Exercise VIA): The purpose of this exercise is to help participants understand their own norms and preferences and to explore strategies for working with patients who have different norms. Relating these cultural values to the concepts of PFCC can highlight the potential for conflict between the provider and the patient. Refer to Figure 4.1.

Review each value, and prompt participants to mark where they fall on the continuum. Discuss and compare how these values reflect the four core concepts of PFCC as identified by the Institute for Patient- and Family-Centered Care (www.ipfcc.org; see Table 4.1). Lead a facilitated discussion

HANDOUT VIA.1

YOUR CULTURAL VALUES

Directions: On each continuum below, place an X indicating where you believe
you fall as an individual. Put parentheses around the area on the continuum
that reflects your comfort zone when interacting with other people.

SOCIAL STATUS

Inherited ·················· Eamed

PRIVACY

Guarded ·················· Open/Shared

FATALISM

Fate determined by ·················· Fate determined by self
outside influence

GROUP/INDIVIDUAL

Health care decisions ·················· Health care decisions
made by family/group   made by Individual

ACCESS TO INFORMATION

Information withhold ·················· Right to know

Figure 4.1 **Your cultural values**. Source: Mutha S, Allen C, and Welch M. Toward Culturally Competent Care:
A Toolbox for Teaching Communication Strategies, 2002, San Francisco: Center for the Health Professions, University
of California-San Francisco, as adapted from Managing Diversity in Health Care, by L. Gardenswartz and A. Rowe,
1999, San Francisco: Jossey-Bass. Reproduced with permission of the Regents of the University of California.

Table 4.1 Cultural values aligned with core concepts of patient/family-centered care.

Cultural Values	Patient/Family-Centered Care Concepts
Social status: inherited or earned	Dignity and respect
Privacy: guarded-open/sharing	Information sharing
Fatalism	
Group/individual: How decisions are made	Participation and independence
Access to information	Collaboration

of how one's personal values might prevent seeing the care situation through the patient's eyes.
An individual who values privacy and independent decision making may fail to recognize a need for
or even reject a request for family presence in a meeting to discuss an elective surgical procedure for
a patient who values family decision making.

Identify organizational values. Values shape health care settings, professional and specialty
practices, and therefore the patient experience (Baggs *et al.*, 2007). Organizational values such as

profit, efficiency, risk reduction, expediency, and compliance may be in play, and core values of the nursing profession "can be challenged or come into conflict when confronted by other values operative within the health care system" (Fowler, 2015). Academic practice settings place value on the generation of new knowledge and education. Staff may be comfortable promoting participation in clinical research and working with students, and may be challenged when patient care priorities conflict. In contrast, in community-based settings where the primary focus may center on the patient care experience, education and research efforts may not be as highly valued. Values may differ between for-profit and not-for-profit organizations. Ensuring that employees understand and reflect organizational values in their practice is challenging (Neumann and Forsyth, 2008). Engage learners in identifying organizational values. An exercise might include a review of health organizations' public web sites for values expressed though content as well as the presentation of information.

Identify professional values. Consider the professional values of nursing as articulated by the ANA and specialty organizations such as the American Association of Critical-Care Nurses and the Oncology Nursing Society. Discuss how these values shape both the individual and their practice setting and therefore influence the patient and family experience. Discuss the interpretations and applications of the ANA Code of Ethics for Nurses in light of partnership- or patient-directed care. Where do values converge and where is there risk of conflict? Consider the ethically controversial issues in intensive care units related to the use of life-prolonging interventions where conflicts do not hinge solely on technical clinical determinations but rather on contested value judgments. Review and discuss the multisociety policy statement that recommends using the term "potentially inappropriate treatments" rather than "futile" in recognition of the underlying value conflict (Bosslet *et al.*, 2015). Nurses may adopt the values of a specialty practice, which in turn may hinder the ability to recognize a patient's alternative value. The promotion of hope in oncology and the use of do-not-resuscitate orders are values reflected in specialty literature. The fields of organ transplantation and neonatology reflect specialty beliefs and values. How can practitioners ensure that the patient's values are respected in light of these well-established specialty values? How does a nurse honor personal values if the patient's values create conflict? How have minority group values shaped or influenced health care in the United States? Consider the diversity in definitions of family. For example, contrast the US Census Bureau (two or more people together related by birth, marriage, or adoptions) with other definitions such as the 1981 White House Conference on Aging, "a family is a system of related and unrelated individuals integrated by patterns of social relationship and mutual help." How might one's definition of family influence care? Topics such as the debate over childhood immunizations or mandatory influenza vaccination for health care workers can be used to illustrate the impact of values on practice. Consider how the rejection of blood transfusions based on spiritual beliefs prompted the development of blood-less surgery (Schaffer, 2015). Pain management is another area where values shape practice. How does the nurse concerned about relief of pain honor a patient or family spiritual belief that suffering is part of the human experience and should not be mitigated?

Care at the end of life is guided by deeply held values concerning the meaning of life, duties to family and friends, beliefs about the significance of pain and suffering, and spiritual considerations. The primacy of patient's values is well recognized in end of life care; yet conflict among providers, patients, and loved ones is evident in public debate and professional literature. Advances in knowledge and technology, such as ventricular assist devices, extracorporeal membrane oxygenation, and hypothermia therapy, make the determination of actual death challenging. Less complex therapies such as placement of gastrostomy tubes for enteral nutrition still prompt conflict over values among all stakeholders. Identifying and communicating individual values and care preferences at the end of life is challenging. Ethics consultations in acute care address value conflicts and often arise around end of life care. Fiester (2015) challenges clinical ethics consultants to guard against values imposition and offers a bioethical positions inventory to prompt identification of strongly held beliefs given the risk of imposing personal or professional values on patients and families. The need to explore values at the end of life increasingly recognized and one highly regarded resource is The Conversation Project (www.theconversationproject.org). This is a national initiative developed by a journalist to promote conversations about preferences for end of life care around the kitchen table with loved ones rather than in a hospital with clinicians (www.theconversationproject.org). Have learners work through one of the starter kits to talk with either family or physician about care preferences.

The phenomenon of moral distress resulting from value conflicts is increasingly recognized in the profession. "Individualized beliefs, values, character traits, cultural background, and life or personal experience will impact the way in which a nurse understands and responds to moral concerns that arise" in practice (Rushton and Kurtz, 2015). An assignment to share preferences for end of life care with the person identified as a surrogate decision maker can help to clarify personal values that will influence their feelings in practice. The focus is communicating preferences and values to another rather than preparing a legal document such as an advance directive. Learners will experience the difficulty of articulating and sharing their values. Another tool to engage learners in reflecting on values is My Gift of Grace, a card game that promotes conversation about values. Game play serves to prompt clinicians to explore personal values as well as experience the deep reflection needed to answer questions commonly asked of patients in the clinical setting (http://mygiftofgrace.com). Direct learners to discover and evaluate the many resources on the web to prepare an advance directive or a Physician Orders for Life-Sustaining Treatment (POLST) (www.nhdd.org).

Teaching What PFCC Looks Like in Action: Examples of Patient-Family Engagement

Engage learners in examining the philosophy and concepts of PFCC as well as what the experience of care in a PFCC organization looks like by introducing them to the myriad resources available in the public domain. Most of them are accessible via organizational web sites. Some examples follow:

- The Joint Commission Roadmaps (2010; 2011) provides many clinical strategies and prescribes actions. This document can be used in a variety of ways to teach the standards as well as how hospitals will be evaluated to determine organizational enculturation during an accreditation survey.
- Planetree offers a self-assessment tool for patient/resident- or client-centered organizations. Core dimensions of patient-centered care are highlighted including structures and functions for culture change, human interactions, promoting patient choice and responsibilities, family involvement, dining and nutrition, and healing environment. These criteria focus on the patient experience as well as the experience of family members, front-line staff, leadership teams, medical staff, patient and family advisors, and board members. The tool is available at http://planetree.org/designation-information-form.
- The Institute for PFCC has materials to develop an understanding of PFCC, for example, *Partnering with Patients and Families to Enhance Safety and Quality: A Mini Toolkit* (2011).
- The 2011 CMS Regulations on Patient Visitation Rights (HHS/CMS, 2010) were prompted by an egregious care situation in a Florida hospital. Learners may research the origin of the regulations and how the media and public have varied in the portrayal of the regulations. Facilitate discussion on how relevant and significant regulations influence the clinical encounter.
- The IHI Organizational Self-Assessment tool allows organizations to understand the range and breadth of elements of patient- and family-centered care and to assess where they are against the

leading edge of practice. This tool is available at http://www.ihi.org/resources/Pages/Tools/PatientFamilyCenteredCareOrganizationalSelfAssessmentTool.aspx.

- "My Patient Passport" (2015) the NQF's Patient and Family Engagement Action Team is a tool to promote dialogue about care preferences and needs. The goal is a conversation rather than answers prompted by routine questions posed by staff (NQF, 2015; Landro, 2015). Create ways to populate and discuss the passport and how its use may promote quality and patient safety (http://www.qualityforum.org/Patient_Passport.aspx).

Exercise: Simulate a Family Meeting

Direct learners to plan a family meeting where information is shared and difficult treatment decisions are discussed. Curtis and White (2008) offer approaches for evidence-based ICU conferences and include a communication component to "explore and focus on patient values and treatment preferences." The Planetree/Picker *Patient-Centered Care Improvement Guide* provides a "Patient Care Conference Form" with nine topics ranging from the hospital's culture of safety to wishes concerning resuscitation (Frampton *et al.*, 2008). Learners can compare and contrast the quality of communication and influence of patient values with two approaches to a family meeting: 1) starting with a medical overview and offering of information from the provider's perspective, versus 2) starting with the patient/family-expressed goals for the meeting and summarizing their current understanding of patient condition/prognosis.

Communication among the patient and the health care team is essential if patients are the source of control and care is based on their preferences, values, and needs. The Joint Commission's SPEAK UP initiative, launched in 2002, offers a variety of materials to promote communication for patients, including videos, for example, "Speak Up: Prevent Errors in Your Care" (www.jointcommission.org/speakup.aspx). Videos focused on engaging individuals in promoting safety are posted on Facebook by the Joint Commission and can be reviewed and discussed for content as well as technique.

Use of Technology to Support PFCC

Barton (2010) examines how technology can enhance patient-centered care and provides two examples that use the computer and equipment alarms. The nurse can place and use the computer in relation to the patient and structure the flow of assessment to allow the patient to tell their story rather than answer a series of questions. Equipment alarms prompt a nurse to respond to the patient, providing an opportunity for meaningful contact and explanation. Discuss the reported differences between clinicians and consumers in their views on the value of new medical technology in terms of impacting patient activation (Boeldt *et al.*, 2015). Consider how personalized technology will enable individuals to control access to their health data and create new care options (Subramanian *et al.*, 2015).

Simulation

Simulation is an effective learning strategy to prepare for clinical practice (Durham and Alden, 2012). McKeon *et al.* (2009) report a pilot study to compare required resources and learning outcomes for prelicensure, intermediate-level nursing students. Faculty developed a pretest-post-test case study design to compare simulation learning methods for achievement of the six QSEN patient-centered care competences. Many of the exercises in this chapter would be considered low fidelity and could be used in the classroom or learning laboratory.

Clinical Strategies

Evaluation of a Clinical Environment

Significant attention has turned toward the importance of the physical environment itself and its impact on health and healing as a component of patient-centered care. Reiling, Hughes, and Murphy (2008) provide a comprehensive review of the impact of facility design on patient safety. The Green Guidelines for Health Care (2010) offer a premier resource for health care leaders as they build new and remodel old facilities. Planetree and the Picker Institute (2008) offer guidelines for designing this environment:

> A patient-centered environment of care is one that is safe and clean, and that guards patient privacy. It also engages all the human senses with color, texture, artwork, music, aromatherapy, views of nature, and comfortable lighting, and considers the experience of the body, mind, and spirit of all who use the facility. Space is provided for loved ones to congregate, as well as for peaceful contemplation, meditation, or prayer, and patients, families, and staff have access to a variety of arts and entertainment that serve as positive diversions. At the heart of the environment of care, however, are the human interactions that occur within the physical structure to calm, comfort, and support those who inhabit it. Together the design, aesthetics, and these interactions can transform an institutional, impersonal, and alien setting into one that is truly healing (Environment of Care section, para. 2).

The Planetree Designation Self-Assessment Tool (2015) offers criteria in the category of Healing Environment: Architecture and Design and is available on request at www.planetree. org. Direct learners to evaluate a practice setting in their community using these criteria as a guide and discuss their findings and recommendations. Entry into the building provides an opportunity to simulate the patient experience through way finding and access to language services. Facilitate discussion of the learner's perceptions and compare to the principles of PFCC. If evaluations of the same practice setting vary, discuss the differing perceptions. Prompt reflection on the impact of environment-patient interaction on the nurse-patient encounter. For example, might a patient's initial interaction with a nurse reflect the experiences in the parking lot, lobby, or admission's office prior to an encounter with the clinician? How does the milieu affect the quality of the patient experience? Consider the Beryl Institute definition of the patient experience, that is, the sum of all interactions that influence patient perceptions (Wolfe *et al.*, 2014). What opportunities can be identified to improve the environment toward the goal of shaping the patient experience? How do they support the patient and family engaging in a partnership for care with clinicians?

Patient-centered Clinical Rounds/Change of Shift Report

In the in-patient setting, practice patterns are well established for care, provider transitions, and physician education. These patterns may present challenges to engaging patients and families as members of their care team. Surgical team rounds are held based on operating room schedules. Medical rounds may focus on education in addition to care review. Meaningful participation of patients and families in interdisciplinary bedside rounds and nursing change of shift report will promote PFCC. AHRQ identifies these as effective strategies promoting patient and family engagement in care (AHRQ, 2014). Review and discuss the implementation of these practices in clinical sites or work settings. Are there innovative approaches to fostering partnerships in the acute care setting if participation in rounds is not feasible?

Reframing Constructive Criticism Using Reflection Based on the QSEN Competencies

Language used in the clinical setting matters and shapes meaning and perspectives. Consider these two examples reflecting family presence: "We allow 24-hour visitation" versus "We welcome you throughout the hospitalization." On the QSEN web site, Altmiller posted examples of reframing constructive criticism based on the QSEN competencies (2010). Consider the shift in perspective from "Your patient needs attention now. You cannot leave him like that" to "If you were that patient lying in that bed, what would be the most important thing the nurse could do for you at this minute?"

When work is challenging, the problem may be identified in relation to the patient and family rather than a deficiency or gaps in the provider or system/organization (Neal *et al.*, 2010). A difficult IV placement may be communicated to a patient as "you have bad veins" versus "I am not skilled enough to place your IV." When family members fill a patient room, a nurse may say, "This is a crowd. Too many people here." rather than "This room is too small to accommodate all those who care about you." Close examination of nursing language may reflect a provider rather than a patient perspective. Analysis and discussion of common language and the perspective it highlights can illustrate PFCC concepts.

Eliciting Patient Preferences and Values

Nurses need to develop skill in listening and eliciting patient values in order to ensure they are reflected in care. Elements of individual variation in communication styles include language fluency, health literacy, degree of directness, use of facial expressions and eye contact, touch, and use of silence. For oral communication, the following is encouraged: using plain language; speaking slowly; providing small amounts of information at one time; and reinforcing with written materials with key points circled. A collaborative style builds from the patient perspective using an "Ask, Tell, Ask" and "Tell Me More" approach (Back *et al.*, 2005). Assessing and responding to communication vulnerabilities is essential, and nurse researchers are studying the communication needs of critically ill patients (Khalaila *et al.*, 2011; Radtke, Tate, and Happ, 2012). Explore the SPEACS-2 training program available on the web and discuss how nurses skilled in these techniques are better prepared to assess patients to create and implement an individualized communication plan for non-vocal ICU patients. Consider how the patient might be able to express values and care preferences when nurses employ assistive and augmentative communication strategies (http://nucleus.con.ohio-state.edu/media/speacs2/speacs.htm).

Eight questions developed by Arthur Kleinman, a Harvard psychiatrist/anthropologist, offer an effective approach for nurses to elicit a patient's illness experience and beliefs. Known as "Kleinman's Questions," they are included in the Joint Commission Roadmap (Kleinman, Eisenberg, and Good, 1978; Joint Commission, 2010):

1) What do you think has caused your problem?
2) Why do you think it started when it did?
3) What do you think your sickness does to you? How does it work?
4) How severe is your sickness? Will it have a short or a long course?
5) What kind of treatment do you think you should receive?
6) What are the most important results you hope to receive from this treatment?
7) What are the chief problems your sickness has caused for you?
8) What do you most fear from your sickness?

In Fadiman's (1997) book *The Spirit Catches You and You Fall Down*, in which a Hmong child is cared for in Western society with disastrous results, the questions are used to illustrate how eliciting the family's explanatory framework would have changed the patient outcome. If care is to reflect a patient's health beliefs and values, the ability to elicit those values is an essential competency for nurses.

Conclusion

Patient-centered care is supported by many individuals, groups, and organizations, but it requires a paradigm shift. The care delivery system in the United States has been largely based on the premise that the health care provider is responsible for providing the care and knows best what works in each situation. There is momentum and support from many to engage patients actively in their care. Achievement requires all health care providers, administrators, and policy makers to recognize the patient-centered value of "nothing about me without me" and act accordingly (Delbanco *et al.*, 2001).

References

Alexander, M., Lenahan, P.A., and Pavlov, A. (2005) *Cinemeducation: A comprehensive guide to using film in medical education.* Oxford: Radcliffe.

Altmiller, G. (2010). *Reframing constructive criticism using reflection based on QSEN competencies.* Retrieved from www.qsen.org.

AHRQ. (2014) Internet citation: Exhibit 9. Strategies to engage patients and families as part of the health care team: Guide to patient and family engagement: Environmental scan report. October. Agency for healthcare research and quality, Rockville, MD. http://www.ahrq.gov/research/findings/final-reports/ptfamilyscan/ptfamilyex9.html.

American Nurses Association (ANA). (2015) *Nursing Scope and Standards of Practice*, 3rd Ed. Silver Spring, MD: Nursebooks.org.

Back, A.L., Arnold, R.M., Baile, W.F., Tulsky, J.A., and Fryer-Edwards, K. (2005) Approaching difficult communication tasks in oncology. *CA: A Cancer Journal of Clinicians*, 55, 164–177.

Baggs, J.G., Norton, S.A., Schmitt, M.H., Dombeck, M.T., Sellers, C.R., and Quinn, J.R. (2007) Intensive care unit cultures and end-of-life decision making. *Journal of Critical Care*, 22, 159–168.

Balik, B., Conway, J., Zipperer, L., and Watson, J. (2011) *Achieving an exceptional patient and family experience of inpatient hospital care.* IHI Innovation Series white paper. Cambridge, Massachusetts: Institute for Healthcare Improvement (available on www.IHI.org).

Balint, E. (1969) The possibilities of patient-centered medicine. *Journal of Royal College of General Practitioners*, 1, 269–276.

Barnsteiner, J., Disch, J., and Walton, M.K. (Eds). (2014) *Person and Family Centered Care.* Indianapolis, IN, Sigma Theta Tau International.

Barton, A.J. (2010) Patient-centeredness and technology-enhanced care. *Clinical Nurse Specialist*, 24, 121–122.

Ber, R., and Alroy, G. (2001) Twenty years of experience using trigger films as a teaching tool. *Academic Medicine*, 76, 656–658.

Berman, A. (2015) A nurse with fatal breast cancer says end-of-life discussions saved her life. The Washington Post, September 28. Available: https://www.washingtonpost.com/national/health-science/a-nurse-with-fatal-breast-cancer-says-end-of-life-duscussions-have-saved-her/2015/09/28/1470b674-5ca8-11e5-b38e-06883aacba64_story.html?postshare=1331443464880688.

Blasco, P.G., Moreto, G., Roncoletta, A., Levites, M.R., and Janaudis M.A. (2006) Using movie clips to foster learners' reflection: Improving education in the affective domain. *Family Medicine*, 38, 94–96.

Boeldt, D.L., Wineinger, N.E., Waalen, J., Gollamudi, S., Grossberg, A., Steinhubl, S.R., Topo, E.J. (2015) How consumers and physicians view new medical technology: a comparative study. *Journal of Medical Internet Research* 19(9):e215. doi: 10.2196/jmir.4456.

Bosslet, G.T., Pope, T.M., Rubenfeld, G.D., Lo, B., Truog, R.D., Rushton, C.H., White, D.B. on behalf of The American Thoracic Society ad hoc Committee on Futile and Potentially Inappropriate Care. (2015) An official ATS/AACN/ACCP/ESICM/SCCM policy statement: responding to requests for potentially inappropriate treatments in intensive care units. *American Journal of Respiratory and Critical Care Medicine, 191*(11), 1318–1330.

Brien, L., Legault, A., and Tremblay, N. (2008) Affective learning in end-of-life care education: The experience of nurse educators and students. *The International Journal of Palliative Nursing, 14*, 610–614.

Brown, S.T., Kirkpatrick, M.K., Mangum, D., and Avery, J. (2008) A review of narrative pedagogy strategies to transform traditional nursing education. *Journal of Nursing Education, 47*, 283–286.

Cantor, M.D., Barach, P., Derse, A., Maklan, C.W., Wlody, G.S., and Fox, E. (2005) Disclosing adverse events to patients. *The Joint Commission Journal on Quality and Patient Safety, 31*(1), 5–12.

Carman, K.L., Dardees, P., Maurer, M., Sofaer, S., Adams, K., Bechtel, C., and Sweeney, J. (2013) Patient and family engagement: a framework for understanding the elements and developing interventions and policies. *Health Affairs, 32*(2) 223–231.

Churchill, L.R., Fanning, J.B., and Schenck, D. (2014) *What Patients Teach—The Everyday Ethics of Health Care.* NY: Oxford University Press.

Cronenwett, L., Sherwood, G., Barnsteiner, J., Disch, J., Johnson, J., Mitchell, P., *et al.* (2007) Quality and safety education for nurses. *Nursing Outlook, 55*, 122–131.

Cronenwett, L., Sherwood, G., Pohl, J., Barnsteiner, Moore, S., Sullivan, D. T., *et al.* (2009) Quality and safety education for advanced practice nurses. *Nursing Outlook, 57*, 338–348.

Curtis, J. R., and White, D. B. (2008) Practical guidance for evidence-based ICU family conferences. *Chest, 134*(4), 835–843.

Daley, L. (1984) The perceived immediate needs of families with relatives in the intensive care setting. *Heart & Lung, 13*, 231–237.

Davidson, J.E., Powers, K., Hedayat, K.M., Tieszen, M., Kon, A.A., Shepard, E., *et al.* (2007) Clinical practice guidelines for support of the family in the patient-centered intensive care unit: American College of Critical Care Medicine Task Force 2004–2005. *Critical Care Medicine, 35*(2), 605–622.

Delbanco, T., Berwick, D.M., Boudfford, J.I., Edgman-Levitan, S., Ollenschlager, G., Plamping, D., and Rockefeller, R.G. (2001) Healthcare in a land called PeoplePower: Nothing about me without me. *Health Expectations, 4*, 144–150.

Department of Health and Human Services, Centers for Medicare and Medicaid Services. (2010) Changes to the hospital and critical access hospital conditions of participation to ensure visitation rights for all patients (42 CFR Parts 482, 485). *Federal Register, 75*(223), Nov. 19, 70831–70844.

Diekelmann, N. (2005) Engaging the students and the teacher: Co-creating substantive reform with narrative pedagogy. *Journal of Nursing Education, 44*, 249–252.

Disch, J. (2010) Patient-centered care. Enhancing quality and safety in nursing education: Preparing nurse faculty to lead curricular change (Vol. 1, Version 7A) [CDROM]. Quality and Safety Education for Nurses/American Association of Colleges of Nursing.

Emergency Nurses Association. (2009) *Emergency nursing resource: Family presence during invasive procedures and resuscitation in the emergency department.* Des Plaines, IL. Retrieved from http://www.ena.org/Research/ENR/Documents/FamilyPresence.pdf.

Erickson, J.I., Ditomassi, M., Sabia, S., and Smith, M.E. (2015) *Fostering clinical success—using clinical narratives for interprofessional team partnerships from Massachusetts General Hospital.* Indianapolis, IN: Sigma Theta Tau International.

Ewing, B., and Hayden-Miles, M. (2011) Narrative pedagogy and art interpretation. *Journal of Nursing Education, 50*, 211–215.

Fadiman, A. (1997) *The spirit catches you and you fall down*. New York: Farrar, Straus and Giroux.

Fiester, A. (2015) Teaching nonauthoritarian clinical ethics: using an inventory of bioethical positions. *Hastings Center Report*, *45*(2) 20–26. doi: 0.1002/hast.428.

Fowler, M.D.M. (2015) *Guide to the Code of Ethics for Nurses with Interpretive Statements. Development, Interpretation, and Application*, 2nd Ed. Silver Spring, MD: American Nurses Association.

Frampton, S.B. (2009) Creating a patient-centered system. *American Journal of Nursing*, *109*, 30–33.

Frampton, S.B., and Guastello, S. (2010) Patient centered care: More than the sum of its parts. *American Journal of Nursing*, *110*, 49–53.

Frampton, S., Guastello, S., Brady, C., Hale, M., Horowitz, S., Bennett Smith, S., and Stone S. (2008) *Patient-centered care improvement guide*. Derby, CT: Planetree; Camden, ME: Picker Institute. Available at http://www.patient-centeredcare.org/inside/practical.html#enviornment.

Frampton, S.B., Wohl, C., and Cappiello, G. (2010). Partnering with patients' families: Three ways hospitals can enhance family members' involvement in health care. *American Journal of Nursing*, *110*, 53–56.

Gazarian, P.K. (2010) Digital stories: Incorporating narrative pedagogy. *Journal of Nursing Education*, *49*, 287–290.

Gerteis, M., Edgman-Levitan, S., Daley, J., and Delbanco, T.L. (1993) *Through the patient's eyes: Understanding and promoting patient-centered care*. San Francisco: Jossey-Bass.

Green Guidelines for Health Care. (2010) http://www.gghc.org.

Gruman, J.C. (2013) Narrative matters–an accidental tourist finds her way in the dangerous land of serious illness. *Health Affairs*, *32*(2) 427–431. doi: 10.1377/hlthaff.2012.1083.

Halm, M. (2005) Family presence during resuscitation: A critical review of the literature. *American Journal of Critical Care*, *14*(6), 494–511.

Health Research and Educational Trust. (2015, March). *Partnering to improve quality and safety: A framework for working with patient and family advisors*. Chicago, IL: Health Research & Educational Trust. Accessed at www.hpoe.org **Accessible at:** www.hpoe.org/pfaengagement.

Henneman, E.A., and Cardin, S. (2002) Family-centered critical care: A practical approach to making it happen. *Critical Care Nurse*, *22*(6), 12–19.

Herrin, J., Harris, K.G., Kenward, K., Hines, S., Joshi, M.S., and Frosch, D.L. (2015) Patient and family engagement: a survey of US hospital practices," *British Medical Journal Quality and Safety* 1–8. doi: 10.1136/bmjqs-2015-004006.

Hickey, M.L., and Leske, J.S. (1992) Needs of families of critically ill patients: State of the science and future directions. *Critical Care Nursing Clinics of North America*, *4*, 645–649.

Howlett, M.S., Alexander, G.A., and Tsuchiya, B. (2010) Health care providers' attitudes regarding family presence during resuscitation of adults: An integrated review of the literature. *Clinical Nurse Specialist*, *24*, 161–174.

Institute for Health Care Improvement (IHI). (2016) About IHI, Retrieved from http://www.ihi.org/about/Pages/default.aspx.

Institute of Medicine. (2001) *Crossing the quality chasm: A new health system for the 21st century*. Washington, DC: National Academies Press.

Institute of Medicine. (2006) *Preventing medication errors*. Washington, DC: National Academies Press.

Institute of Medicine. (2011) *The future of nursing: Leading change, advancing health*. Washington, DC: National Academies Press.

Institute for Patient- and Family-Centered Care. (2010) *Changing hospital "visiting" policies and practices: Supporting family presence and participation*. Retrieved from www.ipfcc.org.

Institute for Patient- and Family-Centered Care. (2011) *Partnering with patients and families to enhance safety and quality: A mini toolkit*. Retrieved from http://www.ipfcc.org/tools/Patient-Safety-Toolkit-04.pdf.

Joint Commission. (2010) *Advancing effective communication, cultural competence, and patient-and family-centered care: A roadmap for hospitals.* Oakbrook Terrace, IL.

Joint Commission. (2011) *Advancing Effective Communication, Cultural Competence, and Patient- and Family-Centered Care for the Lesbian, Gay, Bisexual, and Transgender (LGBT) Community: A Field Guide.* Oak Brook, IL, Oct.

Khalaila, R., Zbidat, W., Anwar, K., Bayya, A., Linton, D.M., and Sviri, S. (2011) Communication difficulties and psychoemotional distress in patients receiving mechanical ventilation. *American Journal of Critical-Care Nurses, 20*(6), 470–479.

Kleinman, A., Eisenberg, L., and Good, B. (1978) Culture, illness and care. *Annals of Internal Medicine, 88,* 251–258.

Koloroutis, M., and Trout, M. (2012) *See me as a person: Creating therapeutic relationships with patients and their families.* Minneapolis, MN: Creative Health Care Management.

Kumagai, A.K. (2008) A conceptual framework for the use of illness narratives in medical education. *Academic Medicine, 83*(7), 653–658.

Landro, L. (2015). *Wall Street Journal: Patient passports.* Feb. 2.

Leske, J.S. (1986) Needs of relatives of critically ill patients: A follow-up. *Heart & Lung, 15,* 189–193.

MacLean, S.L., Guzzetta, C.E., White, C., Fontaine, D., Eichhorn, D.J., Meyers, T.A., and Désy, P. (2003) Family presence during cardiopulmonary resuscitation and invasive procedures: Practices of critical care and emergency nurses. *American Journal of Critical Care, 12*(3), 246–257.

Mangurten, J. A., Scott, S. H., Guzzetta, C. E., Sperry, J. S., Vinson, L. A., Hicks, B. A., *et al.* (2005) Family presence: Making room. *American Journal of Nursing, 105*(5), 40–47.

McKeon, L.M., Norris, T., Cardell, B., and Britt, T. (2009) Developing patient-centered competencies among prelicensure nursing students using simulation. *Journal of Nursing Education, 48*(12), 711–715.

Michalak, J., Schreiner, N.J., Tennis, W., Szekely, L., Hale, M., and Guastello, S. (2010) The patient will see you now. *American Journal of Nursing, 110,* 61–63.

Molter, N.C. (1979) Needs of relatives of critically ill patients: A descriptive study. *Heart & Lung, 8,* 332–339.

Montello, M. (Ed.) (2014). Narrative Ethics: The role of stories in bioethics. *The Hastings Center Report,* Jan.–Feb.

Mundy, C. A. (2010) Assessment of family needs in neonatal intensive care units. *American Journal of Critical Care, 19*(2), 156–163.

Mutha, S., Allen, C., and Welch, M. (2002) *Toward culturally competent care: A toolbox for teaching communication skills.* San Francisco: Center for the Health Professions, University of California. Available at http://futurehealth.ucsf.edu/Public/Leadership-Programs/Program-Details.aspx?pid=155&pcid=88

National Priorities Partnership. (2008) *National priorities and goals: Aligning our efforts to transform America's healthcare.* Washington, DC: National Quality Forum.

National Quality Forum. (2014) *NQF- Endorsed Measures for Person-and Family-Centered Care, Phase 1 Technical Report.* Available at http://www.qualityforum.org/Publications/2015/03/Person-_and_Family-Centered_Care_Final_Report_-_Phase_1.aspx.

Neal, A., Twibell, R., Osborne, K.E., and Harris, D. (2010) Providing family-friendly care—even when stress is high and time is short. *American Nurse Today,* November.

Neumann, J. A., & Forsyth, D. (2008). Teaching in the affective domain for institutional values. *Journal of Continuing Education in Nursing, 39,* 248–254.

The Planetree Designation Self-Assessment Tool. (2015) www.planetree.org.

Planetree and the Picker Institute. (2008) *Patient-centered care improvement guide.* Retrieved from http://www.patient-centeredcare.org/inside/practical. html#environment.

Radtke, J.V., Tate, J.A., and Happ, M.B. (2011) Nurses' perceptions of communication training in the ICU. *Intensive and Critical Care Nursing 28*, 16–25.

Reid-Ponte, P.R., Conlin, G., Conway, J.B., Grant, S., Medeiros, C, Nies, J., *et al.* (2003) Making patient-centered care come alive: Achieving full integration of the patient's perspective. *Journal of Nursing Administration, 33*(2), 82–90.

Reiling, J., Hughes, R.G., and Murphy, M.R. (2008) The impact of facility design on patient safety. In *Patient safety and quality: An evidence-based handbook for nurses* (Prepared with support from the Robert Wood Johnson Foundation, AHRQ publication No. 08-0043). Rockville, MD: AHRQ.

Rossen, E.K. (2004) Media as a teaching tool in psychiatric nursing education. *Nurse Educator, 29*(1), 36–40.

Rushton, C.H., and Kurtz, M.J. (2015) Moral Distress and You—Supporting Ethical Practice and Moral Resilience in Nursing. Silver Spring, MD: American Nurses Association.

Sadler, B.L., Berry, L.L., Guenther, R., Hamilton D.K., Hessler, A., Merritt, C., and Parker D. (2011) Fable hospital 2.0: The business care for building better health care facilities. *Hastings Center Report, 41*, 13–23.

Sakalys, J.A. (2002) Literary pedagogy in nursing: A theory-based perspective. *Journal of Nursing Education, 41*, 386–392.

Sakalys, J.A. (2003) Restoring the patient's voice: The therapeutics of illness narratives. *Journal of Holistic Nursing, 21*, 228–241.

Salmond, S.W. (2011) When a family member is a nurse: The role and needs of nurse family members during critical illness of a loved one. *Intensive and Critical Care Nursing,* 2710–2718.

Savitz, L. and Luther, K. (2015) Patient-Reported Measures. Healthcare Executive. Jan;*30*(1):74–77.

Schaffer, A. (2015) How Jehovah's Witnesses are changing medicine. *The New Yorker,* August 12.

Shattell, M.M. (2007) Engaging students and faculty with diverse first-person experiences: Use of an interpretive research group. *Journal of Nursing Education, 46*(12), 572–575.

Spath, P.L. (2008) *Engaging patients as safety partners.* Chicago: Health Forum.

Subramanian, Dumont, Dankert, and Wong. (2015) Personalized technology will upend the doctor-patient relationship. *Harvard Business Review.* June 19.

Volandes, A. (2007) Medical ethics on film: toward the reconstruction of the teaching of healthcare professionals. *Journal of Medical Ethics, 33*, 678–680.

Wahlert, L. and O'Brien, M.T. (2014) Narrative approaches to understanding patient and family perspectives. In. J. Barnsteiner, J. Disch, and M.K. Walton (Eds.). *Person and Family Centered Care.* Indianapolis, IN. Sigma Theta Tau International.

Wall, B. M. and Rossen, E.K. (2004) Media as a teaching tool in psychiatric nursing education. *Nurse Educator, 29*, 36–40.

Wasson, J.H., Godfrey, M.M., Nelson, E.C., Mohr, J.J., and Batalden, P.B. (2003) Microsystems in health care. Part 4: Planning patient-centered care. *The Joint Commission Journal on Quality and Patient Safety, 29*(5), 227–237.

White House Office of the Press Secretary. (2010) *Presidential memorandum for the Secretary of Health and Human Services: Hospital visitation.* April 15. Retrieved from http://www.whitehouse.gov/the-press-office/presidential-memorandum-hospital-visitation

Wolf, J.A., Niederhauser, V., Marshburn, D., and LaVela, S.L. (2014) Defining patient patient experience. *Patient Experience Journal, 1* (1) Article 3. Available at: http://pxjournal.org/journal/vol1/iss1/3.

Zarubi, K., Reiley, P., and McCarter, B. (2008) Putting patients and families at the center of care. *Journal of Nursing Administration, 38*(6), 275–281.

Resources

Centers for Medicare and Medicaid Services. www.cms.gov
Institute for Healthcare Improvement. www.ihi.org
Institute for Patient- and Family-Centered Care. www.ipfcc.org
National Patient Safety Foundation. www.npsf.org
National Quality Forum. www.qualityforum.org
Planetree. www.planetree.org

5

Teamwork and Collaboration

Joanne Disch, PhD, RN, FAAN

They had worked together for four years, she as the evening charge nurse and he as a critical care attending. They had come to rely on each other's skills and expertise, and enjoyed a collegial relationship, but that had not always been the case. When he first started his rotation as a third year Fellow, he was abrupt and dismissive and could be heard belittling the nursing staff on the unit: "If you want something done right, you've got to do it yourself" or "Their job is to follow the orders." Tensions had escalated until the nursing staff was reluctant to bring problems to his attention, anticipating his response – "Don't you know anything about caring for critically ill patients?" On the other hand, the nursing staff was not without some blame, withholding key information from him and pretending to be busy when he asked for help with a difficult patient. Clearly something had to be done. After one particularly trying evening, the charge nurse asked the Fellow if they could talk. "This has been a really difficult rotation for you with lots going on," she began. "I know that you are committed to doing whatever you can to help these patients. So are the nurses. How can I be helpful?" After a blustery first response, she sat quietly as he calmed down and then said, "I am trying to do my best. You're the first person who acknowledged that. You nurses look at things so differently from what we've been trained to do. Some of the time I have no clue as to what you're trying to tell me." She thought for a moment and said, "So, if we could find a way to improve communication between you and the nurses, especially when exchanging information about vital changes in the patient's condition, could that help?" He replied, "It would certainly be a start."

In 1998, the Institute of Medicine (IOM) alerted the public that 98,000 deaths were occurring annually from medical errors. Since then, however, James (2013) used a more comprehensive methodology and estimated that, actually more than 400,000 individuals were dying from preventable harm each year. There are many factors contributing to this shocking statistic, but one that is increasingly being realized as critically important is the extent and quality of teamwork and collaboration among health care professionals.

For many years, industry leaders have called for improvement in teamwork and collaboration. In 2001, the IOM in its Ten New Rules for delivering safe, effective care stipulated that cooperation among clinicians is essential and, more specifically: "Clinicians and institutions should actively collaborate and communicate to ensure an appropriate exchange of information and coordination of care." In 2010, the IOM in the *Future of Nursing* report reiterated that "Nurses should be full partners, with physicians and other health professionals, in redesigning health care in the United States" (IOM, 2010). However, what has become apparent is that multi-faceted, intentional strategies must be employed within the work setting and, equally important, within health professionals' curricula.

Quality and Safety in Nursing: A Competency Approach to Improving Outcomes, Second Edition.
Edited by Gwen Sherwood and Jane Barnsteiner.
© 2017 John Wiley & Sons, Inc. Published 2017 by John Wiley & Sons, Inc.

This chapter will explore the competency on teamwork and collaboration, with particular emphasis on interprofessional teamwork, and offer suggestions for helping students and clinicians learn the knowledge, skills, and attitudes essential for interprofessional practice.

Teamwork

A team consists of two or more individuals who have specific roles, perform ***interdependent*** tasks, are adaptable, and share a common goal (Salas *et al.*, 1992). However, simply naming or installing a team does not always yield teamwork. According to Xyrichis and Ream (2008), teamwork is "a dynamic process involving ***two or more healthcare professionals with complementary backgrounds and skills***, sharing common health goals and exercising concerted physical and mental effort in assessing, planning, or evaluating patient care." AHRQ (2014) defines teamwork as "a set of ***interrelated knowledge, skills, and attitudes*** (KSAs) that facilitate coordinated, adaptive performance, supporting one's teammates, objectives, and mission." Some of the words above have been highlighted to emphasize that key elements of teamwork are the interdependencies and interconnectedness among people with different backgrounds and perspectives. Eduardo Salas (1997), a renowned expert in the field of teamwork and training, joined with his colleagues in noting that shared mental models are necessary so that members can work under shared assumptions, use common decision-making strategies, and have similar expectations regarding each other's roles and responsibilities.

Teams are the functional groups through which much of health care is delivered. Nelson and colleagues (2002) call this a *microsystem*:

> [the] small, functional, front-line units that provide most health care to most people. They are the essential building blocks of larger organizations and of the health system. They are the place where patients and providers meet. The quality and value of care produced by a large health system can be no better than the services generated by the small systems of which it is composed.

The terms *multidisciplinary* and *interdisciplinary* are often used interchangeably when two or more disciplines are involved. However, within academic health centers, *interdisciplinary* often refers to physicians who are from different specialties or disciplines within the profession of medicine, for example, cardiologists versus nephrologists. Internationally and in many parts of the United States, the term *interprofessional* is increasingly being used to emphasize the inclusion of individuals from different professions.

Several related and overlapping concepts are integral to a full understanding of teamwork. These include collaboration, communication, and mutual support.

Collaboration

A core component of effective teamwork is collaboration, the "process of joint decision making among independent parties involving joint ownership of decisions and collective responsibility for outcomes. The essence of collaboration involves working across professional boundaries" (Liedtka and Whitten, 1998). The parties bring individual areas of expertise to a particular situation, as well as diverse perspectives that are influenced by professional orientation, experience, age, gender, education, and socioeconomic status. Collaboration can occur between two individuals, within a small group, or across a broad coalition. Conditions that enhance collaboration include shared goals, an understanding of the other's roles and responsibilities, mutual respect, clear communication, an openness to learning, and an ability to change one's viewpoint, given new information.

In 2015, the RWJF conducted a national survey on collaboration: *Identifying and Spreading Practices to Enable Effective Interprofessional Collaboration*. They described effective interprofessional collaboration as having the following characteristics:

- promotes the active participation of each discipline in patient care, where all disciplines are working together and fully engaging patients and those who support them, and leadership on the team adapts based on patient needs; and
- enhances patient and family-centered goals and values, provides mechanisms for continuous communication among caregivers, and optimizes participation in clinical decision-making within and across disciplines. It fosters respect for the disciplinary contributions of all professionals.

They then identified 20 organizations that were demonstrating exemplary collaboration and interprofessional practice, and conducted site visits at seven of them. Six common patterns emerged within these organizations:

- *Put patients first.* Although most health care professionals intend to do this, most health care systems are not designed to consistently deliver on this goal. Asking what is best for the patient keeps the focus on the patient and helps to equalize power differentials and authority gradients, helping people "'connect the dots' between their particular role, patient care, and the mission of their organization" (RWJF, 2015).
- *Demonstrate leadership commitment to interprofessional collaboration as an organizational priority through words and actions.* A partnership among clinical leaders at all levels was essential, as was a profound commitment from senior leadership and the board. Talking about this is important, but seeing it actualized on a daily basis is what is really noticed.
- *Create a level playing field that enables team members to work at the top of their license, know their roles, and understand the value they contribute.* The idea of a level playing field was mentioned in almost every organization, reducing unhelpful hierarchy and supporting team members to work together, learning new languages and skills, with the added benefit of learning what each individual brings to the team.
- *Cultivate effective team communication.* This was highlighted as a key strategic imperative, that is, enabling team members who come from disparate backgrounds to share language, tools, and common goals.
- *Explore the use of organizational structure to hardwire interprofessional practice.* Ways in which organizational structure can reinforce collaboration were widely shared, including co-locating of offices and co-chairing key organizational committees. Multiple types of practices and supports are needed; one size does not fit all, even within the same organization.
- *Train different disciplines together so they learn how to work together.* Within the clinical setting, this can happen through orientation, staff development, and continuing education. Given the history of health professions' education occurring in silos, any efforts within educational programs to help students learn and gain experience in teamwork and collaboration before they enter practice will help.

Nurse-Physician Collaboration

Nurse-physician collaboration is a historically important form of collaboration in health care. Baldwin (2007) asserts that the focus of nurse-physician collaboration started in World War II with multidisciplinary medical and surgical teams and expanded in the late President Lyndon B. Johnson's Great Society with the idea that the poor and underserved would be cared for by teams.

Fairman and Lynaugh (1998) in their landmark book on the early days of critical care noted the impact that each profession exerted on the development of the other:

> To gain expertise about the care of complex patients, nurses learned through experience and from physicians. Although many physicians were equally unskilled in the care of physically unstable patients, physicians provided much of nurses' postgraduate education through formal lectures and informal conversations. Nurses learned through slow periods in the intensive care area. During these times, residents (usually) and nurses in the intensive care unit discussed patients in detail, each learning from the other. When cardiac monitors were introduced at one hospital, a nurse remembered nurses and physicians grouped informally around the monitor screen in "pick-up" sessions. ... Unusually close camaraderie developed between nurses and physicians in the units because of the small areas, shared sense of adventure in the new setting, and the selection of the "expert nurses," usually young and "energetic," to staff the unit. "We [nurses and physicians] were all in this together," one nurse noted. "We all learned from each other."

As important as many health care professionals believe collaboration to be, nurses and physicians do not similarly define it. For example, Makary and colleagues (2006) noted that nurses in the operating room described collaboration as having input into decision-making, while physicians described it as having their needs anticipated and directions followed. Fletcher *et al.* (2007) examined nurse practitioner (NP) and physician perceptions of the role of NPs as providers of primary care, noting that NPs saw their role as one of autonomous practice while physicians saw the role similar to a physician extender. Casanova and colleagues (2007) noted that "physicians perceive themselves as the dominant authority in patient care while perceiving nursing's main function as carrying out orders" and that "collaboration is sometimes seen as undermining their [physicians] authoritarian role." Interestingly, in almost every study asking physicians and nurses of their perceptions about collaboration, physicians routinely report the perception of greater levels of collaboration than nurses (Carney *et al.*, 2010; King and Lee, 1994; Mills, Neily, and Dunn, 2008; O'Leary *et al.*, 2010; Rosenstein, 2002; Thomas, Sexton, and Helmreich, 2003).

It is understandable that nurses and physicians would approach collaboration from different viewpoints. They come from different cultures, use specialized languages, face different societal expectations, hold differing viewpoints and goals, and often define success very differently. Increasingly, intergenerational differences about motivation, work ethic, learning styles, authority relationships, and communication patterns are also affecting the harmony of work teams. For collaboration to flourish, however, these differences must be identified, acknowledged, and addressed.

A key question to explore is when does collaboration begin, and what does it look like from the younger physician perspective. In a fascinating qualitative study with 20 residents, Weinberg, Miner, and Rivlin (2009) examined the quality of the nurse/physician relationship from the residents' viewpoint. Through interviews, they found great variability in the experiences and viewpoints of the residents but a few common themes: 1) perception of the nurses' cooperativeness and competence shaped the relationship; 2) most residents initiated communication to tell the nurses which orders to fill or to give instructions, but not to necessarily exchange information with them. As one noted, "I tell them tests that I need, but I don't give them much information. They're not making decisions about treatment or anything."; 3) being trustworthy or 'good' was related to their clinical judgment and ability to identify crucial information; 4) generally the residents were unaware of the educational background of the nurses, including LPNs; and 5) residents repeatedly characterized interdependence as "a pattern in which residents gave orders that nurses carried out."

The Benefits of Collaboration

Even though most health care professionals strongly believe in the merits of some form of collaboration, relatively little evidence exists to definitively connect interprofessional collaborative interventions with improved outcomes. For example, in the most recent Cochrane Review on this topic (Zwarenstein, Goldman, and Reeves, 2009), five studies were found that evaluated the effects of practice-based interventions occurring as a result of interprofessional collaboration. The interventions were categorized as interprofessional rounds, interprofessional meetings, and an externally facilitated interprofessional audit. Three of the studies found improvements in key patient care outcomes, for example, drug use, length of stay, and total hospital charges. One study described mixed outcomes, and one showed no impact. It should be noted, however, that there are hundreds of studies and qualitative reports that examine and/or describe some aspect of collaboration occurring within one organization, or with one population that don't rise to the level of scientific rigor that the Cochrane Review reflects. Examples of these include studies or syntheses on collaboration between nurses and physicians and team collaboration (O'Daniel and Rosenstein, 2008); on ICU patient outcomes (Baggs *et al.*, 1999); on 30-day mortality (Estabrooks *et al.*, 2005); on care providers (Boyle and Kochinda, 2004; Messmer, 2008), and the organizations in which care is provided (Cowan *et al.*, 2006; Mohr, Burgess, and Young, 2008).

In the 2015 RWJF survey mentioned above, several of the leaders in the organizations surveyed or visited expressed their beliefs that the interprofessional collaboration had resulted in positive outcomes. Examples that were given included a reduction in fall rates of 50%, a decreased length of stay of 0.6 days, an increase in bed turns by 20%, an increase in discharges before noon from 10 to 30%, and improved operating room performance (20% decrease in turnover over, and an increase in first-time starts from 33 to 75%).

Communication

Communication is "a process by which information is exchanged between individuals through a common system of symbols, signs, or behavior" (Merriam-Webster, 2009). Communication can occur verbally or nonverbally, and it is widely accepted that effective communication is a precursor to collaboration and teamwork. Poor communication has been identified as a major contributor to patient error. The Joint Commission (2015) cited communication failures as one of the three most frequently identified root causes of sentinel events reported to the Joint Commission between 2004 and the third quarter of 2015.

Barriers to communication in health care are plentiful and arise from the different languages that professionals use among themselves and with patients and families; across gender, age, cultural, and ethnic boundaries; and under conditions of stress that can be experienced by patients, families, and care providers. Communication styles and preferences vary among individuals, and with the escalating pace of society today, forms of communication such as e-mail and text messaging add complexity and potential confusion to the exchange of vital information.

A great deal of effort has gone into strengthening communication during key events in an individual's hospitalization. Situation, Background, Assessment, and Recommendation (SBAR) is a tool that offers a framework to clearly, consistently, and succinctly communicate pertinent information among health care professionals. The tool structures communication and helps clinicians respond to situations with a shared mental model. Given that nurses often use a narrative format to share key information, this has proven tremendously helpful in improving shared understanding of situations.

Transitioning the responsibility for care from one caregiver to another is a major area of communication vulnerability within health care. Hand-offs are a critical time for the transfer of information and accountability for care. It's important to remember that hand-offs are used for a variety of purposes, and the uses need to be differentiated, for example, sharing information, clarifying accountabilities, teaching students, and being clear on the organization's purpose(s) for handoffs.

Many other strategies have also been used to improve communication, such as pre-op checklists, standardized multidisciplinary bedside rounds, and daily goals checklists. Multiple strategies are needed and must be built into underlying processes and student/clinician education. Additionally, as with any new innovation, they must be clear, easy to use, fit within a busy work schedule, and engage all health care professionals involved in the care.

Mutual Support

Critical to effective team functioning is a component that is often overlooked or taken for granted: mutual support. Also called "back-up behavior," it is defined as "the discretionary provision of resources and task-related effort to another member of one's team that is intended to help that team member obtain the goals as defined by his or her role when it is apparent that the team member is failing to reach those goals" (Porter *et al.*, 2003). This can take several forms, for example, helpfully pointing out errors before they occur, volunteering to help out when a colleague is overwhelmed, or speaking up for a colleague when a system error or unintended outcome has occurred. This may appear to some care providers as a 'soft' competency, but mutual support can actually provide a very effective safety net since no one person can know everything. For this reason, AHRQ (2012) now includes it as a fundamental module in team training.

Factors That Compromise Effective Team Performance

Many factors can compromise team performance. Within health care, 1) there are so many individuals involved; 2) each has a different scope of practice, which can result in overlap across the professions; 3) the composition of the team can often change due to factors such as 12-hour shifts, float staff, intern/resident/attending physician rotations; and 4) new roles are emerging at a fast pace. From an organizational standpoint, rigid hierarchical differentiation can occur where hierarchy is forced on situations where differing voices could yield better solutions, and where some team members, such as nurses, have information that is vital to a patient's condition and yet feel unable, or are actively discouraged, from sharing it. Another problem occurs when authority gradients associated with professional status or personal power create a dynamic of control and coercion, and the opinions and decisions of an individual in power supersede those advanced by those perceived as being less powerful. This can occur within teams of physicians or nurses, and between health care providers, in general, and patients and their families.

Disruptive behavior can also impair team performance (Barnsteiner, 2012; Rosenstein and O'Daniel, 2008). Disruptive behavior is "personal conduct, whether verbal or physical, that negatively affects or potentially may affect patient care including, but not limited to, conduct that interferes with one's ability to work with the other members of the health care team" (AMA, 2009). It can take the form of verbal abuse (e.g., profane or disrespectful language, name-calling, failure to respond to concerns about safety, outbursts of anger) and physical (e.g., throwing objects, pushing).

It can also be seen as intimidation and retaliation. Unfortunately, it's fairly common. Budin and colleagues (2013) have studied the phenomenon of bullying in nursing and found that 49% experienced bullying from nursing colleagues within the past three months, while 5% reported a high level of bullying (occurring more than five times in that same period). This figure is lower than Rosenstein (2002) who reported 96% of nurses. These differences may exist because of differing definitions of the behaviors and/or different timelines. Nurses are not the only recipients of abusive behavior. Health care professionals in other professions also experience abusive behavior from senior colleagues, and nurses can actually be the agents of abusive behavior with physicians, other nurses, and nursing students.

The Joint Commission has identified disruptive behavior as a major cause for concern and issued a leadership standard on disruptive behavior (2008):

- EP 4—The hospital/organization has a code of conduct that defines acceptable and disruptive and inappropriate behaviors.
- EP 5—Leaders create and implement a process for managing disruptive and inappropriate behaviors.

Along with these standard statements, the Joint Commission (2008) issued a number of suggested actions, including educating all team members, establishing a zero tolerance approach, and developing organizational processes for monitoring and reporting.

Increasingly, health care organizations and professional organizations are developing policies to address this issue. For example, Barnsteiner, Madigan, and Spray (2001) instituted a Disruptive Physician Conduct policy at the Children's Hospital of Philadelphia, and the American Association of Critical-Care Nurses has just recently issued a second set of Standards for Establishing and Sustaining Healthy Work Environments (2016).

Conflict Resolution

Conflict can exist within a person, occur between two or more people, or within a large group of people who may or may not know each other. There can be actual confrontation, verbal expression, or a conflict that is unexpressed yet apparent through avoidance, denial, or nonverbal signs.

The inability to resolve disagreements among team members is a major impediment to effective team performance. Disagreements can involve minor disputes about an aspect of a particular plan or major conflicts related to the group's direction or performance. Disagreements can also arise from different worldviews or misperceptions. Given the differences cited earlier about characteristics of various health professionals, it is not surprising that one's health profession or role may be associated with a particular response to conflict. For example, Sportsman and Hamilton (2007) studied 126 students in nursing and allied health, and found that, while not significant, the prevalent style for nursing students was compromise, followed by avoidance, whereas for the allied health students, the prevalent style was avoidance, followed by compromise and accommodation. In 2007, Hendel, Fish, and Berger found no difference between 54 head nurses and 75 physicians in five hospitals in their choice of the most frequently used approach, the compromising mode, but collaboration was used next frequently by nurses, while least frequently by physicians.

Conflict can be addressed through avoidance, diffusion, or confrontation. Conflict resolution is a concept that has evolved over the past 50 years, referring to a set of strategies employed to diffuse the conflict and, hopefully, satisfy the wishes of all parties involved. Formal negotiation processes to resolve the conflict are available, but in reality, since conflict or disagreements occur so frequently, this is impractical for daily use. In these situations, a simple process for handling conflict is necessary. Grenny (2009) suggests that a framework of *crucial conversations* is helpful for "talking when the stakes are high." Crucial conversations are discussions that occur when 1) opinions vary, 2) the stakes are high, and/or 3) emotions run strong. Individual responsibility requires that the individual assesses his/her own comfort with conflict, what he/she might have contributed to the situation and develop a respectful approach for addressing the conflict. The group work requires respectful communication, an openness to exploring differences, development of an acceptable plan of action, and turning conversation into action.

Scott and Gerardi (2011a; 2011b) describe the importance of transitioning from an approach of conflict avoidance to one of conflict engagement. To assist organizations in doing this, they outline the steps in developing a strategic approach to conflict management among boards of directors, senior management, and the leaders of the medical staff. They describe how this approach will have "ripple effects throughout the institution. Creating a process that models the type of conflict engagement that is supportive of safe patient care is a powerful means of improving conflict management at all levels of the organization" (2011b).

Creating Expert Teams

A number of success factors have been identified to enhance team performance (O'Daniel and Rosenstein, 2008). They include open communication, a respectful and non-punitive environment, clear direction, clear and known roles and tasks for team members; an acknowledgement and processing of conflict; regular and routine communication and information sharing; and a mechanism for evaluation and adjusting the processes accordingly.

As to the goal of team training, Salas *et al.* (2006) suggest that we should be focusing on preparing expert teams rather than teams of experts, which has been the paradigm within the professions and across professions. They define an expert team as a "set of interdependent team members, each of whom possesses unique and expert-level knowledge, skills, and experience related to task performance, and who adapt, coordinate, and cooperate as a team, thereby producing sustainable and repeatable team functioning at superior or at least near-optimal levels of performance." This contrasts with many teams functioning in health care today that bring together individual experts in their relative fields with little interactive or facilitative competency. A team of experts is evident when clinicians get together and try to trump each other's assessment of a situation or plan of action, or when individual goals supersede those of a collective effort. Expert teams, on the other hand, leverage the skills and expertise of the individual teammates to achieve shared goal(s).

Baker, Day, and Salas (2006) have proposed a set of team components with behavioral examples, drawing from the literature over the past 20 years. These are represented in Table 5.1.

Interestingly, one component that is *not* a prerequisite for effective teams is that they work together on a permanent basis, but rather that they share a commitment to a shared set of KSAs, and that everyone is very clear on who is responsible for what at a given point in time (Baker, Day, and Salas, 2006). Airline flight crews are perhaps the best examples of this reality: As they begin each individual flight, they introduce themselves to each other and are perfectly clear on what everyone's role is for the flight. There is a high degree of trust and mutual respect. An important precursor to this level of performance is that they have trained together with individuals representing the various roles.

Table 5.1 Components of teamwork from a synthesis of the literature. Source: Adapted from Baker DP, Day R, Salas E. Teamwork as an essential component of high-reliability organizations. Health Serv Res. 2006 Aug;41(4 Pt 2). Reproduced with permission of John Wiley & Sons.

Component	Definition	Examples
Team leadership	Ability to direct and coordinate the activities of other team members, assess team performance, assign tasks, develop team KSAs, motivate team members, plan and organize, and establish a positive atmosphere	• Facilitate team problem solving • Clarify team member roles • Synchronize and combine individual team member contributions
Mutual performance monitoring	Ability to develop common understandings of the team environment and apply appropriate task strategies to accurately monitor teammate performance	• Identify mistakes and lapses in other team member actions • Provide feedback to foster self-correction
Back-up behavior	Ability to anticipate other team members' needs through accurate knowledge about their responsibilities; ability to shift workload to achieve balance during periods of high workload or pressure	• Recognition by team members that there's an imbalance • Shifting of work to under-used members
Adaptability	Ability to adjust strategies based on information gathered from the environment; altering a course of action or team repertoire	• Identify cues that change has occurred, assign meaning to the change, and develop a new plan to deal with the situation
Shared mental models	An organizing knowledge structure of the relationships between the task the team is engaged in and how the team members will interact	• Anticipating and predicting each other's needs; identifying changes in the team, task, or teammates and implicitly adjusting strategies
Communication	Exchange of information between a sender and a receiver irrespective of the medium	• Acknowledge that a message was received • Clarify that the message received is the same as that intended
Team/collective organization	Propensity to take other's behavior into account during group interaction and the belief in the importance of team goals over individual member goals	• Considering alternative solutions provided by teammates • Increased task involvement, participatory goal setting
Mutual trust	Shared belief that team members will perform their roles and protect the interests of their teammates	• Information sharing • Willingness to admit mistakes and accept feedback

Team Training

Team training is "a set of theoretically derived strategies and instructional methodologies designed to (1) increase the members' knowledge, skills and attitudes (KSAs) underlying effective communication, cooperation, coordination, and leadership; and (2) give team members opportunities to gain experience using these critical KSAs" (Weaver, Lyons *et al.*, 2010). Points to emphasize here follow: a) It is more than putting people together in a room to hear content or learn tasks; b) There is a base of evidence and experience as to what works best; and 3) Team members must have opportunities for practicing both tasks and teamwork skills. There is growing evidence that this works and makes a measurable difference in patient outcomes, caregiver performance and satisfaction, and organizational performance (Baker, Day, and Salas, 2006; Burke *et al.*, 2004; Weaver, Rosen *et al.*, 2010).

Table 5.2 Instructional strategies for teamwork training. Source: Adapted from Burke 2004. Reproduced with permission of BMJ Publishing Group Ltd.

Instructional strategy	Description
Cross training	Team members develop an understanding of and appreciation for the tasks, duties, and responsibilities of co-workers
Team coordination training	Focuses on teaching team members basic processes in team teamwork; emphasizes mutual performance and 'back-up' behavior
Team self-correction training	Team members learn how to monitor and self-correct their own behaviors, and provide feedback to each other
Assertiveness training	Uses behavioral modeling techniques to demonstrate, and then allow for practice of, assertive and non-assertive behaviors
Metacognition training	Strengthens learner's self-monitoring and regulating behaviors, helping with inductive and deductive reasoning
Stress exposure training	Emphasizes learner's knowledge of potential stressors and coping strategies, and the relationship between these and performance

Much of the content and literature supporting team training arose from the principles and concepts of Crew Resource Management (CRM) (O'Daniel and Rosenstein, 2008), which have been successfully adopted from the aviation and nuclear power industries by the health care sector as a means of improving patient safety. The training emphasizes six key areas: managing fatigue, creating and managing teams, recognizing adverse situations (red flags), cross-checking and communication, decision making, and performance feedback. However, Burke *et al.* (2004) pointed out that CRM training is not enough, and that an array of team instructional strategies have to be employed. Table 5.2 outlines these strategies.

While there is an increasing push for greater team training, just exactly what this entails varies. Weaver, Lyons *et al.* (2010) conducted a comprehensive literature review to examine the findings of 40 peer-reviewed articles related to health care team training evaluations. What they found is that team training is being implemented across many settings and with health care providers caring for diverse populations. The areas that have been primarily targeted for coverage include communication, leadership, role clarity, and situational awareness. There is little information on how training needs were originally established, and while most studies collected data post-training, it was usually done immediately. Fewer than 30% of the studies indicated that evaluation data were collected six months or more. They recommended greater consistency and detail when conducting training evaluations and publishing the results.

Within any training program, one critical factor is the use of debriefing from the learning and experiences (Baker, Day, and Salas, 2006). Many trainers would say that this is possibly the most important aspect, that is, reflecting and sharing what you saw, what you learned, what you would do differently, and to hear and learn from each others' perspectives. Team training is about learning content and also about developing new skills, behaviors, and attitudes.

One of the frequently used and highly regarded training programs is Team Strategies and Tools to Enhance Performance and Patient Safety (TeamSTEPPS) (AHRQ, 2015). Originally developed for work in the military, the Department of Defense and the AHRQ joined together to create TeamSTEPPS for use with physicians, nurses, and other health care providers to reduce clinical errors, improve patient outcomes and improve patient and staff satisfaction. Four key skill areas form the basis for training: leadership, situation monitoring, mutual support, and communication. Learning is achieved through evidence-based content, case studies, simulation, role playing, and debriefing.

The Patient/Family as a Member of the Team

The intersection of the competencies of patient-/family-centered care and teamwork and collaboration is vital if health care is to become safer, more effective, and efficient. The competency of PFCC is covered elsewhere in this text (Walton & Barnsteiner, 2017), as is a description of its evolution to *person- and family-centered care.* The relationship between patients and health care professionals is changing from totally caring *for* patients—and the health care professional making all health care decisions—to a full partnership *with* the patient, and family if that is the patient's wish, in identifying the problem, developing a plan, executing it, and evaluating its success. The IOM in *Crossing the Quality Chasm* (2001) defined patient-centered as "providing care that is respectful of and responsive to individual patient preferences, needs, and values and ensuring that patient values guide all clinical decisions." Thus, the IOM boldly redirected the orientation of the health care industry to one in which full patient engagement is an essential precursor to quality and safety, rather than merely an option.

Wynia, VonKohorn, and Mitchell (2012) examine the challenges at this intersection of team-based and patient-centered care. They offer several examples of how the values and principles of high-functioning health care teams can appropriately be expanded to include active patient/family engagement. Values include honesty, discipline, creativity, humility, and curiosity, while shared principles include clear roles, mutual trust, effective communication, shared goals, and measurable processes and outcomes.

Armstrong *et al.* (2014) make the case that today's health care team *must* include the patient/person and his family as full members of all health care teams. They cite the World Health Organization's (WHO) Framework for Action on Interprofessional Education and Collaborative Practice as a fundamental premise: "Collaborative practice in healthcare occurs when multiple health workers from different professional background provide comprehensive services by working with patients, their families, careers and communities to deliver the highest quality of care across settings" (WHO, 2010). They highlight the importance of collegial trust, humility, and shared decision-making.

Legaré *et al.* (2011) developed a conceptual model to describe six steps for shared decision-making. These include the following: 1) sharing knowledge, 2) exchanging information, 3) clarifying values (and priorities), 4) determining the feasibility and risks and benefits of each option, 5) coming to a decision about the patient's care, and 6) providing ongoing support. This might be considered to be a linear process, however, the dynamic nature of a patient's condition requires various steps to be repeated and refreshed.

The QSEN Competency on Teamwork and Collaboration

In a survey of 629 schools of nursing from prelicensure programs, Smith, Cronenwett, and Sherwood (2007) found that 82% of programs indicated that they had content related to teamwork and collaboration (TWC), with 15% indicating that they had dedicated courses on the topic. Seventy-five percent of educators felt they were "expert/very comfortable" in teaching the content. However, once educator focus groups were asked to critique the KSAs for TWC developed as part of the QSEN project, their reactions were markedly different:

> Although the faculty agreed that they should be teaching these competencies and, in fact, had thought they were, focus group participants did not understand fundamental concepts related to the competencies and could not identify pedagogical strategies in use for teaching the KSAs. An advisory board member led a focus group of new graduates. Not only did the nurses report

that they did not have the learning experiences related to the KSAs, they did not believe their faculties had the expertise to teach the content *(Cronenwett et al., 2007).*

This finding was not isolated to TWC. In a similar vein, educators viewed that they comprehensively covered content on patient-centered care and safety. However, again, the content that had been covered did not reflect that identified with the QSEN competencies.

The prelicensure KSAs that were then developed for the competency on TWC as part of the QSEN project are listed in Appendix A. They reflect a progression from simple to complex and from the individual to the team. This competency more than the others requires joint experiential learning for successfully demonstrating certain KSAs. Although there are KSAs that must be addressed within the nursing curriculum, there are KSAs that require interprofessional effort and integrated learning.

Sequencing the Content

Barton and colleagues from the University of Colorado (2009) conducted a web-based Delphi study to recommend sequencing of the KSAs for all six of the competencies when taught within prelicensure programs. Appendix C includes a recommended sequencing for the TWC KSAs. Sequencing of the KSAs for TWC can also proceed from KSAs an individual must develop to those achieved through group learning. A precursor to becoming an effective team member and collaborating with others is possessing emotional intelligence, or the ability to identify, assess, and manage one's own emotions and the responses to them, as well as to assess and manage our relationships with others. Goleman (2001) offers a simple definition: "The ability to recognize and regulate emotions in self and others."

Some of the KSAs for TWC can be addressed by an individual student, such as:

- Describe own strengths, limitations, and values in functioning as a member of a team
- Demonstrate awareness of own strengths and limitations as a team member
- Initiate plan for self-development as a team member
- Acknowledge own potential to contribute to effective team functioning
- Describe scopes of practice and roles of health care team members

Learning strategies for these KSAs could be enhanced through journaling, use of learning portfolios, dyadic feedback, and personal reflection. Concurrently, there is a growing acceptance that there must be a strong interprofessional component of student and clinician learning if true teamwork and collaboration are to occur.

Thoughts about the best time to introduce the interprofessional content vary. On the one hand, there is some evidence that students enter medical school with preconceived ideas about nurses and physicians so that introducing interprofessional education early and acknowledging the stereotypes may be helpful (Rudland and Mires, 2005). On the other hand, some educators are concerned that socialization to one's own profession has to be sufficiently under way so that students are able to contribute effectively as a member of an interprofessional team.

Interprofessional Education

While there is growing agreement that interpersonal education (IPE) is essential for collaborative practice and, thus, improved patient care, the strength of the evidence lags behind the belief. In 2011, the Cochrane Collaboration identified a total of 15 studies that measured the effectiveness of IPE

Table 5.3 Criteria for full engagement of interprofessional education (IPE). Source: Barnsteiner JH. Promoting Interprofessional Collaboration, 2007, Nursing Outlook, 55, pp. 144–150. Reproduced with permission of Elsevier.

1) Explicit philosophy of IPE that permeates the organization. The philosophy will be well-known, observable, measurable

2) Educators from the different professions co-creating the learning experiences

3) Students having integrated and experiential opportunities to learn collaboration and teamwork, and how it relates to the delivery of safe, quality care delivery

4) IPE learning experiences embedded in the curricula and part of the required caseload for students

5) Demonstrated competence by students with a single set of interprofessional competencies such as those promoted by the Institute of Medicine

6) Organizational infrastructure that fosters IPE, such as support for educator time to develop IPE options, incentive systems for educators to engage in IPE, and integrated activities across schools and professions for students and educators

interventions compared to no educational intervention and found that seven studies reported positive outcomes, four studies reported mixed outcomes, and four reported no impact on either professional practice or patient care (Reeves *et al.*, 2013). That should not be interpreted as a failure of IPE but rather of heterogeneity in study design and outcome measures. The authors made several recommendations for subsequent research: 1) studies that assess the effectiveness of IPE interventions against those of profession-specific interventions; 2) more studies with rigorous methodologies; and 3) cost benefit analyses.

In the absence of definitive research findings, several experts in the field of IPE (Barnsteiner *et al.*, 2007) provided a comprehensive review of the history of IPE and suggested six criteria for effective IPE. These criteria are listed in Table 5.3.

For effective IPE, educators from the schools or colleges involved must be jointly involved in planning and executing the learning; students must be experiencing the learning together; and the learning experiences must be embedded in the formal curricula, not be voluntary or in addition to their normal course loads. Offering opportunities for effective IPE is challenging because of a number of very real factors: conflicting schedules among the schools, differing levels of clinical knowledge, preconceived ideas about other health professions, and educator priorities. However, when successfully offered, they can transform the students' learning and professional socialization.

One misconception about IPE is that it should involve, at a minimum, nursing and medical students. That may not be feasible if a university or college doesn't have a medical school. In that case, IPE can occur with other schools. The important thing is to engage nursing students in learning with and about students from other disciplines and professions. For example, a major grant from the United States Agency for International Development (USAID) partnered the school of nursing and college of veterinary medicine at the University of Minnesota to examine the transmission of infectious diseases between humans and animals. Nursing educators at Grand Valley State University brought together educators from physical therapy, occupational therapy, speech, and the physician assistants' program, in developing a course titled Building Relationships Across Interprofessional Domains (BRAID). Given the vast forces that affect health—and for which nurses would have relevant knowledge—courses could similarly be developed with colleagues in architecture, dietetics, and transportation. The options are endless, limited only by faculty creativity.

Other misconceptions about IPE exist. First is the belief that students have to be at the 'right' level to learn together. Therefore, much effort is targeted toward matching students such as third year nursing with fourth year medical students so that they have comparable backgrounds and clinical experiences. This is admirable, yet the key thing is to bring together students with different professional orientations so that they can learn to appreciate each other's contributions. Learners at very different levels in their respective professions could learn much about communication, authority gradients, power differentials, and collaboration when health care professionals reflect very different levels of experience. This is what the workforce looks like.

A second misperception is that the schedules of the various health schools and colleges must be aligned so that students have similar times available. This presupposes that students learn best in structured learning environments, often in classrooms hearing the same content. As the former dean of the School of Medicine at the University of Minnesota, Deborah Powell, noted: "Sitting together in a classroom does not interprofessional learning make" (Powell, 2004). Discussions, joint interactions, and debriefing are all essential. However, students could be energized by receiving credited time for learning outside traditional classroom hours or beyond single semesters. Suggestions for how this could be handled are provided later in this chapter.

Finally, until academic health centers and organizations charged with providing interprofessional education move toward a philosophy and mission of creating expert teams, and not just teams of expert nurses and physicians, teamwork and collaboration will continue to be suboptimal. How refreshing it would be if an academic health center would proclaim its mission as *Creating expert teams of extraordinary health care professionals who will improve health and health care*, and modify its curricula, schedules and systems to deliver this.

Who Teaches IPE?

An obvious first thought is that faculty from other health professions' schools would be the ideal candidates, but this may be impractical. First, if the school of nursing is situated on a campus where there is no school of medicine or other health professions' school, other disciplines can help nursing students learn about interprofessional or interdisciplinary care. For example, colleagues from the college of engineering can help students think about human factors, and the interface between humans and technology. Colleagues from the arts can help students learn about guided imagery, music therapy, and the role of the arts in healing. Faculty from the communication department can help students learn new methods of communicating and interacting, verbally and nonverbally. The key objective is to expose students to other students and faculty who have different backgrounds and worldviews about health and health care.

Second, clinical partners in the hospital or health system can provide excellent learning opportunities for students. Engaging students in real-time quality improvement activities with quality improvement (QI) specialists, or participating in root cause analyses after Serious Reportable Events can help students appreciate the challenges in delivering safe health care and learn their roles in promoting safe, quality care. Inviting students and nurses to participate in patient rounds, patient care conferences, or relevant committee meetings can provide insights and experiences at seeing how health professionals interact, provide differing perspectives, and reconcile differences.

Third, retired physicians and professionals from other disciplines can be excellent teachers, helping nursing students understand the contributions of various professions and realistically role play in situations that nursing students will encounter.

Fourth, students and other clinicians can assume the roles of different professionals and respond to situations as they would expect the others would respond. That can either strengthen perceptions about others' contributions or provoke lively discussions about inaccuracies and assumptions.

Interprofessional Education and Collaborative Practice

Given the importance of interprofessional collaboration in the health care delivery site, the need for educating tomorrow's professionals in this competency in new ways is tremendously important. For the most part, health care professionals have been educated in professional silos, although this is slowly changing. TWC has always been verbally advocated but rarely practiced. The IOM (2003) accelerated the pace of change when it declared that five competencies should be demonstrated by graduates of all health professions' schools, among them the ability to function effectively in inter-disciplinary teams. Where formerly the goal for teamwork and collaboration was to work effectively with other health care professionals while performing nursing skills, the new definition offers a more dynamic vision: To function effectively within nursing and interprofessional teams, fostering open communication, mutual respect, and shared decision making to achieve quality patient care. The IOM report shaped the work of the nursing profession through the QSEN initiative in its development of competencies for TWC for the prelicensure student (Cronenwett *et al.*, 2007), as well as the graduate student (Cronenwett *et al.*, 2009).

This competency on teamwork and collaboration has implications for practicing nurses and their colleagues. Because many of today's nurses were educated before the IOM recommendations and the QSEN work, they may not be familiar with the new definitions of the six QSEN competencies. We have also found that practicing nurses may have to unlearn what they had previously thought, that is, that teamwork and collaboration relates to shared learning and interdependencies in practice rather than merely working respectfully side by side. Much of this chapter has focused on nursing student education, however, the principles, recommendations, and assignments can either fit or be modified to help practicing nurses strengthen their practice in these areas.

The Interprofessional Education Collaborative

A number of national organizations have emerged to reinforce the need for, and provide resources to support the development of, IPE and collaborative practice (CP). In May 2011, the Interprofessional Education Collaborative released an important document, Core Competencies for Interprofessional Collaborative Practice (2011). The Interprofessional Education Collaborative is a group of leaders from the AACN, the American Association of Colleges of Osteopathic Medicine, the American Association of Colleges of Pharmacy, the American Dental Education Association, the Association of American Medical Colleges, and the Association of Schools of Public Health. The document introduces a set of interprofessional collaborative competencies, with the intent of building on the strengths of the *intra*disciplinary work and creating a paradigm shift toward *inter*professional education whereby students from different professions would learn with and from each other. The document also highlights the concept of *interprofessionality* drawn from the work of D'Amour and Oandasan (2005), who define it as:

> The process by which professionals reflect on and develop ways of practicing that provides an integrated and cohesive answer to the needs of the client/family/population. ... It involves continuous interaction and knowledge sharing between professionals, organized to solve or explore a variety of education and care issues all while seeking to optimize the patient's participation. ... Interprofessionality requires a paradigm shift, since interprofessional practice has unique characteristics in terms of values, codes of conduct, and ways of working.

This concept clearly extends the intended outcome of IPE to incorporate professional socialization.

The Interprofessional Professionalism Collaborative (IPC) is a relatively new group that has been formed to develop a valid and reliable instrument for assessing interprofessional professionalism behaviors and then developing educational materials for use by educators across all health professions. Currently under way is development of an Interprofessional Professionalism Assessment to evaluate the learner's level of professionalism when interacting with other students in the health professions. This tool should be available by the end of 2016.

Another group integrally involved in promoting IPE and CP is The Josiah Macy Jr. Foundation. "Dedicated to improving the health of the public by advancing the education and training of health professionals," it provides publications (e.g., Providing New Curriculum Content for Health Professional Education, Enhancing Health Professions Education through Technology); the Macy Faculty Scholars Program for selecting and strengthening the careers of educational innovators in medicine and nursing; and conferences and special events.

The National Center for Interprofessional Practice and Education was established in 2012 to "provide the leadership, evidence and resources needed to guide the nation on the use of interprofessional education and collaborative practice as a way to enhance the experience of health care, improve population health and reduce the overall cost of care." Housed at the University of Minnesota, the Center is supported by the United States Department of Health and Human Services, Health Resources and Services Administration, the Josiah Macy Jr. Foundation, the Robert Wood Johnson Foundation, and the Gordon and Betty Moore Foundation. It offers a wealth of resources including publications, conferences and events, and faculty development.

The IHI is perhaps one of the most active and best known leaders in IPE and CP. Its National Forum is highly regarded and offers special opportunities for student involvement. IHI also offers an array of programs, publications, conferences, and events. Its Open School connects more than 250,000 learners around the world in designing and executing strategies to improve the quality and safety of health care.

In addition to the above-mentioned national organizations and many others, a growing number of individual colleges and universities are establishing centers and collaboratives for contributing to the science behind IPE and CP, for educating tomorrow's health professions, and for providing opportunities for conversations on how to collaborate to improve health care, provider satisfaction and organizational performance.

Strategies for Learning TWC

As was mentioned above, the content in this chapter and the following strategies are applicable for nursing students and practicing nurses who want to refresh or strengthen their performance in TWC. Drawing from the vast literature on teams, teamwork and team training, initiatives for promoting IPE should consider the following principles:

1) While some of the learning can be done by the individual, achieving competency in TWC requires integrated, experiential, and concurrent learning by students from more than one discipline or profession.
2) The goal is to learn content and develop new skills, attitudes, and behaviors.
3) Learning needs to be multi-faceted and aim to improve performance in tasks and teamwork.
4) The learning experiences need guided practice and debriefing.

Suggested Learning Experiences

The following list provides suggested learning experiences:

- Educators could assign an interprofessional cohort of students to follow a multigenerational family and their health status changes, needs for health care, and experiences with the health care system throughout the course of the students' educational programs. Students would get credit for work done outside of the traditional academic schedule.
- Educators in two or more schools or colleges could jointly develop and conduct a course available to students in at least two health professions' schools on a topic of mutual relevance, for example, ethics or health economics. Students could be given shared assignments and jointly develop and give presentations on selected topics.
- CLARION is a student organization that originated at the University of Minnesota through its Center for Health Interprofessional Programs (2010) and is dedicated to improving health care through interprofessional collaboration. A national organization since 2005, it promotes local student case competitions for health professional students, enabling them to achieve a 360-degree perspective on patient safety in today's health care system and learn how it might be improved. Student teams, consisting of four students, comprising at least two disciplines, are given a case and are charged with creating a root cause analysis. The team presents their analysis to a panel of interprofessional judges that evaluates their analysis in the context of real world standards of practice. Local winners advance to the national competition. The center's web site also offers numerous other suggestions for engaging students in interprofessional activities (www.chip.umn.edu).
- Students might be able to establish and manage a community-based clinic with faculty support. The Philips Neighborhood Clinic (www.phillips.neighborhoodclinic.com) is a student-run community clinic that provides accessible, culturally appropriate, interdisciplincary health care services and education to health professional students on the skills they need to effectively and compassionately serve people who are underinsured and/or unstably housed. Students are supervised by licensed clinicians. In addition to routine clinic times, they also schedule special sessions such as Foot Care Night for individuals who have problems associated with diabetes such as ulcers and/or necrosis.
- The Immunization Tour is a partnership between the nursing and pharmacy schools at the University of Minnesota to plan and implement a mass immunization clinic for the campus during flu season. Engaging approximately 60 students in four interprofessional teams, they administer approximately 4500 doses of vaccine. Students learn leadership principles, organization, how to give injections, teamwork, and collaboration (University of Minnesota Office of Student Affairs, 2011).
- Assign pairs of medical and nursing students to see patients together in a clinic or ambulatory setting, jointly gathering the patient's history, and debriefing as to what each saw as the patient's problems, and what each discipline would address in working with the patient/family to prioritize issues to tackle.
- At Virginia Commonwealth University (VCU), medical, nursing, and pharmacy students see patients at a free clinic in an underserved community one day per week. On another day each month, students from the health professions join with students from social work, biomedical engineering, and the VCU Dietetic Internship Program at a local Kroger's grocery store to talk about healthy eating and conduct some health screening.
- Establish a shared governance council of students from the health professions' schools to create learning experiences for students and community initiatives to provide care and services to local groups.

- Nursing students and nurses could participate in medical staff orientation to a patient care unit. To improve teamwork and collaboration on her unit at the Mayo Clinic, Linnea Bineke, DNP, RN designed an orientation program for new medical staff and, working with the medical leadership of the unit, offered it to incoming medical staff. Feedback from them indicated that they appreciated someone taking the time to help them know their way around and better understand key unit processes.

- Several options exist for practicing communication:
  - *Engaging in a SBAR interaction.* Patient scenarios can be developed that require the nursing student to communicate with a physician about a change in patient status. Medical students, medical staff, or retired physicians can portray the physician.
  - *Practicing a handoff.* This is a time when information is transferred, along with authority and responsibility, during transitions in care across the continuum and includes an opportunity to ask questions, clarify, and confirm responses. Examples include shift changes, physicians transferring off from a patient's care, and patient transfers to other facilities; or a *call-out* to communicate important or critical information, for example, during resuscitations; or a *check-back*, using closed-loop communication to ensure that information conveyed by the sender is understood by the receiver as intended. Verbal orders are a situation when check-backs are helpful.

- Create a Joint Practice Committee within a patient care area with a diverse membership of individuals from the disciplines and professions who practice there.

- Assign a staff nurse to serve as a buddy to each new medical student and intern, serving as a resource and providing orientation to the physical layout of the unit, and the policies and practices that are critical to the area.

- Post pictures of employees and medical staff members on the unit bulletin board with each person's name and role.

- Develop a business case for investing in TeamSTEPPS training and present to senior administration.

- Engage in role playing of actual situations that have occurred or simulating new ones. The increasing use of high-fidelity simulation offers extremely rich learning experiences, but the lack of expensive equipment doesn't preclude this from being an effective tool. According to Ironside, Jeffries, and Martin (2009), what's needed is active and diverse learning, feedback, student/educator interaction, collaboration, and high expectations. Role playing shouldn't be reserved only for use with patients and families. Helping students effectively communicate with physicians and nurses in simulated work encounters is critically important. Also helping health care professionals interact more effectively with each other is key.

- An exercise used at the University of Missouri by Hall (2007) took the learner through a simulated conversation between a nurse and a physician regarding a patient who is deteriorating. The nurse is challenged to find effective means of assertively yet professionally escalating the dialogue on behalf of a patient whose condition does not allow for delay.

- Design a menu of interprofessional learning experiences (ILE) from which students could choose to participate over the course of their program. These could include volunteering in clinical sites, joining interprofessional case study teams, completing an IHI Open School module, co-designing a course or project with students from another discipline, participating in patient care rounds and jointly debriefing with students from other disciplines, etc. Each experience would be assigned a certain number of ILE points, and, at the end of their program, students would receive credit for their independent work that occurred over the course of their program

- Create assignments that require students to create small work teams from diverse disciplines and professions, examine a health care issue that threatens patient safety in their community, gather evidence as to a recommended approach, and present their findings and recommendations to fellow students and faculty. Again, the students would receive credit for work that is outside traditional classrooms.

Finally, the QSEN web site (www.qsen.org) offers dozens of learning experiences that relate to teamwork, collaboration, and the other competencies.

Conclusion

Serving as a member of a dynamic, effective team is a rewarding experience that can enrich one's own personal and professional life, as well as enhance the work of a group and, in the case of health care, save lives. Given the complexity of the health care environment and the threats to patient safety and quality care, collaboration with other members of the health care team is vital. Cooke *et al.* (2000) pointed out the obvious: "The growing complexity of tasks frequently surpasses the cognitive capabilities of individuals and, thus, necessitates a team approach."

References

Agency for Healthcare Research and Quality. (2015) Mutual support—good teamwork. Retrieved 12/9/2015 from http://www.ahrq.gov/professionals/education/curriculum-tools/teamstepps/primarycare/3_mutual_support_good/index.html.

Agency for Healthcare Research and Quality. (2014) TeamSTEPPS Fundamentals course: Module 1. Retrieved 12/9/2015 from http://www.ahrq.gov/professionals/education/curriculum-tools/teamstepps/instructor/fundamentals/module1/m1evidencebase.html.

Agency for Healthcare Research and Quality. (2015) TeamSTEPPS. Retrieved 12/9/2015 from http://www.ahrq.gov/cpi/about/otherwebsites/teamstepps/teamstepps.html.

American Association of Critical-Care Nurses. (2016) *AACN standards for establishing and sustaining healthy work environments*, 2nd Ed. Aliso Viejo, CA: AACN.

American Medical Association (AMA). (2009) Report of the Council on Ethical and Judicial Affairs. Physicians with Disruptive Behavior. Chicago, IL: American Medical Association.

Armstrong, G.E., Barton, A.J., Nuffer, W., and Yancey, L. (2014) Patient- and family-centered care and the interprofessional team. In J. Barnsteiner, J. Disch, and M.K. Walton, *Person and family centered care* (pp. 365–388). Indianapolis, IN: Sigma Theta Tau International.

Baggs, J.G., Schmitt, M.H., Mushlin, A.I., Mitchell, P.H., Eldredge, D.H., Oakes, D., Hutson, A.D. *et al.*, (1999) Association between nurse-physician collaboration and patient outcomes in three intensive care units. *Critical Care Medicine*, 27(9), 1991–1998.

Baker, D.P., Day, R., and Salas, E. (2006) Teamwork as an essential component of high-reliability organizations. Health Res and Ed Trust. doi: 10.1111/j.1475-6773.2006.00566.x.

Baldwin, D.C. (2007) Some historical notes on interdisciplinary and interprofessional education and practice in health care in the USA. *Journal of Interprofessional Care*, 21(SI), 23–37.

Barnsteiner, J.H., Disch, J.M., Hall, L., Mayer, D, and Moore, S. (2007) Promoting interprofessional collaboration. *Nursing Outlook*, 55(3), 144–150.

Barnsteiner, J.H., Madigan, K., and Spray, T.L. (2001) Instituting a disruptive conduct policy for medical staff. *AACN Clinical Issues*, 12, 378–382.

Barnsteiner, J. (2012) Workplace abuse in nursing: Policy strategies. In D. Mason, J.K. Leavitt, and M.W. Chafee (Eds.), *Politics and policy in nursing and health care*, 6th Ed. St. Louis, MO: Elsevier.

Barton, A., Armstrong, G., Preheim, G., Gelman, S.B., and Andrus, L.C. (2009) A national Delphi to determine developmental progression of quality and safety competencies in nursing education. *Nursing Outlook, 57*, 313–322.

Boyle, D. and Kochinda, C. (2004) Enhancing collaborative communication of nurse and physician leadership in two intensive care units. *Journal of Nursing Administration, 34*(2), 60–70.

Budin, W.C., Brewer, C.S., Chao, Y., and Kovner, C. (2013) Verbal abuse from nurse colleagues and work environment of early career registered nurses. *J of Nsg School, 45*(3), 308–316.

Burke, C.S., Salas, E., Wilson-Donnelly, K., and Priest, H. (2004) How to turn a team of experts into an expert medical team: Guidance from the military and aviation communities. *Qual Saf Health Care 13*[supp], i96–i104. doi: 10.1136/qshc.2004.009829.

Carney, B.T., West, P., Neily, J., Mills, P.D., and Bagian, J.P. (2010) Differences in nurse and surgeon perceptions of teamwork: Implications for use of a briefing checklist in the OR. *AORN Journal, 91*(6), 722–729.

Casanova, J., Day, K., Dorpat, D., Hendricks, B., Theis, L., and Weisman, S. (2007) Nurse-physician relations and role expectations. *Journal of Nursing Administration, 37*(2), 68–70.

Center for Health Interprofessional Programs. (2010) Retrieved from http://www. chip.umn.edu/clarion/home.html.

Cooke, N.J., Salas, E., Cannon-Bowers, J.A., and Stout, R.J. (2000) Measuring team knowledge. *Human Factors, 42*, 151–173.

Cowan, M.J., Shapiro, M., Hays, R.D., Afifi, A., Vazirani, S., Ward, C.R., and Ettner, S.L. (2006). The effect of a multidisciplinary hospitalist/physician and advanced practice nurse collaboration on hospital costs. *Journal of Nursing Administration, 36*(2), 79–85.

Cronenwett, L., Sherwood, G., Barnsteiner, J., Disch, J., Johnson, J., Mitchel, P., Warren, J. (2007) Quality and safety education for nurses. *Nursing Outlook, 55*(3), 122–131.

Cronenwett, L., Sherwood, G., Pohl, J., Barnsteiner, J., Moore, S., Sullivan, D.T., Warren, J. (2009) Quality and safety education for advanced nursing practice. *Nursing Outlook, 57*(6), 338–348.

D'Amour, D. and Oandasan, I. (2005) Interprofessionality as the field of interprofessional practice and interprofessional education: An emerging concept. *Journal of Interprofessional Care, 19* (Supplement 1), 8–20.

Estabrooks, C.A., Midodzi, W.K., Cummings, G.G., Ricker, K.L., and Giovannetti P. (2005) The impact of hospital nursing characteristics on 30-day mortality. *Nursing Research, 54*(2), 74–84.

Fairman, J. and Lynaugh, J. (1998) *Critical care nursing: A history*. Philadelphia: University of Pennsylvania Press.

Fletcher, C.E., Baker, S.J., Copeland, L.A., Reeves, P.J., and Lowery, J.C. (2007) Nurse practitioners and physicians' views of NPs as providers of primary care to veterans. *Journal of Nursing Scholarship, 39*(4), 358–362.

Goleman, D. (2001) Issues in paradigm building. In C. Cherniss and D. Goleman (Eds.), *The emotionally intelligent workplace: How to select for, measure, and improve emotional intelligence in individuals, groups, and organizations*. San Francisco: Jossey-Bass.

Grenny, J. (2009) Crucial conversations: The most potent force for eliminating disruptive behavior. *Health Care Manager, 28*(3), 240–245.

Hall L. (2007) Nurse-physician communication exercise. Retrieved from http://www.qsen.org/search_strategies.php?id=50)

Hendel, T., Fish, M., & Berger, O. (2007). Nurse/physician conflict management mode choices: Implications for improved collaborative practice. *Nursing Administration Quarterly, 31*(3), 244–254.

Institute for Healthcare Improvement. (2015) *Achieving competence today*. Retrieved from http://www. ihi.org/IHI/Programs/IHIOpenSchool/TeachingResourceACT.htm? tabId = 0.

Institute of Medicine. (1998) *To err is human.* Washington, DC: National Academies Press.

Institute of Medicine. (2001) *Crossing the quality chasm: A new health system for the 21st century.* Washington, DC: National Academies Press.

Institute of Medicine. (2003) *Health professions education: A bridge to quality.* Washington, DC: National Academies Press.

Institute of Medicine. (2010) *The future of nursing: Advancing health, leading change.* Washington, DC: National Academies Press.

Interprofessional Education Collaborative Expert Panel. (2011) *Core competencies for interprofessional collaborative practice: Report of an expert panel.* Washington, DC: Interprofessional Education Collaborative.

Interprofessional Professionalism Collaborative. (2015) What is interprofessional professionalism? Retrieved at http://www.interprofessionalprofessionalism.org/

Ironside, P., Jeffries, P.R., and Martin, A. (2009) Fostering patient safety competencies using multiple-patient simulation experiences. *Nursing Outlook, 6,* 332–337.

James, J.T. (2013) A new, evidence-based estimate of patient harms associated with hospital care. *J of Pat Safety, 9*(3), 122–128.

Josiah Macy Jr Foundation (2015) Retrieved December 28 from http://macyfoundation.org/.

King, L. and Lee, J.L. (1994) Perceptions of collaborative practice between Navy nurses and physicians in the ICU setting. *American Journal of Critical Care, 3*(5), 331–336.

Legaré, F., Stacey, D., Pouliot, S., Gauvin, F-P, Desroches, S., Kryworuchko, J., Graham, I.D. (2011) Interprofessionalism and shared decision-making in primary care: A stepwise approach towards a new model. *J of Interprof Care, 25*(1), 18–25.

Liedtka, J.M. and Whitten E. (1998) Enhancing care delivery through cross-disciplinary collaboration: A case study. *Journal of Healthcare Management, 43*(2), 185–205.

Makary, M.A., Sexton, J.B., Freischlag, J.A., Holzmueller, C.G., Millman, E.A., Rowen, L., et al. (2006) Operating room teamwork among physicians and nurses: Teamwork in the eye of the beholder. *Journal of the American College of Surgeons, 202*(5), 746–752.

Merriam-Webster. (2009) Communication. Retrieved from http://www.merriamwebster.com/dictionary/communication.

Messmer, P.R. (2008) Enhancing nurse-physician collaboration using pediatric simulation. *Journal of Continuing Education in Nursing, 39*(7), 319–327.

Mills, P., Neily, J., and Dunn, E. (2008) Teamwork and collaboration in surgical teams: Implications for patient safety. *Journal of the American College of Surgeons, 206*(1),107–112.

Mohr, D.C., Burgess, J.F., and Young, G.J. (2008) The influence of teamwork culture on physician and nurse resignation rates in hospitals. *Health Services Management Research, 21*(1), 23–31.

National Center for International Practice and Education. (2015) Retrieved December 28, 2015 from https://nexusipe.org/.

Nelson, E.N., Batalden, P.B., Huber, T.P., Mohr, J.J., Godfrey, M.M., Headrick, L.A., Wasson, J. H. (2002) Microsystems in health care: Part l. Learning from high-performing front-line clinical units. *Joint Commission Journal on Quality Improvement, 28*(9), 472–497.

Nielsen, P.E., Goldman, M.B., Mann, S., Shapiro, D.E., Marcus, R.G., Pratt, S.D., *et al.* (2007) Effects of teamwork training on adverse outcomes and process of care in labor and delivery: A randomized control trial. *Obstetrics and Gynecology, 109,* 48–55.

O'Daniel, M. and Rosenstein, A.H. (2008) Professional communication and team collaboration. In R. Hughes (Ed.), *Patient safety and quality: An evidence-based handbook for nurses* (Prepared with support from the Robert Wood Johnson Foundation). AHRQ Publication No. 08–0043. Rockville, MD: Agency for Healthcare Research and Quality.

O'Leary, K.J., Ritter, C.D., Wheeler, H., Szekendi, M.K., Brinton, T.S., and Williams, M.V. (2010) Teamwork on inpatient medical units: Assessing attitudes and barriers. *Quality and Safety in Health Care*, *19*, 117–121.

Porter, C.O., Hollenbeck, J.R., Ilgen, D.R., Ellis, A.P.J., West, B.J., and Moon, H.K. (2003) Backing up behaviors in teams: The role of personality and legitimacy of need. *J Appl Psychol*, *88*(3), 391–403.

Powell, D. (2004) Personal communication.

Reeves, S., Perrier, L., Goldman, J., Freeth, D., and Zwarenstein, M. (2013) Interprofessional education: Effects on professional practice and healthcare outcomes. doi: 10.1002/14651858.CD002213.pub3.

Robert Wood Johnson Foundation. (2015) Lessons from the field: Promising interprofessional collaboration practices. Princeton, NJ: Robert Wood Johnson Foundation.

Rosenstein, A.H., (2002) Nurse-physician relationships: Impact on nurse satisfaction and retention. *American Journal of Nursing*, *102*(6), 26–34.

Rosenstein, A.H., and O'Daniel, M. (2008) A survey of the impact of disruptive behaviors and communication defects on patient safety. *Jt Comm J Qual Pat Saf*, *34*(8), 464–471.

Rudland, J.R., and Mires, G.J. (2005) Characteristics of doctors and nurses as perceived by students entering medical school: Implications for shared teaching. *Medical Education*, *39*, 448–455.

Salas, E., Almeida, S. A., Salisbury, M., King, H., Lazzara, E. H., Lyons, R., *et al.* (2009) What are the critical success factors for team training in health care? *Joint Commission Journal on Quality and Patient Safety*, *35*(8), 398–405.

Salas, E., Cannon-Bowers, J.A., and Johnston, J.H. (1997) How can you turn a team of experts into an expert team? Emerging training strategies, Chapter 33. In C.E. Zsambok and G. Klein (Eds.), Naturalistic Decision Making. Mahwah, NJ: Erlbaum.

Salas, E., Dickinson, T.L., and S.A. Converse. (1992) Toward an understanding of team performance and training. In teams: Their training and performance, R. W. Swezey and E. Salas (Eds), 3–29. Norwood, NJ: Ablex.

Salas, E., Rosen, M.A., Burke, C., Rosen, M.A., Burke, S.C., Goodwin, G.F., and Fiore, S.M. (2006) The making of a dream team: When expert teams do best. In K. A. Ericsson, N. Charness, P.J. Feltovish, and R.R. Hoffman (Eds.), *The Cambridge handbook of expertise and expert performance* (pp. 439–453). New York: Cambridge University Press.

Scott, C., and Gerardi, D. (2011a) A strategic approach for managing conflict in hospitals: Responding to the Joint Commission leadership standard, Part 1. *Joint Commission Journal on Quality and Patient Safety*, *37*(2), 59–69.

Scott, C., and Gerardi, D. (2011b) A strategic approach for managing conflict in hospitals: Responding to the Joint Commission leadership standard, Part 2. *Joint Commission Journal on Quality and Patient Safety*, *37*(2), 70–80.

Smith, E.L., Cronenwett, L., and Sherwood, G. (2007) Current assessments of quality and safety education in nursing. *Nursing Outlook*, *55*(3), 132–137.

Sportsman, S., and Hamilton, P. (2007) Conflict management styles in the health professions. *JProfNsg*, *23*(3), 157–166.

The Joint Commission. (2008) Sentinel event alert, Issue 40. Behaviors that undermine a culture of safety. Retrieved December 28, 2015 from http://www.jointcommission.org/sentinel_event_alert_issue_40_behaviors_that_undermine_a_culture_of_safety/.

The Joint Commission. (2015) Most Frequently Identified Root Causes of Sentinel Events Reviewed by The Joint Commission by Year. Retrieved Dec 28, 2015 at http://www.jointcommission.org/sentinel_event_statistics/.

Thomas, E.J., Sexton, J.B., and Helmreich, R.L. (2003) Discrepant attitudes about teamwork among critical care nurses and physicians. *Critical Care Medicine*, *31*(3), 956–959.

University of Minnesota Office of Student Affairs. (2011) Immunization Tour. Retrieved December 28, 2015 from http://www.osa.umn.edu/documents/Issue42.html.

Walton, M.K., and Barnsteiner, J. (2017) Patient-centered care. In G. Sherwood and J. Barnsteiner (2nd ed), *Quality and safety in nursing: A competency approach to improving outcomes*. Hoboken, NJ: Wiley-Blackwell.

Weaver, S.J., Lyons, R., DiazGranados, C., Rosen, M.A., Salas, E., Oglesby, J., King, H.B. (2010) The anatomy of health care team training and the state of practice: A critical review. *Acad Med*, *85*(11), 1746–1760. DOI: 10.1097/ACM.0b013e3181f2e907.

Weaver, S.J., Rosen, M.A., DiazGranados, D., Lazzara, E.H., Lyons, R., Salas, E., King, H.B. (2010) Does teamwork improve performance in the operating room? A multilevel evaluation. *Joint Commission Journal on Quality and Patient Safety*, *36*(3), 133–142.

Weinberg, D.B., Miner, D.C., and Rivlin, L. (2009) It depends: Medical residents' perspectives on working with nurses. *AJN*, *109*(7), 34–43.

World Health Organization (WHO). (2010) *Framework for action on interprofessional education and collaborative practice*. Geneva, Switzerland: World Health Organization.

Wynia, M.K., VonKohorn, I., and Mitchell, P.M. (2012) Challenges at the intersection of team-based and patient-centered health care. *JAMA*, *308*(13), 1327–1328.

Xyrichis, A., and Ream, E. (2008) Teamwork: A concept analysis. *J Adv Nsg*, *61*(2), 232–241.

Zwarenstein, M., Goldman, J., and Reeves, S. (2009) Interprofessional collaboration: Effects of practice-based interventions on professional practice and healthcare outcomes. *Cochrane Database of Systematic Reviews*, Issue 3. Art. no. CD000072. doi: 10.1002/14651858.CD000072.

Resources

AHRQ. (2014) Teamwork training. Retrieved from https://psnet.ahrq.gov/primers/primer/8/teamwork-training

Eisler, R. and Potter, T.M. (ongoing online journal) *The interdisciplinary journal of partnership studies*. Retrieved from http://pubs.lib.umn.edu/ijps/

Korner, M., Butof, S., Muller, C., Zimmermann, L., Becker, S., and Bengel, J. (2016) Interprofessional teamwork and team interventions in chronic care: A systematic review. *J Interprof Care*, *30*(1), 15–28.

Oster, C.A. and Braaten, J.S (2016) High reliability organizations: A healthcare handbook for patient safety and quality. Indianapolis, IN: Sigma Theta Tau International.

Potter, T.M. and Eisler, R. (2014) *Transforming interprofessional partnerships: A new framework for nursing and partnership-based health care*. Indianapolis, IN: Sigma Theta Tau International.

Robert Wood Johnson Foundation. (2011) Transforming care at the bedside. Retrieved from http://www.rwjf.org/en/library/research/2011/07/transforming-care-at-the-bedside.html

6

Quality Improvement

Jean Johnson, PhD, RN, FAAN

Having expertise in quality improvement is important for nurses. A nurse working with a large Midwest-based health system is a Six Sigma Master Black Belt, one of the highest levels of accomplishment. She has led a broad range of quality improvement efforts within her system including very complex projects. A challenge was brought to her by a VP of the organization who recognized that there was an emerging problem with delivering guaranteed clinical outcomes to customers. (An example of a performance guarantee is guaranteeing that an agreed-upon percentage of customer members having coronary artery disease will be taking an ace inhibitor or the health system will pay the customer an agreed-upon amount for not meeting the benchmark.) Creating accountability for hitting the benchmark involved bringing together several different units, all of which were blaming each other for failures to meet the benchmark. The nurse was able to use her skills to get the units past the blame phase and into problem solving phase, a key step to moving beyond the problem to better patient care and a more efficient system.

Background of Quality Improvement

As the profession comprising the largest percentage of the health care workforce in the United States, nursing has both the opportunity and the obligation to lead efforts to improve care. Who better to lead the effort to improve health care delivery and outcomes than the professionals delivering the majority of health care in America? In order to lead those efforts, however, nurses need to know how to use data to measure quality of care and implement improvement processes. While there have been gains in a number of areas in health care quality, studies suggest that much progress remains to be made. A study of hospitals in Colorado found that from 2006 to 2008, the same number of patients died each year as a result of medical errors, similar to the findings of the IOM studies of a decade ago (IOM, 2000; IOM, 2001; Landrigan *et al.*, 2010). A more sensitive but controversial measure of medical errors has been developed that suggests that between 250,000 and 400,000 patients may die of medical error per year. This number would make medical error the third leading cause of death in the United States (James, 2013). In order to be a major force that makes a difference in the lives of millions of patients, nurses need tools to measure the quality of care they provide as well as skills to create and implement transformational change (Berwick, 2011). Providing nurses with these skills and tools offers new opportunities for success in improving health care quality and outcome.

Quality and Safety in Nursing: A Competency Approach to Improving Outcomes, Second Edition.
Edited by Gwen Sherwood and Jane Barnsteiner.
© 2017 John Wiley & Sons, Inc. Published 2017 by John Wiley & Sons, Inc.

Quality improvement as defined by the QSEN project is the "use of data to monitor the outcomes of care processes and use improvement methods to design and test changes to continuously improve the quality and safety of health care systems" (Cronenwett *et al.*, 2007a). Before they can improve care, nurses must assess how well they are doing. Data reflecting the important elements of care are the only credible way of demonstrating the quality of care nurses provide. Thus, it is essential that nurses be taught systematic processes and methods for defining problems, identifying potential causes of those problems, and testing possible solutions to improve care. It is critical that nurses lead the changes that need to be made.

Leadership in Quality by Florence Nightingale

Nurses have a historic role model as an inspiration to improve care. Florence Nightingale was the first health professional to outline a comprehensive approach to health care quality improvement. She called for the collection and analysis of statistical data to ascertain patient outcomes beyond simple mortality. In her seminal work *Notes on Hospitals*, first published in 1859, Nightingale (1863) notes the need to understand the ways in which multiple factors interact with one another:

> The first step in the way of improvement is to obtain a terse and accurate registration of the elements of the problem. Every well-kept hospital record ought to contain these. But for the sake of uniformity, I enumerate them as follows: 1. Age; 2. Sex; 3. Occupation; 4. Accident or disease leading to operation; 5. Date of accident and of operation, or date of operation if from disease; 6. Nature of operation; 7. Constitution of patient; 8. Complications occurring after operation; 9. Date of recovery or of death; 10. Fatal complication, a. Resulting directly from the accident, b. Occurring after the operation *(Nightingale, 1863)*.

Nightingale not only understood the issues related to outcomes of care but also the economics of care as demonstrated in the following excerpt:

> These methods ... would enable us to ascertain how much of each year of life is wasted by illness—what diseases and ages press most heavily on the resources of particular hospitals. ... The relation of the duration of cases to the general utility of a hospital requires also to be shown, because it must be obvious that if, by any sanitary means or improved treatment, the duration of cases could be reduced to one-half, the utility of the hospital would be doubled, so far as its funds are concerned *(Nightingale, 1863)*.

Nightingale's vision was that rigorous data collection would yield a "uniform record of facts from which to deduce statistical results" (1863). Her prescient treatise on the value of collecting and analyzing health care outcomes data is remarkable when one reflects on the social and financial costs incurred as a direct result of her guidance being largely ignored.

The Evolution and Activities of Quality Improvement Organizations

Since the mid-1990s, several independent organizations have been established to focus on quality measurement and have contributed to the healthcare quality landscape (Aquaviva and Johnson, 2014). The NCQA was one of the first, with the development of the HEDIS measures used to assess the quality of health plans as well as provide accreditation (NCQA, 2015). Additional measures and recognition programs have been developed by NCQA including diabetes management, case management, wellness and health promotion, patient-centered medical homes, and others. Although the

HEDIS and other program measures are not specific to nursing, they are important measures of quality of care that provide useful information to purchasers of health care such as employers in order to choose high value care. The Joint Commission, known primarily for hospital accreditation, also has several accreditation and certification programs (Joint Commission, 2015).

The NQF was chartered in 1999 and became operational in 2000 as the result of recommendations by President Clinton's Commission on Consumer Protection and Quality Health Care Industry (RWJF, 2015). The forum has been established as the endorser of measures and has over 600 endorsed measures (NQF, 2015a). The NQF endorsement process examines the evidence to support the use of measures and acts as the final arbiter of measures being recognized as valid, reliable and useful (NQF 2015b). NQF is playing a critical role as endorsed measures are intended for use by Medicare and private payers as well as public reporting. However, not every endorsed measure is integrated into a reporting system. In efforts to streamline reporting and not overwhelm providers or consumers only select measures are included in reporting systems.

At the beginning of the quality improvement movement, several alliances of health care providers emerged with an initial mission to review and endorse measures. The most active alliance was the HQA, a partnership of providers, purchasers, CMS, and others that provided the impetus to establish hospital measures for public reporting. Another active alliance, the Ambulatory Quality Alliance, was initiated by the American Academy of Family Physicians, the American College of Physicians, America's Health Insurance Plans, and the Agency for Healthcare Research and Quality in 2004 (Ambulatory Quality Alliance, 2014). The focus of this alliance has been on measures related to outpatient care. With measurement evolving to having a fairly robust though not exhaustive set of measures, the alliances have had a more limited role.

Nursing also has an alliance that was started in 2010 with funding from the RWJF and currently managed by the ANA (NAQC, 2015). The focus of the NAQC is to ensure that patients get the right care at the right time from the right providers. This alliance differs from others in that its mission is to improve patient care through advocating for use of existing measures, ensuring that nursing has a voice at policy tables, and focusing on improving nursing's impact on care coordination and patient engagement.

CMS is the largest force in moving quality improvement forward. The Medicare and Medicaid programs are federally funded (either in full or in part) and have a large market impact. CMS has a significant interest in making sure that the care they pay for is effective and efficient; the current cost of health care was about $3 trillion in 2013, with about a third of the cost being paid from public funds (Chantrill, 2015; Centers for Disease Control and Prevention [CDC], 2015a). CMS has many rules and regulations governing payment for care and has aggressively moved to link payment to quality. In addition, CMS initiated The Center for Medicare and Medicaid Innovation to generate and test new ideas to deliver more efficient, high quality care. For instance, among the many different models being tested by CMS, one example is the Medicare Care Choices Model that will allow patients to keep their curative care as well as receive palliative care. Currently, the hospice regulations prevent continuation of curative care (CMS, 2015a). There are many different models being tested. Importantly, regulations and practices established by CMS are often implemented by private payers.

Value-based Purchasing as an Impetus for Quality

The United States has the most expensive health system in the world but is ranked last among 11 developed nations (Mahon and Fox, 2014). Even though there are several important drivers to improve the quality of care in the United States, a strong impetus to quality improvement efforts has been through the concept of value-based purchasing, particularly by the federal government.

Value-based purchasing is defined by the National Business Coalition on Health's Value-based Purchasing Council and adopted by CMS as a "demand-side strategy to measure, report, and reward excellence in health care delivery, taking into consideration access, price, quality, efficiency, and alignment of incentives" (National Business Coalition on Health, 2011). The intended outcome is that there is value for every dollar spent and includes both the cost and quality aspects of health care. Value-based purchasing has largely focused on hospitals and more recently outpatient as well as long-term care settings. There are several types of value-based purchasing approaches including pay for performance, accountable care organizations, and bundled payment (Danberg *et al.*, 2014).

Pay for Performance

CMS has already begun to implement pay for performance policies that link payment levels to specific measures of quality. One specific policy is to not pay for specific adverse events occurring to hospitalized patients, such as surgery on the wrong body part or development of stage III or IV pressure sores. Currently, there are 14 categories of conditions for non-payment (Centers for Medicare and Medicaid, 2015b). Hospitals are increasingly looking to nursing to prevent the adverse events (Kurtzman, Dawson, and Johnson, 2008). Another policy that has captured the attention of hospitals is CMS refusing to pay for readmission within 30 days for the same diagnosis as the initial hospitalization. For 2015, a little over 2400 hospitals will get a lower payment due to readmission measures, amounting to approximately $420 million in the aggregate (Rau, 2015).

In the acute care sector, CMS is giving each of the hospitals that receive Medicare or Medicaid payment a "total performance score" that is a basis for either incentive payments or a reduction in payments. The score is comprised of four categories of measures including clinical process of care, patient experience of care, outcomes, and efficiency (CMS, 2015c). Many hospitals are looking to enhance their payments by improving their patient experience rating particularly as related to nursing care.

In the ambulatory care sector, practices that successfully implement patient-centered medical homes and meet the quality measure benchmarks are getting incentive payments. There is also a large ongoing Comprehensive Primary Care Initiative (CPC) that involves more than 2400 providers caring for over 2.6 million patients as well as 38 payers (CMS, 2015d). The initiative is designed to be a shared savings program that also includes a monthly care coordination payment. In return, the primary care practices must deliver on five functions: "1) risk-stratified care management; 2) access and continuity; 3) planned care for chronic conditions and preventive care; 4) patient and caregiver engagement; 5) coordination of care across the medical neighborhood" (CMS, 2015c). In addition to the CPC initiative, there are many payers who are providing incentive payers to primary care practices that have met the requirements of being a recognized or accredited patient centered medical home. There is considerable data about pay for performance related quality improvement; however, the data are mixed. The study by the Rand Corporation and funded by the HHS has a detailed summary of pay for performance research findings (Danberg *et al.*, 2014).

Case Example

An example of a nurse practitioner as leader as well as partner in becoming an NCQA-recognized patient-centered medical practice is a pediatric practice in the mid-Atlantic states in which the nurse practitioner and physician collaborated to meet the standards established for NCQA recognition. The nurse practitioner developed continuous quality improvement, population-based care, flexible access, and care coordination systems within the practice as a physician colleague implemented an electronic health record. Together they coordinated the electronic health record (EHR), which is also known as an electronic medical record (EMR), to support the changes in the practice to set up registries and monitor select patient care processes and outcomes as well as enhance their health promotion and chronic care management of populations. They included all members of their team in moving the quality improvement forward. Over a three-year period the practice was recognized at the highest level of patient-centered care. As a result, they get an increase in their payment from select insurers.

Accountable Care Organizations

The Patient Protection and Affordable Care Act included language that recognizes ACOs (Social Security Administration, 2010). CMS defines an ACO as "groups of doctors, hospitals, and other health care providers, who come together voluntarily to give coordinated high quality care to their Medicare patients" (Centers for Medicare and Medicaid, 2015e). There are different types of ACOs, but the incentive to become an ACO includes sharing of the savings obtained through more efficient and effective care. A key factor is for ACOs to work across settings so that care will not be fragmented. While working to control costs, ACOs also must provide high quality care as demonstrated by achieving specific quality benchmarks. Although shared savings is an incentive to become an ACO, there is also increased risk assumed by providers. If providers are not efficient in attaining high quality outcomes, they will assume the costs of inefficiency.

Findings related to ACOs are beginning to be reported. One study examining quality measures related to diabetes and coronary artery disease found no differences between care provided within ACOs and that by physician group practices (Singh, Khosla, and Sethi, 2015).Many ACOs have recognized the importance of engaging patients and families in care and are developing a variety of strategies to better engage patients and families in care (Shortell *et al.*, 2015). In addition, ACOs compared to traditional fee-for-service payment-based care have demonstrated lower costs and utilization but comparable patient satisfaction, as with traditional Medicare fee-for-service payment (Nyweide *et al.*, 2015). A study comparing a pediatric ACO, managed care, and Medicaid fee-for-service in Ohio found that the ACO model had the lowest cost growth of the three models while maintaining quality of patient care and satisfaction (Kelleher *et al.*, 2015). Because of the nature of ACOs, there is evidence to suggest that partnerships with high quality post-acute care facilities are important in managing the total care of a patient (Lage *et al.*, 2015). A recent study exploring changes in the role of nurses in ACOs found that nursing roles were changing along several dimensions, namely, using nurses to coordinate care between settings, increasing the number of nurses, and establishing different patterns of delegation (Pittman & Forrest, 2015).

Bundled Payment

As part of the value-based purchasing movement, there were early demonstrations to test the concept of "bundled payments" for specific conditions or treatments (Birkmeyer *et al.*, 2010; Cromwell, Dayhoff, and Thoumaian, 1997; Hackbarth, Reischauer, and Mutti, 2008). Bundled payment (also referred to as episode-of-care based payment) requires a seamless approach to care that crosses settings, such as that provided through an ACO. For instance, bundled payment for a person needing hip replacement would include all of the services needed as part of the hip replacement such as pre-surgery care, surgery, rehabilitation, and health provider visits. CMS has begun the Bundled Payment and Care Improvement Initiative in which organizations select the conditions for which they will be paid under the bundled payment model (Centers for Medicare and Medicaid, 2015f). Examples of conditions include acute myocardial infarction, diabetes, congestive heart failure, major joint replacement of the lower extremity, and 45 others (Centers for Medicare and Medicaid, 2015b). There are currently four bundled payment models that include retrospective payment for a hospitalization only (physician payment is separate); retrospective payment for acute care and post-acute episode of care; retrospective payment for post-acute care only; and a prospective payment for acute care only including all costs.

Quality Improvement Approaches

Over the years, there have been numerous quality improvement approaches and philosophies embraced by a variety of industries. Most of these approaches have been based on measurement of performance. Well-known approaches include the Deming method, which uses 14 principles to improve quality and reduce costs (Deming, 1986; Neuhauser, 1988). Deming is best known for his work with Japanese industries in the 1950s and is credited with beginning the Total Quality Management approach to quality improvement. Nurses are increasingly being certified in a variety of methods, including the Deming method.

Six Sigma is another approach to quality, focused on reducing variation in order to improve quality. It was developed by Motorola Company in 1981 and widely adapted as a strategy to improve products and customer service. The concept of Six Sigma is that 99.99966% of products are free of defects. Individuals can become expert in the approach, with one of the most accomplished levels being a "master black belt." Six Sigma has been applied to numerous health care issues, including decreasing Methicillin-resistant Staphylococcus aureus (MRSA), improving efficiency in an interventional radiology suite, improving screening for Genetic Syndrome, reducing postsurgical problems, improving efficiency in an adult infusion clinic, improving hand hygiene, and addressing many other challenges (Dineen *et al.*, 2015; Glasgow, Scott-Caziewell, and Kaboli, 2010; Lamm *et al.*, 2015; Murphree, Vath, and Daigle, 2011; Wannemuehler *et al.*, 2015). Nurses with expertise in Six Sigma play a major role in improving quality and efficiency.

Another perspective is the lean production philosophy, largely based on the Toyota Production approach to quality (Lean Enterprise Institute, 2015; Lewis *et al.*, 2014). Dr. Jim Womack who was the director of research at the Massachusetts Institute of Technology (MIT) International Motor Vehicle Program first coined the term lean in his *The Machine That Changed the World* (1990). Lean focuses on value to the customer; anything that is not of value to the customer is waste and should be eliminated. This approach has also been used to improve system efficiency in health care (Ajami *et al.*, 2015; Dickson *et al.*, 2009; Improta *et al.*, 2015; Merguerian *et al.*, 2015; Ng *et al.*, 2010; Sinnott *et al.*, 2015; Sugianto *et al.*, 2015). The Deming, Six Sigma, and Lean approaches have similarities in terms of overall concept and are often combined (e.g., Lean Six Sigma), and these approaches have demonstrated improvement in health care (Chassin, Mayer, and Nether, 2015; Domato and Rickard, 2015).

The International Organization for Standardization (ISO) has a strong influence on quality for many different industries as well as health care. The ISO has developed 19,500 standards since 1946 when it was established by engineers who were committed to developing and harmonizing standards for all countries. It is an organization of 162 member countries that establishes standards to be used across the world. The intent is to create high reliability regardless of where in the world a product is made or a service occurs (ISO, 2013). Within the health care sector, 1200 standards have been created (ISO, 2013).

All of these quality improvement approaches can be found in health care. A common thread for each of these approaches is the use of statistical monitoring techniques to monitor variation in production or services in order to identify and then correct problems as quickly as possible with the goal to be a high reliability organization with high quality standards.

Measuring Nursing Care Quality

Framework for Quality Measures

As part of the IOM series of reports on quality, *Crossing the Quality Chasm* established an "aim" for quality measurement (IOM, 2001). There are six aims marking high-quality health care: safe, timely, efficient, effective, equitable, and patient-centered care. These six aims define the areas that are

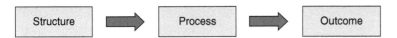

Figure 6.1 Structure, process, outcome framework (Donabedian framework).

important for measurement development. The measurement framework most used in developing and monitoring measures is the structure/process/outcome framework developed by Avedis Donabedian (Donabedian, 1966). The theoretical underpinning of this framework is that the right structure will support the right processes, which will in turn result in the desired patient outcomes. The Donabedian framework can be applied to the IOM aims. All measures related to one of the aims fall into structure, process, or outcome measures, as shown in Figure 6.1.

To provide a policy framework to improve quality, the IHI recognized that there needed to be a broad framework of goals to improve health care. This was followed by an article by Berwick, Nolan, and Whittington (2008) stating the need for overarching goals for the nation to improve health care. These goals have been broadly adopted as a national policy and are referred to as the triple aim: 1) improve health of populations; 2) control costs; and 3) improve the experience of care. The triple aim has become the framework for a national approach to improving quality and is shown in Figure 6.2 below.

Measures Reflecting Nursing Care

There are hundreds of endorsed measures as noted above, including several sets of quality measures that have been developed to directly reflect nursing care. In the early 2000s, the ANA began critical work to develop quality measures that reflect nursing care that became known as the NDNQI. The "nursing sensitive measures" currently include patient falls and pressure sores that are among outcomes that CMS will withhold payment. Approximately 2000 health care institutions, primarily acute care institutions and 98% of magnet facilities, report measures to a central data repository for benchmarking and reporting back to institutions (Press Ganey, 2015). The ANA recently sold the measures to Press Ganey, a business that is well known for its work on patient satisfaction as well as work with thousands of health care entities to improve care. The NDNQI is the only database that provides benchmarking comparisons regionally and nationally for participating hospitals.

In 2004, the NQF released a report recognizing 15 measures specifically as "nursing sensitive measures." Since that time NQF has integrated many of those measures into other categories of endorsed measures including a series of measures related to falls, the practice environment, and skill mix that reflect the quality of nursing care (NQF, 2015b). However, the Joint Commission has maintained endorsement of 12 of the 15 original measures with hospital reporting requirements. There is ongoing work with CMS to have select nursing sensitive measures included in required Medicare reporting.

Figure 6.2 Triple aim goals.

Healthy populations

Affordable care

Patient experience

The HCAHPS is a set of measures that CMS requires all hospitals to report. Of the total 32 questions, 18 are considered "substantive," meaning they relate directly to care experience compared to other questions related to demographic information. Of the18 substantive measures, 11 are reported in the Hospital Compare web site with seven of the measures reflecting nursing care (Centers for Medicare and Medicaid, 2015g). The HCAHPS is the only set of measures collected uniformly and nationally from all accredited acute care facilities that provides information related to nursing. See Textbox 6.1 for a summary of the nursing-related HCAHPS questions.

Validity, Reliability, and Risk Adjustment of Measures

It is important that measures are useful for either internal use to improve care or for public reporting in order for the public to be able to make judgments about the quality of care provided by an institution or specific provider. Public reporting is intended to guide consumers to the best care. In addition, measures need to be reliable so that anyone who measures a particular event, set of events, or phenomenon measures it in the same way using the same specifications for the measure. For instance, if one facility measures falls based on people who only hit the ground when they fall

---

Textbox 6.1 Nursing-related HCAHPS survey questions

Nursing Specific Questions

During this hospital stay …

- How often did nurses communicate well with patients?
- How often did nurses treat you with courtesy and respect? (Q1)
- How often did nurses listen carefully to you? (Q2)
- How often did nurses explain things in a way you could understand? (Q3)
- After you pressed the call button, how often did you get help as soon as you wanted it? (Q4)
- Did you need help from nurses or other hospital staff in getting to the bathroom or in using a bedpan? (Q 10)
- How often did you get help in getting to the bathroom or in using a bedpan as soon as you wanted (Q11)

Nursing Related Questions

During this hospital stay…

- How often was the area around your room quiet at night? (Q9)
- How often was your pain well controlled? (Q13)
- How often did the hospital staff do everything they could to help you with your pain? (Q14)
- Before giving you any new medicine how often did the hospital staff tell you what the medicine was for? (Q16)
- Before giving you any new medicine how often did hospital staff describe possible side effects in a way that you could understand? (Q17)
- Did doctors, nurses, or other hospital staff talk with you about whether you would have the help you needed when you left the hospital? (Q19)
- Did you get information in writing about what symptoms or health problems to look out for after you left the hospital? (Q20) (CMS, 2015d)

and another facility counts a fall even if someone caught the patient before he or she hit the ground, falls will be counted in very different ways.

Measures also need to be valid and assess the event or phenomena that they are intended to assess. For measures to be useful in measuring quality of care, there has to be variation in the measure, with that variation being influenced by the provision of good or bad care. If there is no variation, a measure lacks usefulness to improve care because everyone performs the same. Measures also need to be risk adjusted. This means that some institutions or providers will appear to perform worse than others because of factors that are related to the population cared for and not the quality of care provided. For instance, hospitals that have sicker patients will have a higher likelihood of an increased mortality rate than hospitals with less sick patients. The mortality rate needs to be risk adjusted based on the severity of patient conditions in order to compare their mortality rate with hospitals that have less acutely ill patients (Jerant, Tancredi, and Franks, 2011; Joynt, Orav, and Jha, 2011).

In addition, as part of specifying a measure, there has to be the inclusion of the total population at risk (denominator) and the number of events that occurred in that population (numerator) to determine a rate. The populations have to be defined in the same way. For measures to be useful, valid, and reliable, the number of events is critical. Measures of rare events do not produce enough data to create valid and reliable measures.

Quality Measures and Health Information Technology

Technology and electronic health records are revolutionizing how data are collected and used. Health care has been slower than many other industries to integrate electronic data into the workflow. Integration of electronic health records was greatly enhanced by an investment of $20+ billion through the Health Information Technology for Economic and Clinical Health Act (HITECH) program of 2009. The goal of this initiative was to provide an incentive to physicians and hospitals to integrate electronic health records. Currently about 50% of physician offices and nearly 80 of hospitals have some form of EHR (Adler-Milstein, 2014; CDC, 2015b; US Department of Health and Human Services, 2015). Having robust EHRs makes the collection of patient-level clinical data much easier and is accelerating the use of data to improve care.

To ensure that health care institutions use health information technology (HIT) to improve care, the Office of the National Coordinator for Health Information Technology (ONC) (a federal agency that is part of the Department of Health and Human Services) has begun to require institutions to collect data related to specific measures before they receive federal funds for HIT implementation. The required measures are called "meaningful use." The ONC has identified five intended outcomes from the meaningful use requirements: 1) improve quality, safety, and efficiency; 2) engage patients and families; 3) improve care coordination; 4); improve population health; and 5) ensure security of personal health data (US Department of Health and Human Services, 2015). Meaningful use is focused on eligible providers (physicians) and hospitals with each needing to report core measures and then measures from a list of optional measures. An example of a required meaningful use core measure is that 60% of medication orders, 30% of lab orders, and 30% of radiology orders use computerized physician order entry (CPOE).

ONC is implementing meaningful use in three stages. Stage 1 was to generate data through incentive and required reporting initiatives. Stage 2 is focusing on improving clinical processes. Stage 3 is to improve outcomes. Stage 3 is planned to begin in 2017. For data to be useful, there needs to be advances in analytics, data sharing through exchanges, and dissemination and use of the information. Health information is a way to better inform consumers as well as providers in order to improve the health of individuals and populations.

Table 6.1 HCAHPS Survey Questions Example of Benchmarking for "Patients Who Reported That Their Nurses "Always" Communicated Well.

Average of all hospitals in United States	79%
Average of hospitals in Maryland (example of a state-level data source)	76%
Hospital A	84%
Hospital B	74%
Hospital C	71%

Publically Reported Measures and Benchmarking

Measures have maximum utility when they can be compared with measures that have been established as standards or best practice measures. This allows an organization to know how their performance compares with others. Common benchmarks are based on national and/or state averages as well as highest scoring and lowest scoring institutions, agencies, or providers. CMS publically reports many measures for hospitals, nursing homes, and home care through a series of web sites referred to collectively as the Compare web sites. In the Compare web sites, each institution is benchmarked against state and national comparisons. For instance, CMS has created a web site called Hospital Compare for consumers to use in choosing hospitals based on quality. The categories of information include general information, survey of patient experiences, timely and effective care, complications, readmissions and deaths, use of medical imaging, payment and value of care (Centers for Medicare and Medicaid, 2015h). Information about specific hospitals compared to the state and national averages for each measure is included in Hospital Compare. An example of benchmarking for the question in the patient experience of care section related to "How well do nurses communicate with patients?" is provided in Table 6.1.

The Nursing Home Compare web site presents information from the state survey process (Centers for Medicare and Medicaid, 2015i). Every nursing home is reviewed by onsite surveyors on a periodic basis with no longer than 18 months between surveys. Nursing Home Compare organizes data from each facility's inspections as well as the minimum data set (MDS) that is derived from data collected on each resident. The Compare site has detailed information in several categories including report of deficiencies, self-report with verification on nurse staffing, and quality measures. CMS has a five-star rating for nursing homes based on these categories of information. The best rating is five stars, and the worst rating is one star. The Nursing Home Compare web site also has benchmarking of state and national data for each measure reported.

Similar to Hospital Care and Nursing Home Compare, the Home Health Compare web site reports quality measures for specific home health agencies compared with state and national data (Centers for Medicare and Medicaid, 2015j). The Home Health Compare site provides information about services offered by each agency using a five-star rating for quality of care and data about patient experience of care. Quality of care ratings include managing pain, managing daily activities, preventing harm, preventing unplanned hospital care, treating wounds, and preventing pressure sores (Centers for Medicare and Medicaid, 2015e). As with the other Compare sites, there is benchmarking for state and national measures.

The ACA required that CMS set up the Physician Compare web site (Centers for Medicare and Medicaid, 2014). Any provider who is a Medicare-recognized provider including nurse practitioners is incorporated in this site. Currently the web site includes very basic data such as name, location, and clinical affiliation. CMS plans to incorporate quality data from incentive reporting programs such as the Physician Quality Reporting System. In addition, Yelp has developed an online review of physician and nurse practitioner practices based on consumer reviews of their experience. These reviews are often detailed but can also reflect providers who provide appropriate care but not what patients want, such as antibiotics for a viral infection. As measures related to the quality of care provided by individual clinicians evolve, advanced practice registered nurses will need to make sure that they are recognized in data by being recognized providers by Medicare.

Quality Improvement Process

Monitoring and Improving Quality

Monitoring care through the use of valid and reliable measures is foundational to the quality improvement process. The quality improvement process begins with monitoring the specific measures that are part of a care process to identify variations and compare findings with benchmarks. If monitoring indicates that a particular measure is outside of the expected performance level, a problem is identified. Once a problem is noted, the cause(s) of the problem, or root cause, needs to be determined. Once causes are determined, a small test of change using the plan, do, study, act (PDSA) process is then implemented. PDSA is a process used for many different problems worldwide (Crowl *et al.*, 2015; Donnelly and Kirk, 2015; Jones, 2015; Lehman *et al.*, 2011; Montella and Pelegano, 2015; Nakayama *et al.*, 2010).

For example, a hospital unit may be monitoring patient falls as part of a required measure. After monitoring falls for months, one week of data indicates that the number of falls far exceeds the unit average, the hospital average, and the national average. A problem is then identified as a fall rate that is too high. A root cause or other type of analysis such as brainstorming is then done, followed by the PDSA process.

Quality Improvement Tools

There are now many tools available to improve quality. Some of the richest resources are on the AHRQ Innovation Exchange web site that has tools for many disease-specific entities as well as a variety of situations (AHRQ, 2015). In addition to these tools, the web site has articles and programs related to implementation of best practices. The IHI also has many resources and educational modules available online (Institute for Healthcare Improvement, 2015). Numerous measures as noted above are being collected in all settings of health care. These measures can be the basis for monitoring high priority quality concerns and taking action to correct quality concerns.

Quality improvement is based on collecting, analyzing, and making decisions about data. Data can be organized in many different ways, some more useful to practicing nurses than others. Many clinical sites use unit-level dashboards that provide data in charts, bar graphs, and other ways of organizing information (Jeffs *et al.*, 2014; Jeffs *et al.*, 2015). Dashboards are an efficient way of organizing critical information and show trend data so changes in quality can be quickly observed. The events to follow should be determined by the unit to address the issues specific to that unit. However, all units may need to track the required reporting events such as falls, pressure ulcer development, or use of restraints.

These tools include line graphs, histograms, run charts, scatter grams, and ways to visually show frequency of events. All nurses should know how to use a dashboard that includes different ways of portraying data. Examples of data potentially displayed on dashboards are presented in

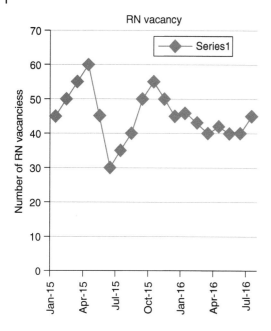

Figure 6.3 Line graph of RN vacancy.

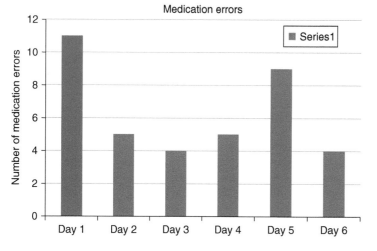

Figure 6.4 Histogram of medication errors.

Figures 6.3 through 6.5. Figure 6.3 is a basic line graph that shows the number of RN vacancies in a provider institution at the beginning of each month. The vacancy rate goes down in the late spring that reflects the availability and hiring of new graduates. Figure 6.4 is a column chart that shows the number of medication errors per day in an institution. There are two spikes in medication errors that would warrant examination. Figure 6.5 is a bar graph that represents the number of catheter-associated urinary tract infections (CAUTI) based on 1000 device days. There is a decrease in the infections from January to July representing efforts on the part of the institution to reduce the incidence of CAUTI. Each of the graphs is a way of showing trends of data. It is useful to monitor change to continually compare performance against benchmarks.

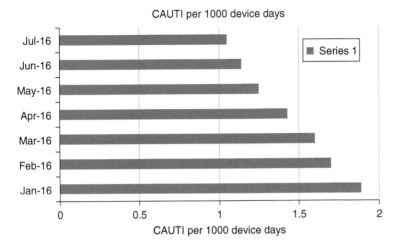

Figure 6.5 Bar graph of CAUTI per 1000 device days.

Identifying Reasons for Problems

In identifying the reason for the problem, a root cause analysis is useful. Root cause analysis is a systematic approach to get to the root causes of the problem. The use of a fishbone diagram was originated in the 1960s by Kaoru Ishikawa, a leader in modern quality management. The diagram is used to reflect the results of brainstorming and/or the use of "five whys" to get to the root cause of a problem. The process of five whys is simply to keep asking why for each problem statement related to an overall problem identified. For instance, a problem identified is that residents of a nursing home have more pressure ulcers than the national average. The first why is 'Why do residents of a nursing home have more pressure ulcers than the national average?' One possible reason is that pressure ulcer risk assessments are not being done or done correctly. The second why then asks 'Why isn't the risk assessment being done or done correctly?' The group keeps going through this exercise until they have answered "five whys." After identifying all the possible reasons for a problem, the one or two most likely reasons for the problem are then the presumed root cause.

An example of the fishbone diagram is provided in Figure 6.6. The problem statement is at the tip of the fishbone. The fishbone usually has several organizing categories that provide a guide to identifying problems. The categories commonly used include people, equipment, processes, environment, materials, and management. All six categories, or as few as two categories, may be applicable to a specific problem. For each category, everyone involved in the quality improvement team brainstorms possible reasons for the problem. Brainstorming and/or the five whys are applied to each category used in the fishbone.

After all of the most likely causes have been considered and the top two have been identified, the PDSA is initiated. The PDSA process can be guided by the questions and/or information noted for each phase of the PDSA in Table 6.2.

Figure 6.7 summarizes the complete quality improvement process. The process begins with monitoring. There are specific measures that are required to be monitored. However, monitoring can also include being vigilant about possible problems that are not being measured. The frequency of events that are being measured can be put into a histogram or control chart for ease in tracking the events. If a problem is identified, then a root cause analysis is conducted to determine the most likely root cause of the problem, and then a PDSA to do a small test of change to fix the problem is conducted. Then the process continues.

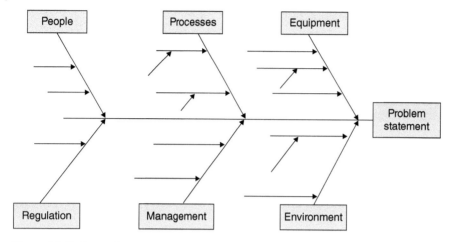

Figure 6.6 Fishbone diagram.

Table 6.2 Questions related to Plan, Do, Study, Act.

Plan	Do	Study	Act
What is the objective? What do you think will happen? What is the plan for the test of change (who, what, where, when)?	Conduct the test. Document unexpected observations and problems.	Analyze the data. How do the findings compare with predictions? What was learned from the test?	What modifications should be made? What is the next test?

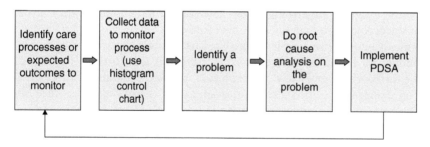

Figure 6.7 Summary of the quality improvement process. PDSA = plan, do, study, act.

Case Example

A hospital in the mid-Atlantic region of the United States recognized that many of their nurses in the intensive care units did not know how to do a PDSA process to use small tests of change to improve care. The Director of Education held educational sessions for all the intensive care nurses teaching the PDSA process and combined that with requiring the nurses to review specific data on their units. The supervising nurse of the four intensive care units had also gone through more extensive training and was asked to work with the unit leaders to implement a PDSA process. Each unit identified a problem to work on and used the PDSA process to improve care.

Teaching Quality Improvement

The IOM issued a report in 2003 identifying competencies that all health care providers should know about patient safety and health care quality (IOM, 2003). Based on these competencies, the RWJF supported the development of a program identifying entry level and graduate knowledge, skills, and attitudes. Every nurse learner should be able to attain these competencies called QSEN (Barnsteiner *et al.*, 2013; Barnsteiner *et al.*, 2013; Cronenwett *et al.*, 2007; Cronenwett, Sherwood, and Gelmon, 2009; Johnson *et al.*, 2015; Sullivan, Hirst, and Cronenwett, 2009).

Nurse educators are integrating these competencies across all of nursing and continue to identify innovative teaching approaches. Strategies for teaching quality improvement, whether to new nurses or experienced nurses, include classroom, online, case study, and clinical simulation methods. The following are strategies for teaching nurse learners various aspects of quality improvement. These suggestions are examples and not meant to be comprehensive.

- Ask nurse learners to review the Medicare Compare web sites for all hospital, nursing home, or home care agency clinical sites in their area to review the measures reported, assess the quality of care of the provider, and identify the strengths and weaknesses of the public reporting. The learners should have the opportunity to discuss their findings. The following questions could be used to structure the discussion:
  - Could you make a decision about choosing where to get care from the Compare site?
  - How did nursing care related measures in the clinical agency you work compare to state/national benchmarks? How would you explain the difference?
  - How do you think patients will use the information you just reviewed?
  - Do you agree with the rating of the institution/agency by the Compare site? Explain and give examples.
  - Does the institution/agency have quality improvement programs that you observed or participated in? If so, describe.
- Ask the learner to assess the philosophy of quality improvement of their clinical site. The learners should base their assessment on talking with nurses, physicians, and others throughout the facility about the philosophy and observe signs and messages that are in the facility that convey the presence of a commitment to quality and patient safety. Questions of providers could include:
  - Does the leadership of the organization prioritize quality improvement and patient safety?
  - In what ways is this commitment demonstrated?
  - How are all staff included in quality improvement efforts?
  - What type of patient outcome information is shared with staff?
  - How do you know that patients are getting the best care possible?
- Use a case study method in which students are asked to do a root cause analysis using a fishbone diagram and five whys. Learners can then engage in the PDSA process to define a small test of change. A root cause analysis can also be integrated into a simulation lab using the fishbone in which the "patient" develops a central line infection, fall with injury, or any one of the non-payment adverse patient experiences. The case study would include data related to the "problem," and learners would be expected to apply the PDSA process as above.
  - Partner with health care delivery settings to enable nurse learners to join QI teams so that they experience first hand the steps for identifying the problem, measure steps to determine the gap, and find solutions to improve.
  - Have learners interview the Director of Quality Improvement or Performance Improvement to learn the projects under way in a particular setting and discuss observations of situations students see during their clinical practice.

- Invite a panel of nurses who are engaged in QI to present in the classroom, in a post-clinical conference, or continuing education offering for staff nurses to share projects, strategies, challenges, and imperatives for change, and illustrate how nurses can speak up about process breakdowns that would benefit from a QI project.
- Assign learners to work in small groups on a selected item from the NDNQI list to do a literature search to determine best practices, inquire for the status in their clinical site for the selected item (e.g., what is the falls data on the unit where they are assigned?).
- Learners can also practice QI by identifying a problem in their world, such as sleep deprivation for nursing students. They can survey their classmates to determine hours of sleep per night over a week's time, search the literature for the ideal amount of sleep for college students, and share strategies for improving sleep with their class.
- Integrate research article on quality improvement in a class for student nurses or as part of effort to enhance staff nurses to do engage in research/quality improvement.
- Ask the learners to consider the differences between research and quality improvement projects based on data, and how they can integrate quality improvement into evidence-based care.
- Ask learners to consider how they would build a culture of quality in a specific clinical site. Challenge them to think about how they would engage all staff, how they would know they were successful, and what specific activities they would initiate.
- Have the learners compare the health care industry efforts in quality with one other non-health related industry. Key areas for comparison could include historic roots of quality efforts, approaches to quality, and the impact of efforts on quality.

Bridging Education and Clinical Practice

Marrying educational efforts to teach quality improvement to the realities and challenges of clinical practice is critical to having a nursing workforce able to keep patients safe regardless of the setting or circumstance. The partnership needs to be a shared effort to educate not only new nurses but also experienced nurses. Clinical nurses are living the challenges of quality as they are often expected to collect data, implement change, and evaluate outcomes.

Faculty are also living quality improvement as they teach quality, take students into clinical settings, and may be involved in research about quality. The challenge is often how to create the best relationships for partnership to thrive and use everyone's strengths to benefit all. A critical element of developing this partnership is the commitment of deans and nurse executives to the partnership. One way to assure a shared approach is for the dean to have an appointment in the clinical site and the nurse executive likewise have a faculty appointment. The commitment can be operationalized by deans participating in clinical rounds, sitting on clinical committees, providing the opportunity for joint appointments, and supporting faculty to work with clinical partners on quality improvement projects. Nurse executives can teach select lectures, participate in school committees and events, and provide the opportunity to staff for joint appointments.

Another critical element is equity in the partnership. Clinical sites often feel that educational programs come to them with requests but seldom offer help. Budget constraints are often sited as a reason that one entity cannot help the other. Partnerships are most successful when each party gets something that is important to them and that the reward of the partnership outweighs the cost. Exploring efficiencies that contribute to the value of the partnership is a key to success. One consideration could be that clinical sites integrate students in meaningful ways into their quality improvement activities and faculty members work with clinical staff to enhance their knowledge or confidence in using quality improvement methods. This will result in more knowledgeable existing nurses and better prepared future nurses.

It is important that nurses become leaders for improving quality. Recognition of expertise in quality improvement can be achieved through certification programs. Certification in quality improvement can be obtained from the National Association for Healthcare Quality. In addition, ASQ (originally American Society for Quality) has numerous certification programs.

Conclusion

Nurses are critical to improving quality of care in all health care settings. Nurses can change the landscape of quality and significantly reduce injury and death due to harm caused by errors. In order to be effective, nurses need to know how to use data to measure quality of care and implement improvement processes. Clinical sites expect nurses to know how to apply quality improvemrent processes to patient care improvement. More and more as providers are subject to financial penalties for poor care, nurses will be both held accountable and also looked to for providing high quality care.

References

Acquaviva, K., and Johnson, J. (2014) The quality improvement landscape. In E.R. Ransom, M. Joshi, D.B. Nash, and S.B. Ransom (Eds.), *The healthcare quality book: Vision, strategy and tools* (3rd Ed). Chicago: Health Administration Press.

Adler-Milstein, J., DesRoches, C.M., Furukawa, M.F., Worzala, C., Charles, D., Kralovec, P., *et al.* (2014) More than half of US hospitals have at least a basic EHR, but stage 2 criteria remain challenging for most. *Health Affairs (Project Hope), 33*(9), 1664–1671.

Agency for Healthcare Research and Quality. *AHRQ healthcare innovations exchange: innovations and tools to improve care and reduce disparities.* Retrieved 8/17, 2015, from https://innovations.ahrq.gov.

Ajami, S., Ketabi, S., Sadcghian, A., and Saghaeinnejad-Isfahani, S. (2015) Improving the medical records department processes by lean management. *Journal of Education and Health Promotion, 4,* 48-9531.157244. eCollection 2015.

Ambulatory Quality Alliance. (2014) *About AQA.* Retrieved 8/17/2015, from http://www.aqaalliance.org/about.htm.

Barnsteiner, J., Disch, J., Johnson, J., and McGuinn, K. (2013) The quality and safety education for nurses (QSEN) initiative began in 2005 and has rapidly gained traction in enhancing nursing curricula, practice-academic partnerships, and clinical practice. preface. *Journal of Professional Nursing: Official Journal of the American Association of Colleges of Nursing, 29*(2), 65.

Barnsteiner, J., Disch, J., Johnson, J., McGuinn, K., Chappell, K., and Swartwout, E. (2013) Diffusing QSEN competencies across schools of nursing: The AACN/RWJF faculty development institutes. *Journal of Professional Nursing: Official Journal of the American Association of Colleges of Nursing, 29*(2), 68–74.

Berwick, D.M. (2011) Preparing nurses for participation in and leadership of continual improvement. *The Journal of Nursing Education, 50*(6), 322–327.

Berwick, D.M., Nolan, T.W., and Whittington, J. (2008) The triple aim: Care, health, and cost. *Health Affairs (Project Hope), 27*(3), 759–769.

Birkmeyer, J.D., Gust, C., Baser, O., Dimick, J.B., Sutherland, J.M., and Skinner, J.S. (2010) Medicare payments for common inpatient procedures: Implications for episode-based payment bundling. *Health Services Research, 45*(6 Pt 1), 1783–1795.

Centers for Disease Control and Prevention. (2015a) *Health expenditures.* Retrieved 8/17/2015, from http://www.cdc.gov/nchs/fastats/health-expenditures.htm.

Centers for Disease Control and Prevention. (2015b) *Electronic medical records/electronic health records (EMR/EHR).* Retrieved 9/9, 2015, from http://www.cdc.gov/nchs/fastats/electronic-medical-records.htm.

Centers for Medicare and Medicaid. (2014) *Physician compare overview.* Retrieved 8/17/2015, from https://www.cms.gov/Medicare/Quality-Initiatives-Patient-Assessment-Instruments/physician-compare-initiative/Physician-Compare-Overview.html.

Centers for Medicare and Medicaid. (2015e) *Accountable care organizations (ACO).* Retrieved 9/8/2015, from https://www.cms.gov/Medicare/Medicare-Fee-for-Service-Payment/ACO/index.html?redirect=/aco.

Centers for Medicare and Medicaid. (2015f) *Bundled payments for care improvement (BPCI) initiative: General information.* Retrieved 8/17/2015, from http://innovation.cms.gov/initiatives/bundled-payments/index.html.

Centers for Medicare and Medicaid. (2015d) *Comprehensive Primary Care Initiative.* Retrieved 9/2/2015, from http://innovation.cms.gov/initiatives/comprehensive-primary-care-initiative/.

Centers for Medicare and Medicaid. (2015g) *HCAHPS survey.* Retrieved 8/17/2015, from http://www.hcahpsonline.org/files/HCAHPS%20V10.0%20Appendix%20A%20-%20HCAHPS%20Mail%20Survey%20Materials%20%28English%29%20March%202015.pdf.

Centers for Medicare and Medicaid. (2015j) *Home health compare.* Retrieved 9/1/2015, from https://www.medicare.gov/homehealthcompare/.

Centers for Medicare and Medicaid. (2015h) *Hospital compare.* Retrieved 8/17/2015, from https://www.cms.gov/Medicare/Quality-Initiatives-Patient-Assessment-Instruments/HospitalQualityInits/HospitalCompare.html.

Centers for Medicare and Medicaid. (2015c) *Hospital value-based purchasing.* Retrieved 9/8/2015, from https://www.medicare.gov/hospitalcompare/data/hospital-vbp.html.

Centers for Medicare and Medicaid. (2015b) *Hospital-acquired conditions.* Retrieved 9/1/2015, from https://www.cms.gov/Medicare/Medicare-Fee-for-Service-Payment/HospitalAcqCond/Hospital-Acquired_Conditions.html.

Centers for Medicare and Medicaid. (2015a) *Medicare care choices model.* Retrieved 8/17/2015, from http://innovation.cms.gov/initiatives/Medicare-Care-Choices/.

Centers for Medicare and Medicaid. (2015i) *Nursing home Compare.* Retrieved 8/17/2015, from https://www.medicare.gov/nursinghomecompare/search.html.

Chantrill, C. (2015) *US health spending.* Retrieved 8/17/2015, from http://www.usgovernmentspending.com/us_health_care_spending_10.html.

Chassin, M.R., Mayer, C., and Nether, K. (2015) Improving hand hygiene at eight hospitals in the united states by targeting specific causes of noncompliance. *Joint Commission Journal on Quality and Patient Safety/Joint Commission Resources, 41*(1), 4–12.

Cromwell, J., Dayhoff, D.A., and Thoumaian, A.H. (1997) Cost savings and physician responses to global bundled payments for medicare heart bypass surgery. *Health Care Financing Review, 19*(1), 41–57.

Cronenwett, L., Sherwood, G., Barnsteiner, J., Disch, J., Johnson, J., Mitchell, P., *et al.* (2007) Quality and safety education for nurses. *Nursing Outlook, 55*(3), 122–131.

Cronenwett, L., Sherwood, G., and Gelmon, S.B. (2009) Improving quality and safety education: The QSEN learning collaborative. *Nursing Outlook, 57*(6), 304–312.

Crowl, A., Sharma, A., Sorge, L., and Sorensen, T. (2015) Accelerating quality improvement within your organization: Applying the model for improvement. *Journal of the American Pharmacists Association: JAPhA, 55*(4), e364–76.

Damato, C. and Rickard, D. (2015) Using lean-six sigma to reduce hemolysis in the emergency care center in a collaborative quality improvement project with the hospital laboratory. *Joint Commission Journal on Quality and Patient Safety/Joint Commission Resources, 41*(3), 99–91.

Danberg, C.L., Sorbero, M.E., Lovejoy, S.L., Martsoff, G., Raaen, L., and Mandel, D. (2014) *Measuring success in health care value-based purchasing programs* (Research No. RR-306-ASPE). Santa Monica, CA: Rand Corporation.

Deming, E. (1986) *Out of the crisis*, MIT Press.

Dickson, E. W., Anguelov, Z., Vetterick, D., Eller, A., and Singh, S. (2009) Use of lean in the emergency department: A case series of 4 hospitals. *Annals of Emergency Medicine, 54*(4), 504–510.

Dineen, S., Lynch, P.M., Rodriguez-Bigas, M.A., Bannon, S., Taggart, M., Reeves, C., *et al.* (2015) A prospective six sigma quality improvement trial to optimize universal screening for genetic syndrome among patients with young-onset colorectal cancer. *Journal of the National Comprehensive Cancer Network: JNCCN, 13*(7), 865–872.

Donabedian, A. (1966) Evaluating the quality of medical care. *Milbank Memorial Fund Quarterly, 44*, 166–206.

Donnelly, P., and Kirk, P. (2015) Use the PDSA model for effective change management. *Education for Primary Care: An Official Publication of the Association of Course Organisers, National Association of GP Tutors, World Organisation of Family Doctors, 26*(4), 279–281.

Donnelly, P., and Kirk, P. (2015) Use the PDSA model for effective change management. *Education for Primary Care: An Official Publication of the Association of Course Organisers, National Association of GP Tutors, World Organisation of Family Doctors, 26*(4), 279–281.

Glasgow, J.M., Scott-Caziewell, J.R., and Kaboli, P.J. (2010) Guiding inpatient quality improvement: A systematic review of lean and six sigma. *Joint Commission Journal on Quality and Patient Safety/Joint Commission Resources, 36*(12), 533–540.

Hackbarth, G., Reischauer, R., and Mutti, A. (2008) Collective accountability for medical care–toward bundled medicare payments. *The New England Journal of Medicine, 359*(1), 3–5.

Improta, G., Balato, G., Romano, M., Carpentieri, F., Bifulco, P., Alessandro Russo, M., *et al.* (2015) Lean six sigma: A new approach to the management of patients undergoing prosthetic hip replacement surgery. *Journal of Evaluation in Clinical Practice, 21*(4), 662–672.

Institute for Healthcare Improvement. (2015) *Resources.* Retrieved 9/2/2015, from http://www.ihi.org/resources/Pages/default.aspx.

Institute of Medicine. (2000) In Kohn L.T., Corrigan J., and Donaldson M. (Eds.), *To err is human: Building a safer health system.* Washington, DC: National Academy Press.

Institute of Medicine. (2001) *Crossing the quality chasm: A new health system for the 21st century.* Washington, DC: National Academy Press.

Institute of Medicine. (2003) In Greiner A., Knebel E. (Eds.), *Health professions education: A bridge to quality.* Washington, D.C.: National Academy Press.

International Organization for Standardization. *About ISO.* Retrieved 8/17/2015, from http://www.iso.org/iso/about.htm.

ISO. (2013) *Health.* Retrieved 8/17/2015, from http://www.iso.org/iso/home/news_index/iso-in-action/health.htm.

James, J.T. (2013) A new, evidence-based estimate of patient harms associated with hospital care. *Journal of Patient Safety, 9*(3), 122–128.

Jeffs, L., Lo, J., Beswick, S., Chuun, A., Lai, Y., Campbell, H., *et al.* (2014) Enablers and barriers to implementing unit-specific nursing performance dashboards. *Journal of Nursing Care Quality, 29*(3), 200–203.

Jeffs, L., Nincic, V., White, P., Hayes, L., and Lo, J. (2015) Leveraging data to transform nursing care: Insights from nurse leaders. *Journal of Nursing Care Quality*, *30*(3), 269–274.

Jerant, A., Tancredi, D.J., and Franks, P. (2011) Mortality prediction by quality-adjusted life year compatible health measures: Findings in a nationally representative US sample. *Medical Care.*

Johnson, J., Drenkard, K., Emard, E., and McGuinn, K. (2015) Leveraging quality and safety education for nurses to enhance graduate-level nursing education and practice. *Nurse Educator.*

Joynt, K.E., Orav, E.J., and Jha, A.K. (2011) The association between hospital volume and processes, outcomes, and costs of care for congestive heart failure. *Annals of Internal Medicine*, *154*(2), 94–102.

Kelleher, K. J., Cooper, J., Deans, K., Carr, P., Brilli, R. J., Allen, S., *et al.* (2015) Cost saving and quality of care in a pediatric accountable care organization. *Pediatrics*, *135*(3), e582–9.

Kurtzman, E.T., Dawson, E.M., and Johnson, J.E. (2008) The current state of nursing performance measurement, public reporting, and value-based purchasing. *Policy, Politics & Nursing Practice*, *9*(3), 181–191.

Lage, D.E., Rusinak, D., Carr, D., Grabowski, D.C., and Ackerly, D.C. (2015) Creating a network of high-quality skilled nursing facilities: Preliminary data on the postacute care quality improvement experiences of an accountable care organization. *Journal of the American Geriatrics Society*, *63*(4), 804–808.

Lamm, M. H., Eckel, S., Daniels, R., and Amerine, L.B. (2015) Using lean principles to improve outpatient adult infusion clinic chemotherapy preparation turnaround times. *American Journal of Health-System Pharmacy: AJHP: Official Journal of the American Society of Health-System Pharmacists*, *72*(13), 1138–1146.

Landrigan, C.P., Parry, G.J., Bones, C.B., Hackbarth, A.D., Goldmann, D.A., and Sharek, P.J. (2010) Temporal trends in rates of patient harm resulting from medical care. *The New England Journal of Medicine*, *363*(22), 2124–2134.

Lean Enterprise Institute. (2015) *A brief history of lean*. Retrieved 8/17/2015 from http://www.lean.org/whatslean/History.cfm

Lehman, W.E., Simpson, D.D., Knight, D.K., and Flynn, P.M. (2011) Integration of treatment innovation planning and implementation: Strategic process models and organizational challenges. Psychology of Addictive Behaviors*: Journal of the Society of Psychologists in Addictive Behaviors.*

Lewis, V.A., Colla, C.H., Schpero, W.L., Shortell, S.M., and Fisher, E.S. (2014) ACO contracting with private and public payers: A baseline comparative analysis. *The American Journal of Managed Care*, *20*(12), 1008–1014.

Lippincott, J.B. (2014) *NDNQI measures aim to improve health care safety and quality*. Retrieved 9/8/2015, from http://lippincottsolutions.com/blog/12302014/ndnqimeasuresaimtoimprovehealthcaresafetyandquality.

Mahon, M., and Fox, B. (2014) *US health system ranks last among eleven countries on measures o, access, equity, quality, efficiency and healthy lives* No. 2015). New York: Commonwealth Fund.

Merguerian, P.A., Grady, R., Waldhausen, J., Libby, A., Murphy, W., Melzer, L., *et al.* (2015) Optimizing value utilizing toyota kata methodology in a multidisciplinary clinic. *Journal of Pediatric Urology.*

Montella, J.M., and Pelegano, J.F. (2015) Improving the rate of colposcopy in an urban population of patients with known abnormal pap smears. *American Journal of Medical Quality: The Official Journal of the American College of Medical Quality.*

Murphree, P., Vath, R. R., and Daigle, L. (2011) Sustaining lean six sigma projects in health care. *Physician Executive*, *37*(1), 44–48.

Nakayama, D.K., Bushey, T.N., Hubbard, I., Cole, D., Brown, A., Grant, T. M., *et al.* (2010) Using a plan-do-study-act cycle to introduce a new or service line. *AORN Journal*, *92*(3), 335–343.

National Business Coalition on Health. (2011) *Value-based purchasing: A definition*. Retrieved 8/24/2015, from http://www.nbch.org/Value-based-Purchasing-A-Definition.

National Committee for Quality Assurance. (2015) *HEDIS and quality measurement*. Retrieved 8/17/2015, from http://www.ncqa.org/tabid/59/Default.aspx.

National Quality Forum. (2015a) *About NQF*. Retrieved 8/17/2015, from http://www.qualityforum.org/About_NQF/About_NQF.aspx.

National Quality Forum. (2015b) *NQF-endorsed measures*. Retrieved 8/17/2015, from http://www.qualitymeasures.ahrq.gov/browse/nqf-endorsed.aspx.

Neuhauser, D. (1988) The quality of medical care and the 14 points of Edward Deming. *Health Matrix*, 6(2), 7–10.

Ng, D., Vail, G., Thomas, S., and Schmidt, N. (2010) Applying the lean principles of the Toyota production system to reduce wait times in the emergency department. *CJEM: Canadian Journal of Emergency Medical Care, JCMU: Journal Canadien De Soins Medicaux d'Urgence*, 12(1), 50–57.

Nightingale, F. (1863) *Notes on hospitals* (3rd Ed). London: Longman, Green, Longman, Roberts and Green.

Nursing Alliance For Quality Care. (2015) *Nursing alliance for quality care*. Retrieved 8/17/2015, from http://www.naqc.org/

Nyweide, D.J., Lee, W., Cuerdon, T.T., Pham, H.H., Cox, M., Rajkumar, R., *et al.* (2015) Association of pioneer accountable care organizations vs traditional medicare fee for service with spending, utilization, and patient experience. *Jama*, 313(21), 2152–2161.

Pittman, P., and Forrest, E. (2015) The changing roles of registered nurses in pioneer accountable care organizations. *Nursing Outlook*.

Press Ganey. (2015) *Turn nursing quality insights into improved patient experiences*. Retrieved 8/17/2015, from http://pressganey.com/ourSolutions/performance-and-advanced-analytics/clinical-business-performance/nursing-quality-ndnqi.

Rau, J. (2015) *Half of nation's hospitals fail again to escape medicare's readmission policies*. Retrieved 9/1/2015, from http://khn.org/news/half-of-nations-hospitals-fail-again-to-escape-medicares-readmission-penalties/.

Robert Wood Johnson Fondation. (2015) *Quality forum*. Retrieved 8/20/2015, from http://www.rwjf.org.proxygw.wrlc.org/en/how-we-work/grants/grantees/national-quality-forum.html.

Shortell, S.M., Colla, C.H., Lewis, V.A., Fisher, E., Kessell, E., and Ramsay, P. (2015) Accountable care organizations: The national landscape. *Journal of Health Politics, Policy and Law*.

Shortell, S.M., Sehgal, N.J., Bibi, S., Ramsay, P.P., Neuhauser, L., Colla, C.H., *et al.* (2015) An early assessment of accountable care organizations' efforts to engage patients and their families. *Medical Care Research and Review: MCRR*.

Singh, S., Khosla, S., and Sethi, A. (2015) Comparison of healthcare quality outcomes between accountable care organizations and physician group practices. *The Journal of Medical Practice Management: MPM*, 30(4), 261–264.

Sinnott, P.L., Breckenridge, J.S., Helgerson, P., and Asch, S. (2015) Using lean management to reduce blood culture contamination. *Joint Commission Journal on Quality and Patient Safety/Joint Commission Resources*, 41(1), 26–22.

Social Security Administration. (2010) *Social security act, section 1899, 2010*. Retrieved 9/1/2015, from http://www.ssa.gov/OP_Home/ssact/title18/1899.htm.

Sugianto, J.Z., Stewart, B., Ambruzs, J.M., Arista, A., Park, J.Y., Cope-Yokoyama, S., *et al.* (2015) Applying the principles of lean production to gastrointestinal biopsy handling: From the factory floor to the anatomic pathology laboratory. *Laboratory Medicine*, 46(3), 259–264.

Sullivan, D.T., Hirst, D., and Cronenwett, L. (2009) Assessing quality and safety competencies of graduating prelicensure nursing students. *Nursing Outlook, 57*(6), 323–331.

The Joint Commission. (2015) *Facts about the joint commission.* Retrieved 8/17/2015, from Facts about The Joint Commission http://www.jointcommission.org/facts_about_the_joint_commission/2015 July.

US Department of Health and Human Services. (2015) *Achieving meaningful use.* Retrieved 9/7, 2015, from http://www.healthit.gov/providers-professionals/ehr-implementation-steps/step-5-achieve-meaningful-use.

Wannemuehler, T.J., Elghouche, A.N., Kokoska, M.S., Deig, C.R., and Matt, B.H. (2015) Impact of lean on surgical instrument reduction: Less is more. *The Laryngoscope.*

Womack, J.P., Jones, D.T., and Ross, D. (1990) *The machine that changed the world.* New York: Rawson Associates.

Zarbo, R.J., Varney, R.C., Copeland, J. R., D'Angelo, R., and Sharma, G. (2015) Daily management system of the henry ford production system: QTIPS to focus continuous improvements at the level of the work. *American Journal of Clinical Pathology, 144*(1), 122–136.

Resources

Agency for Healthcare Research and Quality. https://innovations.ahrq.gov

Ambulatory Quality Alliance. http://www.aqaalliance.org/about.htm

Institute for Healthcare Improvement. http://www.ihi.org/resources/Pages/default.aspx

National Committee for Quality Assurance. http://www.ncqa.org/tabid/59/Default.aspx

National Quality Forum. http://www.qualityforum.org/About_NQF/About_NQF.aspx

SQUIRE 2.0: Standards for Quality Improvement Reporting Excellence http://www.squire-statement.org/index.cfm?fuseaction=page.viewpage&pageid=471

SQUIRE 2.0 Explanation and Elaboration of Guidelines. http://www.squire-statement.org/index.cfm?fuseaction=page.viewpage&pageid=504

7

Evidence-based Practice

Mary Fran Tracy, PhD, RN, APRN, CNS, FAAN and Jane Barnsteiner, PhD, RN, FAAN

A group of six prelicensure nursing students have their clinical rotation in a busy medical intensive care unit (ICU). In a postclinical conference, one of the students mentions how noisy the ICU is— something she did not anticipate—and states that much of the noise is related to what seems like the constant number of alarms chiming. The other students agree and one states that she is surprised how, at times, the nurses seem to "ignore" the alarms. The clinical instructor discussed with them the current literature related to alarm fatigue and the impact that "nuisance" alarms can have on a nurse's ability to differentiate between alarms that are false and those that need to be quickly addressed. The students agreed that this was an interesting area for further exploration and as a group committed to look at the latest evidence surrounding the appropriate use of alarms and the concept of alarm fatigue by asking the question "What interventions can be used by staff nurses to reduce the number of ventilator and electrocardiogram alarms in medical intensive care unit patients?"

As the students explored the evidence, it became clear that addressing the number of alarms in this ICU setting would require partnership with nurses in the clinical setting including the staff nurses, the Clinical Nurse Specialist (CNS), and the critical care educator. In addition, the academic clinical instructor believed that additional work in alarm management could be appropriate for an in-depth graduate nursing student project. The prelicensure students approached the unit's clinical leadership about a partnership to evaluate the current alarm situation and implement a project for the semester on decreasing the number of inappropriate ventilator alarms. In addition, a doctor of nursing practice (DNP) student agreed to partner on a more in-depth year-long project to decrease the number of electrocardiogram alarms in the ICU. It was agreed that both the prelicensure students and the DNP student would work with the ICU's Nursing Practice Council and the CNS to identify and implement the latest evidence on alarm fatigue and alarm management into the daily practice of the ICU nurses.

Health care in the United States is at the brink of unprecedented transformation. The public is concerned with obtaining quality preventive and acute care in the most effective and cost efficient manner at the same time that patients and patient care are becoming increasingly complex. Successful evolution of this health care transformation depends on a variety of factors, one of them being the provision of education that prepares health care providers to optimally function in this new era.

The groundbreaking Institute of Medicine (IOM) (2001) report *Crossing the Quality Chasm* outlined 10 rules to redesign and improve health care. Rule 5 for improving health care in the United States is using evidence-based decision-making. However, it is estimated that there is a significant lag of 17 years between the time patient care evidence is generated and the time it is fully embedded into clinical practice (Balas and

Quality and Safety in Nursing: A Competency Approach to Improving Outcomes, Second Edition.
Edited by Gwen Sherwood and Jane Barnsteiner.
© 2017 John Wiley & Sons, Inc. Published 2017 by John Wiley & Sons, Inc.

Boren, 2000). Why does this gap exist? Is it because health care providers are unaware the evidence exists? Are providers unable to critically evaluate the evidence? Is it easier to continue to practice as you were originally taught, and tradition is difficult to alter? It would seem that the purpose of the education in the academic and practice setting is to instill the value of using current best evidence to guide practice.

The 2003 report by the IOM, *Healthcare Professions Education: A Bridge to Quality*, calls for competencies for all health care professionals in the areas of safe and quality care. Competencies outlined by the IOM call on academic institutions to advance the education of health care professionals in order to have highly functioning interdisciplinary teams focused on patient-centered care. It is essential that this safe care be guided by evidence, continuous quality improvement outcomes, and optimal use of informatics (IOM, 2003).

The Affordable Care Act of 2010 emphasizes evidence-based policies and interventions when making recommendations about health care prevention strategies. In addition, the Centers for Medicare and Medicaid Services (CMS) are increasingly focused on hospitals, nursing homes, home health care agencies, and dialysis facilities to meet standards for providing evidence-based care (CMS, 2014; Department of Health and Human Services, 2015) and are adjusting reimbursement accordingly. For 2015 there are 14 hospital-acquired conditions (HACs) for which hospitals will not receive additional payment for cases in which one of the selected conditions was not present on admission. These include Stage III and IV pressure ulcers, central line associated blood stream infection (CLABSI), and catheter-associated urinary tract infection (CAUTI). They are improving consumer access to performance data from agencies and guiding consumers on how to make informed decisions based on that data (CMS, 2014; Department of Health and Human Services, 2015). In this way, evidence-based practice (EBP) becomes an important link to continuous quality improvement. The Agency for Healthcare Research and Quality (AHRQ) has provided evidence-based practice guidelines to assist clinicians in the prevention of HACs (http://www.guideline.gov/resources/hospital-acquired-conditions.aspx).

Since the time of Nightingale, nursing as a profession has been committed to providing safe and quality care for our patients. However, it is clear there is a gap in relation to the IOM recommendations related to performance competencies and competency preparation in nursing education. The Robert Wood Johnson Foundation funded the Quality and Safey Education for Nurses (QSEN) project to initiate dialogue and develop recommendations for closing that gap. The QSEN faculty and advisory board leaders explored the literature and adapted the IOM competencies to fully explicate competency expectations for all registered nurses. These competencies include patient-centered care, teamwork and collaboration, evidence-based practice, quality improvement, safety, and informatics. In addition to defining the competencies, the QSEN group also delineated the knowledge, skills and attitudes (KSA) components that are essential for each of the competencies. This work is a foundation for promoting advances in nursing education to address the gap in competency achievement (Cronenwett *et al.*, 2007; Cronenwett *et al.*, 2009; Cronenwett, Sherwood, and Gelmon, 2009).

This chapter will explore the competency related to EBP—what it is, a description of the KSAs that make up the competency for EBP, the state of the science, and innovative approaches for teaching strategies to achieve the EBP competency. The chapter includes application to student learners in academic settings, both prelicensure and graduate, as well as clinicians in clinical settings.

Definition and Description of Evidence-Based Practice

EBP is defined as practice based on the best available evidence that also incorporates patient values and preferences and clinician judgment and expertise (Sackett *et al.*, 2000; Cronenwett *et al.*, 2007; Cronenwett *et al.*, 2009). As many as 33 different terms have been used to describe EBP and translational research (Tetroe *et al.*, 2008). Over time, the concept of using evidence to guide nursing practice has evolved from simple research utilization to more broad-based and inclusive EBP. Some experts have chosen to modify the EBP definition to one focusing specifically on nursing. Scott and McSherry (2009) defined evidence-based nursing (EBN) as "an ongoing process by which evidence, nursing theory, and the practitioner's clinical expertise are critically evaluated and considered, in conjunction with patient involvement, to provide the delivery of optimum nursing care for the individual." Their definition adds to that of EBP by adding the need to critically evaluate the practitioner's judgment and research and incorporate the use of a theoretical framework relevant to nursing practice.

It has been estimated that approximately 15% of health care is actually research based (McKenna, Cutcliffe, and McKenna, 2000). The remainder of care interventions fall into three other categories: 1) interventions supported by other types of evidence such as expert opinion or quality improvement, 2) interventions based on tradition in which it is not clearly known whether they do more harm or good, and 3) interventions that we know cause more harm than good but practitioners either refuse or are slow to change practice. The goal of EBP should be to advance practice so interventions are based on the best available evidence and eliminate any interventions that we know cause more harm than good (McKenna *et al.*, 2000; Newhouse and Spring, 2010).

Although the purpose of research utilization is to disseminate and translate research findings as the basis for sound clinical practice, EBP recognizes the value of the gamut of evidence that can be incorporated into decision-making about best care for the individual patient. The randomized, controlled trial has traditionally been considered the gold standard for guiding health care practice, but from an EBP paradigm we should recognize the value that controlled nonrandom, quasi-experimental, and descriptive studies can contribute to decision making along with quality improvement data, program evaluation data, and expert consensus opinions (Ferguson and Day, 2005). Significant skill on the part of the health care provider is required to be able to analyze and synthesize the evidence based on the credibility of the source, while simultaneously exploring and acknowledging the patient's values in relation to that evidence and the clinician's judgment as to the fit of the body of evidence with the particular individual's situation.

The KSAs developed for the six competences as related to prelicensure education were initially drafted by the QSEN group through workshops and e-mail communication (Cronenwett *et al.*, 2007; Cronenwett *et al.*, 2009) to reach consensus. The KSAs for EBP range from basic to increasingly complex and are intended to guide the EBP curriculum (see Appendices A and B). Critical thinking skills are essential in having an evidence-based practice and developing alternative interventions as needed to achieve the best outcome for the individual patient (Ferguson and Day, 2005). It is these analytical and critical thinking skills that nurse educators are being challenged to develop in nursing students at all educational levels.

Evidence-Based Practice–Models and Process

Numerous models have been developed to guide nurses through the EBP process (Mitchell *et al.*, 2010). The most commonly known models are the Colorado, Iowa, STAR, Hopkins, and University of Arizona (Goode *et al.*, 2011; Melnyk and Fineout-Overholt, 2004; Newhouse *et al.*, 2005a; Rosswurm and Larrabee, 1999; Stetler, 2003; Stevens, 2004; Titler *et al.*, 2001). While models may take slightly different approaches, all essentially guide nurses through the EBP process utilizing the Planned Action theoretical approach (Straus, Tetroe, and Graham, 2009).

There are five basic steps to the EBP process. Each needs to be thoroughly addressed in order to have sound decision making for patient care (Fineout-Overholt, Melnyk, and Schultz, 2005; Johnston and Fineout-Overholt, 2005). The case study provided at the beginning of the chapter highlights an example of using the steps of the EBP process in the inpatient clinical setting. This example provides ideas of how multiple nursing roles, both clinical and academic, can partner to use evidence in improving patient care. See Table 7.1 for information on the roles of each of the participants in these EBP projects.

Table 7.1 Roles of students, faculty, and clinical staff in a student-led clinical alarm management evidence-based practice project.

Step of EBP Process	Who is Involved? (Roles of students, nurse residents, and clinical staff can be interchanged dependent on who is leading project and skill level.)	Actions

Develop a searchable question	• Prelicensure students/nurse residents
	  – Gather and compile baseline data
	  – Utilize clinical setting resources for validation and agreement to partner on the project
	  – Determine focus/scope of the EBP project
	
	• Masters/DNP student
	  – Gather and compile baseline evidence
	  – Utilize clinical setting resources for validation and agreement to partner on project
	  – Determine focus/scope of the project
	
	• Clinical staff
	  – Commitment to partnership
	  – Answer questions of students
	  – Identify barriers/facilitators of alarm management
	  – Provide context/perspective
	
	• Clinical faculty
	  – Teaching
	  – Mentorship
	
	• Clinical nurse specialist
	  – Provision of clinical setting data and confirmation of practice issue
	  – Commitment to Partnership
	  – Mentorship
		• Prelicensure students/nurse residents
		  – Count number and types of ventilator alarms they hear during two clinical days in the medical intensive care unit (MICU)
		  – Question preceptors about their perceptions of the validity of the alarms they hear throughout their shift
		  – Meet with MICU CNS to determine extent and prioritization of the problem
		  – Write a PICOT question focusing on ventilator alarm management
		
		• Masters/DNP student
		  – Develop a tool and method for observational direct data collection of all ECG alarms over defined period of time
		  – Develop a tool for staff satisfaction related to frequency of alarms and perception of alarm accuracy
		  – Request a report/query of the ECG system to list number and type of alarms over a set period of time
		  – Meet with MICU CNS to determine extent and prioritization of the problem
		  – Write a PICOT question focusing on ECG alarm management
		
		• Clinical staff
		  – Partner in finding evidence
		  – Confirm evidence found
		
		• Clinical faculty
		  – Mentor students on the scope of their project for the semester/year
		  – Facilitate learning as needed on compilation of and analysis of data collected
		  – Facilitate development of a PICOT question
		  – Help students prepare for their presentation/interaction with CNS for project partnership
		
		• Clinical nurse specialist
		  – Review data with students
		  – Provide advice regarding regulatory and policy requirements related to alarm use in the clinical setting
		  – Provide overview of clinical setting in relation to staff openness to change

Search for evidence	• Prelicensure students/nurse residents – Work with medical librarian to refine PICOT question and identify appropriate search terms and databases – Contact ventilator vendor to obtain manufacturer information on device function – Search for regulatory requirements related to alarms and institutional policies • Masters/DNP student – Search for evidence on electrocardiogram (ECG) alarm management – Contact ECG vendor to obtain manufacturer information on device function – Search for regulatory requirements related to alarms and institutional policies • Clinical nursing staff – Provide experiential evidence – Search for evidence • Clinical faculty – Connect students with medical librarian – Review findings to mentor in appropriateness and completeness • Clinical nurse specialist – Review findings for appropriateness to setting and completeness	• Prelicensure students/nurse residents – Perform search for evidence • Masters/DNP student – Perform search for evidence • Clinical nursing staff – Assist with search using literature, etc., depending on extent of partnership • Clinical faculty – Teaching – Mentorship • Clinical nurse specialist – Mentorship – Partnership
Critical analysis and synthesis	• Prelicensure students/nurse residents – Divide evidence among students for analysis using grading model(s) and evaluation tools – Compile findings • Masters/DNP student – Utilize grading model(s) and evaluation tools to evaluate evidence – Compile findings • Clinical nursing staff – Utilize grading model(s) to evaluate evidence – Provide experiential perspective • Clinical faculty – Evaluate strength and completeness of analysis • Clinical nurse specialist – Evaluate strength and completeness of analysis	• Prelicensure students/nurse residents – Perform analysis of evidence • Masters/DNP student – Perform analysis of evidence • Clinical nursing staff – Partner in analysis of evidence • Clinical faculty – Teaching – Mentorship • Clinical nurse specialist – Mentorship – Partnership

(Continued)

Table 7.1 (Continued)

Step of EBP Process	Who is Involved? (Roles of students, nurse residents, and clinical staff can be interchanged dependent on who is leading project and skill level.)	Actions

Recommendations for practice	• Prelicensure students/nurse residents
	  – Make recommendations for practice in partnership with clinical staff
	
	• Masters/DNP student
	  – Make recommendations for practice in partnership with clinical staff
	
	• Clinical nursing staff
	  – Make recommendations in partnership with nursing students
	
	• Clinical faculty
	  – Teaching
	  – Mentorship
	
	• Clinical nurse specialist
	  – Mentorship
	  – Partnership
		• Prelicensure students/nurse residents
		  – Based on strength of evidence, make recommendations for practice to reduce false ventilator alarms
		  – Present findings to CNS and ICU Nursing Practice Council to garner stakeholder buy-in for practice changes
		
		• Masters/DNP student
		  – Based on strength of evidence, make recommendations for practice to reduce false ECG alarms (e.g., changing ECG patches every day, setting appropriate alarm parameters at beginning of each shift, working with biomed to optimize default settings in the ECG monitors, etc.)
		  – Develop a cost analysis of proposed practice changes
		  – Present findings to CNS and ICU Nursing Practice Council to garner stakeholder buy-in for practice changes
		
		• Clinical nursing staff
		  – Confirm appropriateness of recommendations in context of setting and populations
		  – Verify recommendations with staff nurse colleagues
		  – Partner with nurse manager, CNS, and clinical educator for implications of education and implementation
		
		• Clinical faculty
		  – Review recommendations for practice to ensure alignment with analysis of evidence
		  – Facilitate presentation of findings and recommendations to CNS and ICU Nursing Practice Council
		
		• Clinical nurse specialist
		  – Review recommendations for practice to ensure alignment with analysis of evidence
		  – Partner with students and staff to ensure recommendations are feasible for implementation in practice setting
		  – Partner with students and staff to develop an implementation plan including education and appropriate resources needed

Evaluate the outcomes	• Nurse manager	• Nurse manager
	– Partnership	– Review analysis of practice recommendations in terms of potential operational costs related to time for staff education, potential budget increases in supply costs
	• Critical care educator	• Critical care educator
	– Partnership	– Partner with students/nurse residents/clinical staff to develop and implement educational plan for staff
	• Prelicensure students/nurse residents	• Prelicensure students/nurse residents
	– Gather and compile post practice change data	– Count number and types of ventilator alarms they hear during two clinical days in the MICU post implementation
	– Analyze outcomes	– Question preceptors about their perceptions about the validity of the alarms they hear throughout their shift post implementation
		– Analyze findings
		– Write up findings and present to staff
	• Masters/DNP student	• Masters/DNP student
	– Gather and compile post practice change data	– Collect post implementation observational direct data collection of all ECG alarms over defined period of time
	– Analyze outcomes	– Collect post implementation staff satisfaction data related to frequency of alarms and perception of alarm accuracy
		– Request a report/query of the ECG system to list number and type of alarms over a set period of time
		– Analyze outcomes including patient, staff, and financial outcomes
	• Clinical nursing staff	• Clinical nursing staff
	– Assist with collection and analysis of outcomes data	– Collect post implementation data
		– Identify experiential outcomes post implementation
	• Clinical faculty	• Clinical faculty
	– Teaching	– Evaluate and oversee analysis
	– Mentorship	– Facilitate presentation of findings to staff and nursing leadership
	• Clinical nurse specialist	• Clinical nurse specialist
	– Mentorship	– Assist with analysis of outcomes as needed
	– Partnership	– Assist with dissemination of findings to other appropriate clinical areas, e.g., surgical ICU, cardiovascular ICU

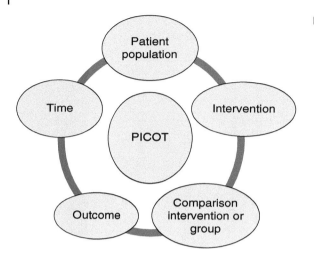

Figure 7.1 Five components of a PICOT question.

Develop a Searchable Question

Inquiry is the driving force to questioning why nurses practice as they do. Developing a question that accurately reflects the practice to be evaluated will start the EBP process down a sound path. Students can use the PICOT format to structure the question: **P**atient population; **I**ntervention; **C**omparison intervention or group; **O**utcome; **T**ime (Fineout-Overholt *et al.*, 2005). The more refined and explicit the question, the easier the search is to find relevant evidence. An example of a PICOT question would be: Do patients in a skilled nursing facility (P) who are restrained (I) experience higher rates of confusion or delirium (O) than those patients who are not restrained (C)? See Figure 7.1 for the five components of a PICOT question.

Search for the Best Evidence Available

The PICOT question components will provide guidance for the databases and keywords to search. Performing a database search can require multiple strategies. Since the PICOT question may have already been asked and answered by others, starting with sites that provide systematic reviews (e.g., Cochrane Collaboration, The Joanna Briggs Institute) or evidence-based care guidelines (AHRQ, National Guideline Clearinghouse) is prudent. Reviews may also be indexed in databases such as Medline and Cumulative Index to Nursing and Allied Health Literature (CINAHL). If no systematic reviews or guidelines are found, then individual articles must be searched and retrieved. The assistance of a medical librarian who is skilled at searching the health care literature can be invaluable.

Critical Analysis and Synthesis of the Evidence

A critical appraisal and synthesis of the evidence is the next step. What are the results of the evidence you've found? How closely does the population and evidence match the question you are asking?

Several models for grading of evidence exist, ranging from four to eight levels of evidence strength. Many of these models originated from medicine and therefore posit that the randomized controlled trial is the gold standard from which all subsequent levels are based. Models differ in what and how evidence is graded. For example, the American Heart Association uses both Level A, B, C and Class I, IIa, IIb, III to describe certainty and size of the treatment effect (Gibbons, Smith, and Antman, 2003). There are nursing grading models as well (Rosswurm and Larrabee, 1999; Stetler, 2001).

It is important for nursing students to learn that just because a study is not a randomized controlled trial does not mean it has no value in influencing nursing practice. The clinical question to be answered dictates the research design (Barnsteiner, 2010; Barnsteiner *et al.*, 2010). Tools for systematically evaluating various types of evidence (including randomized controlled trials, qualitative research studies, case control studies, systematic reviews, etc.) are readily available (EBM Librarian, 2013; Moher *et al.*, 2009; Newhouse *et al.*, 2005b; University of South Australia, 2014).

The new paradigm of evidence analysis and synthesis allows for the possibility that the strength of evidence does not need to be an "all or nothing" proposition. In other words, either all of the evidence from one source is strong and can be incorporated into the synthesis, or none of it can be utilized. It is rare that any evidence has no limitations. We need to critically evaluate all evidence to determine if even minor components of the evidence can contribute to decision making for patient care (Fineout-Overholt *et al.*, 2005).

Develop Recommendations for Practice

The health care provider will take the synthesis of evidence to determine if there is sufficient validity and strength to incorporate it into practice. The evidence may be applicable to an entire patient population or the provider may incorporate specific clinical judgment and patient preferences to make care decisions for an individual patient. Providers must have the insight to determine whether they alone have adequate expertise to make the patient care decision with the available evidence or whether they need to consult with other experts.

Evaluate the Outcome of Evidence-based Practice Changes

The final step in the EBP process is to evaluate the practice change. Evaluation of the change includes impact to patient outcomes, provider practice, and the cost effectiveness of the practice. To effectively evaluate the outcome, one must know the expected outcomes, the baseline performance prior to the change, and how and when to collect the evaluation data (Barnsteiner, 2010). Understanding the outcomes of the changes we make offers opportunities for continual improvement as well as for nurses to own accountability for our EBP.

An additional component to the evaluation step is to recognize that, with today's pressure in health care to rapidly and continually implement evidence, there may be times when evidence is implemented prior to it being truly generalizeable. In these instances, the evaluation step is key to determining when evidence must be "de-implemented" (Prasad and Ioannidis, 2014). Elimination of practices that can be harmful or non-productive can also decrease health care costs and optimize outcomes (Prasad and Ioannidis, 2014).

These five steps are an overview of the EBP process. Each of these steps is frequently divided into further additional components in order to successfully accomplish the complicated process of implementing and maintaining practice changes.

The extent of knowledge development and level of expert skill attainment expected related to the EBP competency will vary based on the educational level of the student. For instance, the associate degree and baccalaureate-prepared nurse can be expected to identify searchable questions, develop beginning analysis and synthesis skills, formulate initial recommendations for practice based on the synthesis, and participate as members of implementation and evaluation teams. Master's and DNP-prepared nurses should have more extensive skill at developing practice recommendations, taking into account patient populations, organizational priorities, and stewardship of resources; developing detailed implementation plans for practice changes based on change theory; and developing processes to fully evaluate the impact on patient and organizational outcomes of the EBP changes (see Appendix B).

The Evidence for Evidence-based Practice

Evidence-based Practice Skills in Students and New Graduates

As the QSEN group delineated the KSAs for the six competencies for prelicensure education, they sought feedback from faculty and leaders in nursing specialty organizations. Nurse educators initially believed they were teaching to all six of the identified competencies. However, in reviewing the details of the expectations, many agreed that students were not being adequately prepared at the identified competency level (Cronenwett *et al.*, 2007). This was corroborated by perspectives of new graduates who stated they were not receiving significant learning experiences in the competency areas and to some extent that they were not taught by nurse educators with expertise in these areas (Cronenwett *et al.*, 2007). In fact, a survey of all member schools of the AACN as well as a convenience sample of community college associate degree programs in North Carolina showed that more than 50% of schools reported that nurse educators had only "some" comfort in teaching EBP. Eleven percent of schools considered them "novice" in that area. Schools that had BSN and graduate programs were more likely to rate nurse educators as "expert" in EBP, though that rating was still only 47% of nurse educators (Smith, Cronenwett, and Sherwood, 2007).

Sullivan, Hirst, and Cronenwett (2009) reported that although there has been increasing awareness of EBP terms and the concept of EBP over time, new graduates reported they felt the least prepared/skilled in EBP and quality improvement. In addition, they believed that having an attitude of valuing the competencies was least important in these same two areas when compared with the other four competencies. This brings unique challenges to nurse educators to instill KSAs in these areas that nursing students and new graduates may feel are "optional" competencies rather than "essential" competencies (Moch and Cronje, 2010; Moch, Cronje, and Branson, 2010).

The findings surrounding faculty comfort and expertise in teaching EBP have recently been replicated in a study of faculty in New York State Associate and Baccalaureate nursing degree programs (Pollard *et al.*, 2014). Through an online survey and two smaller focus groups, the researchers reported that faculty did not feel as comfortable teaching EBP nor had as much confidence about student competence in this area as they did for the patient-centered care, teamwork and collaboration, and safety competencies. In fact, nearly half of participants in the focus group arm of the research stated they relied heavily on use of textbooks for teaching EBP.

Teaching Evidence-based Practice

EBP is identified by the AACN as an essential component of all levels of nursing education for their member schools—baccalaureate, master's, and DNP preparation. Entry-level nurses should be prepared to differentiate between research and EBP, understand models of EBP, demonstrate retrieval of all types of evidence and evaluate credibility of the source, critique and synthesize the evidence and be able to propose evidence-based solutions, and collaborate in the implementation and dissemination of that evidence into practice (AACN, 2008). The master's prepared nurse should be prepared to perform rigorous evaluation of multiple sources of evidence in relation to clinical judgment and perspectives of all health care providers; participate and/or lead teams in practice change implementation; articulate to broad audiences the rationale for EBP changes; and evaluate the impact on quality of EBP changes in a systematic fashion (AACN, 2011). The DNP graduate would ideally function at the highest level of EBP—designing and implementing quality improvement activities to improve care; lead substantive EBP changes to practice; collect, analyze, and synthesize evidence; and propose changes for patient populations (AACN, 2006).

McCurry and Martins (2010) examined the effect of teaching research terminology, research critique, and EBP process using innovative approaches aimed at the "millennial" learner. The innovative strategies were interactive, group focused, or experiential as compared with more traditional teaching methods such as textbook readings, quizzes, library orientation, and didactic content. At the end of the course, students rated the innovative approaches as more effective, and instructors found increased classroom participation, more collaborative learning, and greater mastery of the content compared to traditional approaches.

The effectiveness of small group work has been demonstrated in teaching EBP at the undergraduate level, particularly as it relates to significantly improving the EBP knowledge and skill level of the student (Balakas and Sparks, 2010; Kim *et al.*, 2009; Kruszewski, Brough, and Killeen, 2009; Oh *et al.*, 2010). Results regarding the improvement of attitudes toward EBP and the likelihood of future use of EBP, however, were inconsistent in some of those studies (Oh *et al.*, 2010; Kim *et al.*, 2009).

Adequate preparation of nursing students to use and understand EBP in the clinical setting relies on the staff nurses who precept them to be well versed and proficient in EBP as well. A study by Hagler and colleagues found that focused preceptor education about EBP resulted in stronger belief in EBP by the preceptors. This education was effective regardless of the role of the nurse, educational preparation, or level of experience, though more research is needed to determine whether this improved understanding of and belief in EBP results in better outcomes for student competency (Hagler *et al.*, 2012).

Barriers to Evidence-based Practice in Clinical Practice

It has been said that for practicing RNs EBP is an "abstraction whose benefits are neither immediately visible nor necessarily compatible with existing practice values, needs, and experiences" (Cronje and Moch, 2010). Practicing RNs lack basic EBP knowledge and skills, which will continue to impede the integration of new evidence into practice (Duffy, Culp, Yarberry, *et al.*, 2015; Pravikoff, Tanner, and Pierce, 2005; Sciarra, 2011; Yoder, Kirkley, McFall, *et al.*, 2014).

Practicing nurses are more likely to seek advice from a colleague rather than utilize research or journals (Pravikoff *et al.*, 2005). A significant majority (<gt> 80%) have never used a hospital library or sought assistance from a librarian. This is not surprising because 77% report they have never learned to use electronic databases. Disappointingly, only 46% of practicing nurses state that they are even familiar with the term *evidence-based practice* (Pravikoff *et al.*, 2005).

Barriers to the use of EBP in the clinical setting have changed little over recent years. Barriers cited by practicing nurses include lack of value for research in the clinical setting, lack of understanding of electronic databases, and difficulty gaining access to research (Melnyk *et al.*, 2012; Pravikoff *et al.*, 2005; Solomons and Spross, 2011; Yoder *et al.*, 2014). Additionally, practicing nurses do not feel they have the skills to search for, analyze, or synthesize the evidence (Melnyck *et al.*, 2012; Solomons and Spross, 2011; Yoder *et al.*, 2014). They also cite a lack of organizational resources or support for use of research. It may be as basic as having a computer available on the unit with access to a digital library. Nurses have also consistently identified a lack of time and a lack of autonomy to actually change practice as barriers (Solomons and Spross, 2011; Yoder, *et al.*, 2014). These barriers exist at both the individual nurse level and at the organizational level. Similar to faculty comfort with teaching EBP, if nurse leaders in the clinical setting are not educated in or using EBP, it is unlikely they will be able to support the staff in the EBP process or resources.

Nurses working in settings other than acute care facilities such as ambulatory and primary care clinics, physician offices, and other delivery areas may have added challenges to assure their practice is based on current evidence. These challenges may include even less evidence available on which to base practice improvement decisions, fewer nurses prepared at an advanced level of EBP, lack of EBP mentors familiar with these settings, and fewer colleagues to form EBP teams. However, the process of EBP is essentially the same regardless of setting. The use of today's technology may be particularly helpful for nurses practicing in these settings because it can facilitate long-distance mentoring and multisite teams from similar settings in evaluating evidence and finding support/advice in implementing EBP.

Examination of these barriers creates an even stronger imperative to set a strong foundation in nursing curricula because new graduates will encounter challenges and barriers as they transition into practice in the "real world." Based on the current evidence about EBP, nursing education in all settings should focus on preparing nurses who see the value and moral imperative to be life-long consumers of evidence in the quest to provide best care for our patients. The educational environment can be the leader for instilling in learners the value and required skills needed for EBP (Ferguson and Day, 2005).

Teaching Strategies for Students

The QSEN project serves to advance competency achievement in nursing to support this new era of health care quality and engages nurse educators to examine the competencies in a new light. Education of learners about EBP is more than teaching the steps of the process and where to find the evidence; it also helps learners explore more deeply. For example, it helps students to develop understanding of formal and informal grading of evidence, differentiate between evidence and consensus opinion, to look at the use of evidence and related patient preferences from an ethics perspective, and to develop care plans utilizing not just research evidence but also patient values and clinical judgment. But when is the best time to introduce EBP into the nursing curriculum?

Traditionally, nursing curriculum has been built on a progression of simple to complex concepts— from discrete skills to the increasing complexity of families, organizations, and systems (Barton *et al.*, 2009). It is not unusual for EBP to be introduced later in the nursing program, often as late as the last semester of the senior year in the form of an EBP project.

Barton and colleagues (2009) conducted a web-based modified Delphi study to recommend when the KSAs for the six quality and safety competencies should be introduced and emphasized in a prelicensure program (see Appendix C). The study goal was to reach two-thirds consensus with three survey rounds. Consensus among nurse educator experts was that many of the KSAs for EBP should be introduced primarily in the beginning and intermediate phases of nursing programs, which would allow students time to gain experience in evidence-based applications. Examples of recommended timing for EBP KSAs include the following:

Beginning phase introduction:

- Knowledge of scientific methods/processes
- Description of EBP and sources of evidence
- Skill in developing patient care plans with evidence, patient values, and clinical judgment
- Promotion of the value of EBP to clinical practice

Intermediate phase introduction:

- Knowledge in determining the strength of evidence
- Developing skill in data collection and analysis in reading research and evidence reports
- Skill in finding evidence

- Questioning traditional care practices
- Appreciating the strengths and weaknesses of types of evidence

Advanced phase introduction:

- Differentiate when it's appropriate to use patient requests or clinical judgment to deviate from EBP guidelines
- Skill in preparing the environment to integrate new evidence into practice

It is important to set the stage early for development of KSAs for EBP. Start introduction of the concepts early and expand each year on the competency in order to facilitate building of the foundation (Barton *et al.*, 2009; Rolloff, 2010). Education requires a multipronged approach threaded throughout the curriculum, reinforcing and linking EBP concepts with patient encounters. As students develop critical thinking skills, their critical thinking related to EBP will also develop in relation to the judgment needed to critically evaluate the evidence with a new appreciation of the impact of patient values and the judgment needed to seek advice when considering deviating from guidelines. Providing opportunities for students to learn about organizational structures and institutional culture regarding attitudes toward and support for change will assist new graduates as they transition to practice and apply what they have learned about EBP.

Finally, it is important to also teach students that they need to be prepared to relearn information about their nursing practice throughout their careers and to be committed to life-long learning. It has been noted that clinical behavior is originally based on beliefs, attitudes, and intention, but over time that behavior becomes based on repetition triggered by situation and context (Nilsen *et al.*, 2012). In the fast-paced health care environment, this development of habits is helpful to being efficient and is natural in becoming expert, not having to think through every step of practices and skills in each situation. However these habits may result in nurses over time seeing what they expect to see and behaving accordingly, leaving them less open to and aware of new information (Nilsen *et al.*, 2012).

The QSEN Learning Collaborative was a seven-year project (2005–2012) funded by the RWJF to develop the next steps in revising curricula for quality and safety education, trialing innovative teaching strategies, and promoting future educator development (Cronenwett *et al.*, 2009). Innovative teaching strategies continue to be posted on the QSEN web site (www.QSEN.org), or faculty and clinical educators share and explore new educational approaches related to evidence-based practice. Below are examples of teaching strategies that can be applied and adapted for the classroom, simulation, and clinical settings.

Didactic Strategies

Exposure to Evidence-based Practice Models

Using EBP models can guide students through the EBP process. Students can form small groups, each choosing different EBP models to explore. Examples of common EBP models include the Iowa, STAR, Hopkins, and University of Arizona models (Melnyk and Fineout-Overholt, 2004; Newhouse *et al.*, 2005a; Rosswurm and Larrabee, 1999; Stetler, 2003; Stevens, 2004; Titler *et al.*, 2001). Assign clinical practice questions to the groups and have them work through the EBP process using their models. Group presentations can be used to discuss the models and results. After all groups have presented, have the entire group compare and contrast differences between the models and evaluate the ease of use of each of the models.

Grading of Evidence

Small groups of students can choose both a nursing and a non-nursing grading model. Have the groups compare and contrast differences between the rating models. Using a nursing research study, have the groups explore the feasibility of grading the study using both a nursing and non-nursing grading model (Levin and Chang, 2014). Small group presentations can be used to describe the different grading models and what study designs would best be used with each grading model.

Evaluation of Web Site Resources

Small groups of students can be assigned to explore and critically evaluate EBP web sites (Nadelson, 2014). Have students evaluate web sites for information such as ease of navigation, what disciplines could use the information posted, and for what patient populations the information could be used. Have the small groups present their findings to their peers to broaden student exposure to the numerous web sites available for EBP.

Journal Clubs

Assign research articles relevant to current clinical rotations and provide students with a research critique tool. In small groups, have one or two students lead the group through the critique process.

Evidence-based Project

An EBP project can be used at both the graduate and undergraduate levels. Have students select an EBP question they have identified from the clinical setting and work through the steps of the EBP process. This can be done in small groups with undergraduates and as an individual project with graduate students (Sullivan, 2010a). Course instructors could collaborate by forming groups with members from both undergraduate and graduate students, adding a library student to the group, or having interdisciplinary groups of students. Criteria for evaluating the project could be more stringent for graduate student projects. Objectives would vary based on the formation of the small groups. For instance, having a graduate student facilitate an undergraduate EBP project could prepare them for the practice setting where they will be leading staff in working through a clinical question and implementation of a practice change. Interdisciplinary teams could take similar questions from their discipline perspective and compare the evidence between disciplines, noting how the entire evidence base could be used in an interdisciplinary approach in care of a patient. Involving a library student could allow for development of finding evidence sources on the part of nursing students while giving the library student an opportunity to look at the utility of the literature from a health care perspective.

Simulation or Skills Lab Strategies

Utilize Evidence-based Practice Simulation Scenarios

Patient scenarios utilized in a simulation lab should be based on evidence with purposeful EBP concepts woven in. Student preparation for the simulation scenario can include reading relevant guidelines, determining the source of the evidence, encouraging students to write down questions of how scenarios and the corresponding evidence may differ from practice in the clinical setting, and review of evidence-based tools for the skill development (e.g., Confusion Assessment Method [CAM] or

Confusion Assessment Method for the Intensive Care Unit [CAM-ICU] for delirious patients, hand-washing guidelines, continuous passive motion (CPM) for knee replacement surgery, ventilator-associated pneumonia (VAP) prevention guidelines for suctioning in mechanically ventilated patients, diabetes mellitus guidelines, asthma guidelines in pediatrics) (Jarzemsky, 2010).

Student-led Simulation Scenarios

Using the previous example, students could be assigned to lead the discussion about the EBP components of the simulation scenario.

Clinical Strategies

Use of Journals for Reflection

Encourage students to use journals to reflect on discrepancies between evidence and practices they note in the clinical setting. Nursing students can query preceptors and practicing nurses about the discrepancies they note (Sullivan, 2010b). Graduate students can utilize journals to document EBP decision-making used when caring for patients and how they applied the evidence to practice and how they accommodated patient values, beliefs, and preferences according to patient-centered care (Winters and Echeverri, 2012).

Sacred Cows Contest

Leake (2004) had nursing students ask three questions of practicing nurses when they were in the clinical setting: 1) What is the most traditional nursing practice being done?; 2) What is the least logical nursing practice?; and 3) What is the most time-consuming practice on the unit? Nurses then formed small groups and searched the evidence surrounding the practices they identified. Frequently the evidence found did not support the practice being observed. The assignment could be turned into an EBP project where results are presented to the hospital nursing staff and a practice change implemented if feasible.

Use of Technology

Ideally clinical settings would provide easy access to technology for obtaining evidence at the point of care, both internal resources such as policies/procedures, and electronic nursing skills and care planning resources. This would include computers and Internet access to well respected web sites at or close to the bedside. Many students also have access to handheld mobile devices and tablets. Clinical instructors can teach students how to evaluate and use mobile applications to gather evidence to their practice questions in real time (Williamson *et al.*, 2011).

Postclinical Discussion and Debrief

EBP discussions can occur through the routine postclinical discussion and debrief sessions. "Students need opportunities to discuss the credibility of the research-generated evidence from both quantitative and qualitative paradigms and to explore the relative weighting of particular evidence in specific patient situations" (Ferguson and Day, 2005). Students could be encouraged to comment on their journal notes if they feel comfortable or the discrepancies they note in their clinical rotations. The instructor can lead students in looking at all the evidence in patient situations and how to deal with the dilemma of preceptors performing interventions that are not evidence based. Frontline nurses could be encouraged to apply similar opportunities to their daily work, for example, use of journal clubs, opportunities for reflection on differences in practice between staff nurses at forums such as nursing practice or research committees, and facilitated discussions about differences between preceptors on what they teach.

Attendance at Nursing Practice or Research Committee Meetings

Students could be offered the opportunity to attend health care institutions' nursing practice or research committee meetings. They could evaluate the extent of EBP utilized and any models for guiding the work of the committee.

Role Playing

Learners can discuss and role play interactions they may have as both students and new graduates in initiating a dialogue with more experienced nurses or physicians about practices that are not evidence based. This develops skill in effective communication, teamwork and collaboration when differing opinions exist, consensus reaching in providing optimal care for patients, role modeling EBP, and approaching a situation in a way that minimizes a defensive reaction.

Teaching Strategies for Clinical Staff

Several of the teaching strategies for nursing students can easily be utilized for clinical staff in the practice setting. Examples include using a sacred cows contest (i.e. practices that seem to be treasured by nurses but upon inspection may not be based on evidence) to evaluate current nursing practice, teaching staff how to use technology at the point of care to find evidence, and using EBP scenarios in simulation exercises. Journal clubs can be held jointly with students, faculty, and clinical staff participation (Winters and Echeverri, 2012). There are additional strategies that can be used for staff at the bedside.

Organizational Evidence-based Practice Models

If the institution has chosen a model as a framework for the EBP process, ensure nurses have formal and informal opportunities to learn about the model and how it is or can be used both for major projects and in daily practice. This model should be prominently utilized whenever nursing policies are revised and procedures are updated or implemented. When education is provided to staff about these revised and new policies and procedures, emphasize the evidence that was evaluated and the rationale for the EBP decision, not simply what the new skill or practice entails. This can help nurses to recognize the value of the EBP decision and may assist in embedding the practice more readily, particularly if the new practice appears to staff to be contrary to what they perceive to be their anecdotal experiences.

Teach Through Council and Committee Projects

Teach about the EBP process through the work of nursing councils and committees in real time as staff identify and work through problems that are pertinent to their daily practice. Utilize resources such as CNSs and medical librarians to role model and guide in the EBP process steps. Group and one-on-one mentoring throughout the process can be invaluable in raising the knowledge level of staff and improving staff confidence in their EBP skills.

Broadening the Evidence-based Practice Perspective

It is imperative that nurse leaders in the clinical setting also understand and utilize EBP to role model for staff and to ensure quality decision making in nursing operations decisions. EBP is not just for clinical bedside practice but should also be used for operational questions such as staffing decisions, scheduling, and creating a healthy work environment and supportive culture. To accomplish this, nurse leaders may need EBP education that is specifically tailored for their practice.

Academic and Clinical Partnerships

There are many reasons to foster the partnership between academic and clinical settings, particularly facilitating the ability for students and practicing nurses to promote and cultivate EBP. The academic instructor should be cognizant that preceptors for nursing students may be skilled and experienced practicing nurses but may not be familiar with the concepts of EBP. The academic-clinical partnership can be maximized to ensure openness of the preceptor toward EBP to help both the preceptor and student and provide optimal patient care. Ideally the academic and clinical organizations have similar philosophies regarding the use and approach to EBP, allowing for use of similar language to lessen confusion and a common process for EBP projects.

Academic instructors should know the organizational structure of the clinical setting where students have rotations as it relates to advancing EBP student objectives. For instance, does the organization have advanced practice nurses who are accountable for EBP in the clinical setting? Who is accountable for implementing change and for education of the staff if an EBP project is to be fully carried out in the clinical setting? How will a student navigate the system if there are multiple nursing roles accountable for pieces of an EBP implementation in the setting? What are the current organizational priorities that will impact the ability of any particular unit to be involved in an EBP implementation? What is the feasibility of any one unit to absorb multiple EBP projects at one time versus having one student group project for the semester? Who ultimately oversees the content and process of the EBP project to be implemented in the clinical setting? Is it the academic instructor or the nursing leadership from the clinical setting?

In setting goals and plans, be realistic about the extent of the project that can be feasibly implemented in the time frame of a nursing course. Priorities in a health care organization can change quickly, meaning resources can be quickly diverted to other initiatives.

Ideally, the academic and health care organizational leadership will develop a comprehensive approach to EBP projects completed in the clinical setting. This ensures that course instructors and the organizational leadership have an overview of all projects planned for the semester, including both undergraduate and graduate work. An institution may have multiple levels of students from several academic institutions all needing to complete EBP projects in the same time frame. Student placement managers are acutely aware of the number of students being matched to preceptors by unit throughout the hospital; however, they may not be aware of the course project expectations for those preceptors, students, and nursing leadership and the resulting impact that can have on units, nursing leadership, and the institution. Just as course instructors from the same academic institution may not be aware of other course requirements for students in the clinical setting, nursing leaders at the health care institution may not be aware of projects that are occurring throughout the institution.

This academic and clinical collaboration can include a discussion about organizational priorities during the semester and the learning objectives required for the nursing students. A consistent approach among students and units throughout the organization will help students have the support needed to meet their objectives, and units will not have discrepancies in either benefit from student projects or burden from multiple student projects at the same time.

When there is a lack of EBP experts in the healthcare organization, faculty can serve as mentors to the clinical staff and to develop experts for the clinical setting to ensure the ongoing sustainment and importance of EBP. Use of faculty mentors can result in improved knowledge and skills of staff nurses, encourage the use of evidence to improve patient care and outcomes, and promote a 'spirit of inquiry' while also contributing back to the organization (Roe and Whyte-Marshall, 2012).

Conclusion

This is both a challenging and an exciting time to be a health care professional. There are great opportunities to make significant strides in providing excellent evidence-based care, both through nursing practice and as part of an interdisciplinary team that can contribute to improved quality of care. The competencies identified by the IOM and adapted by the QSEN group are the next steps in ensuring patients receive the care they deserve and expect. Nursing has a unique opportunity to be at the front of this health care transformation by preparing nurses who are ready to accept the challenge of providing exceptional evidence-based patient care.

References

American Association of Colleges of Nursing. (2006) *The essentials of doctoral education for advanced nursing practice*. Retrieved September 15, 2015, from www.aacn.nche.edu/publications/position/ DNPEssentials.pdf.

American Association of Colleges of Nursing. (2008) *The essentials of baccalaureate education for professional nursing*. Retrieved September 15, 2015, from www.aacn.nche.edu/education-resources/ BaccEssentials08.pdf.

American Association of Colleges of Nursing. (2011) *AACN's essentials of master's education in nursing*. Retrieved September 15, 2015, from www.aacn.nche.edu/Education/pdf/ Master'sEssentials11.pdf.

Balakas, K., and Sparks, L. (2010) Teaching research and evidence-based practice. *Journal of Nursing Education, 49*(12), 691–695.

Balas, E.A., and Boren, S.A. (2000) Managing clinical knowledge for healthcare improvements. In V. Schattauer (Ed.), *Yearbook of medical informatics* (pp. 65–70). New York: Stuttgart.

Barnsteiner, J. (2010) *Evidence based practice. Enhancing quality and safety in nursing education: Preparing nurse faculty to lead curricular change*. [CDROM] Vol. 1, Version 7A. Quality and Safety Education for Nurses/American Association of Colleges of Nursing.

Barnsteiner, J., Palma, W., Preston, A., Reeder, V., and Walton, M. (2010) Fueling a love of knowledge: Promoting evidence-based practice and translational research. *Nursing Administrative Quarterly, 34*, 217–235.

Barton, A.J., Armstrong, G., Preheim, G., Gelmon, S.B., and Andrus, L.C. (2009). A national Delphi to determine developmental progression of quality and safety competencies in nursing education. *Nursing Outlook, 57*, 313–22.

Centers for Medicare and Medicaid Services. (2014) Linking quality to payment. Retrieved September 15, 2015 from http://www.hhs.gov/programs/social-services/health-care-facilities/index.htm

Cronenwett, L., Sherwood, G., Barnsteiner, J., Disch, J., Johnson, J., Mitchell, P., *et al.* (2007) Quality and safety education for nurses. *Nursing Outlook, 55*, 122–131.

Cronenwett, L., Sherwood, G., and Gelmon, S.B. (2009) Improving quality and safety education: The QSEN learning collaborative. *Nursing Outlook, 57,* 304–312.

Cronenwett, L., Sherwood, G., Pohl, J., Barnsteiner, J., Moore, S., Sullivan, D., T., *et al.* (2009) Quality and safety education for advanced practice nurses. *Nursing Outlook, 57,* 338–348.

Cronje, R.J., and Moch, S.D. (2010) Part III. Re-envisioning undergraduate nursing students as opinion leaders to diffuse evidence-based practice in clinical settings. *Journal of Professional Nursing, 26*(1), 23–28.

Department of Health and Human Services. (2015) Retrieved September 15, 2015, from http://www.hhs.gov/programs/social-services/health-care-facilities/index.html.

Duffy, J.R., Culp, S., Yarberry, C., Stroupe, L., Sand-Jecklin, K., and Coburn, A.S. (2015) Nurses' research capacity and use of evidence in acute care: Baseline findings from a partnership study. *Journal of Nursing Administration, 45*(3), 158–164.

EBM Librarian. (2013) Appraising the evidence. Retrieved September 15, 2015 from https://sites.google.com/site/ebmlibrarian/appraising-the-evidence.

Ferguson, L. and Day, R.A. (2005). Evidence-based nursing education: Myth or reality? *Journal of Nursing Education, 44*(3), 107–115.

Fineout E., Melnyk, B.M., and Schultz, A. (2005) Transforming health care from the inside out: Advancing evidence-based practice in the 21st century. *Journal of Professional Nursing, 21,* 335–344.

Gibbons, R.J., Smith, S., and Antman, E. (2003) American College of Cardiology/American Heart Association clinical practice guidelines: Part I. Where do they come from? *Circulation, 107,* 2979–2986.

Goode, C., Fink, R., Krugman, M., Oman, K., and Traditi, L. (2011) *The Colorado patient-centered interprofessional evidence-based practice model: A framework for transformation. Worldviews on Evidence-Based Practice. 8*(2), 96–105.

Hagler, D., Mays, M.Z., Stillwell, S.B., Kastenbaum, B., Brooks, R., Fineout-Overholt, E., Williamson, K.M., and Jirsak, J. (2012) Preparing clinical preceptors to support nursing students in evidence-based practice. *Journal of Continuing Education in Nursing, 43*(11), 502–508.

Institute of Medicine. (2001) *Crossing the quality chasm: A new health system for the 21st century.* Washington, DC: National Academies Press.

Institute of Medicine. (2003) *Health professions education: A bridge to quality.* Washington, DC: National Academics Press.

Jarzemsky, P. (2010) Integration of QSEN competencies when designing simulation scenarios. Retrieved September 15, 2015 from http://qsen.org/integration-of-qsen-competencies-when-designing-simulation-scenarios/.

Johnston, L. and Fineout-Overholt, E. (2005) Teaching EBP: Getting from zero to one. Moving from recognizing and admitting uncertainties to asking searchable, answerable questions. *Worldviews on Evidence-Based Nursing, 2,* 98–102.

Kim, S.C., Brown, C.E., Fields, W., and Stichler, J.F. (2009) Evidence-based practice-focused interactive teaching strategy: A controlled study. *Journal of Advanced Nursing, 65*(6), 1218–1227.

Kruszewski, A., Brough, E., and Killeen, M.B. (2009) Collaborative strategies for teaching evidence-based practice in accelerated second-degree programs. *Journal of Nursing Education, 48*(6), 340–342.

Leake, P.Y. (2004) Teaming with students and a sacred cow contest to make changes in nursing practice. *Journal of Continuing Nursing Education, 35*(6), 271–277.

Levin, R.F. and Chang, A. (2014) Tactics for teaching evidence-based practice: Determining the level of evidence of a study. *Worldviews on Evidence Based Nursing, 11*(1), 75–78.

McCurry, M.K., and Martins, D.C. (2010) Teaching undergraduate nursing research: A comparison of traditional and innovative approaches for success with millennial learners. *Journal of Nursing Education, 49*(5), 276–279.

McKenna, H., Cutcliffe, J., and McKenna, P. (2000) Evidence-based practice: Demolishing some myths. *Nursing Standard, 14*(16), 39–42.

Melnyk, B.M. and Fineout-Overholt, E. (2004) *Evidence-based practice nursing and healthcare: A guide to best practice*. Hagerstown, MD: Lippincott Williams and Wilkins.

Melnyk, B.M., Fineout-Overholt, E., Gallagher-Ford, L, and Kaplan L. (2012) The state of evidence-based practice in US nurses. *JONA*, *42*(9), 410–419.

Mitchell, S., Fischer, C., Hastings, C., Silverman, L., and Wallen, G. (2010) A thematic analysis of theoretical models for translational science in nursing: Mapping the field. *Nursing Outlook*, *58*(6), 287–300.

Moch, S.D., and Cronje, R.J. (2010) Empowering grassroots evidence-based practice: Part II. A curricular model to foster undergraduate student-enabled practice change. *Journal of Professional Nursing*, *26*(1), 14–22.

Moch, S.D., Cronje, R.J., and Branson, J. (2010) Undergraduate nursing evidence-based practice: Part I. Envisioning the role of students. *Journal of Professional Nursing*, *26*(1), 5–13.

Moher, D., Liberati, A., Tetzlaff, J., and Altman, D.G. The PRISMA Group (2009) Preferred reporting items for systematic reviews and meta-analyses: The PRISMA statement. *PLoS Med*, *6*(6): e1000097. doi:10.1371/journal.pmed1000097 http://www.prisma-statement.org/2.1.2%20-%20PRISMA%20 2009%20Checklist.pdf.

Nadelson, S.G. (2014) Online research: Fostering students' evidence-based practice through group critical appraisals. *Worldviews on Evidence-Based Nursing*, *11*(2), 143–144.

Newhouse, R., Dearholt, S., Poe, S., Pugh, L. C., and White, K.M. (2005a) Evidence-based practice: A practical approach to implementation. *Journal of Nursing Administration*, *35*(1), 35–40.

Newhouse, R., Dearholt, S., Poe, S., Pugh, L.C., and White, K. (2005b) *The Johns Hopkins Nursing Evidence-based Practice Rating Scale*. Baltimore, MD: The Johns Hopkins Hospital and Johns Hopkins University School of Nursing.

Newhouse, R.P., and Spring, B. (2010) Interdisciplinary evidence-based practice: Moving from silos to synergy. *Nursing Outlook*, *58*, 309–317.

Nilsen, P., Roback, K., Brostom, A., and Ellstrom, P.E. (2012) Creatures of habit: Accounting for the role of habit in implementation research on clinical behaviour change. *Implementation Science*, *7*(53), 1–6.

Oh, E.G., Kim, S., Kim, S. S., Kim, S., Cho, E., Yoo, J., *et al.* (2010) Integrating evidence-based practice into RN-to-BSN clinical nursing education. *Journal of Nursing Education*, *49*(7), 387–392.

Pollard, M.L., Stapleton, M., Kennelly, L., Bagdan, L., Cannistraci, P., Millenbach, L., and Odondi, M. (2014) Assessment of quality and safety education in nursing: A New York State perspective. *Nursing Education Perspectives*, *36*(4), 224–229.

Prasad, V. and Ioannidis, J.P. (2014) Evidence-based de-implementation for contradicted, unproven, and aspiring healthcare practices. *Science*, *9*(1), 5908–5909.

Pravikoff, D.S., Tanner, A.B., and Pierce, S.T. (2005) Readiness of US nurses for evidence-based practice. *American Journal of Nursing*, *105*(9), 40–51.

Roe, E.A., and Whyte-Marshall, M. (2012) Mentoring for evidence-based practice. *Journal for Nurses in Staff Development*, *28*(4), 177–181.

Rolloff, M. (2010) A constructivist model for teaching evidence-based practice. *Journal of Nursing Education Perspectives*, *31*(5), 290–293.

Rosswurm, M.A., and Larrabee, J.H. (1999) A model for change to evidence-based practice. *Image: Journal of Nursing Scholarship*, *31*(4), 317–322.

Sackett, D.L., Strauss, S.E., Richardson, W.S., Rosenberg, W., and Haynes, R.B. (2000) *Evidence-based medicine: How to practice and teach EBM*. Edinburgh, UK: Churchill Livingstone.

Sciarra, E. (2011) Impacting practice through evidence-based education. *Dimensions of Critical Care Nursing*, *30*(5), 269–275.

Scott, K., and McSherry, R. (2009) Evidence based nursing: Clarifying the concepts for nurses in practice. *Journal of Clinical Nursing*, *18*, 1085–1095.

Smith, E.L., Cronenwett, L., and Sherwood, G. (2007) Current assessments of quality and safety education in nursing. *Nursing Outlook, 55*, 132–137.

Solomons, N.M., and Spross, J.A. (2011) Evidence-based practice barriers and facilitators from a quality improvement perspective: An integrative review. *Journal of Nursing Management, 10*(1), 109–120.

Stetler, C.B. (2001) Evidence-based nursing: What it is and what it isn't. *Nursing Outlook, 49*(6), 286.

Stetler, C.B. (2003). Role of the organization in translating research into evidence-based practice. *Outcomes Management, 7*(3), 97–105.

Stevens, K.C. (2004) *ACE star model of EBP: Knowledge transformation.* San Antonio, TX: Academic Center for Evidence-Based Practice, University of Texas Health Science Center. Retrieved September 15, 2015, from www.acestar.uthscsa.edu.

Straus, S.E., Tetroe, J., and Graham, I.D. (Eds.). (2009) *Knowledge translation in health care: Moving evidence to practice.* Oxford, UK: Wiley-Blackwell.

Sullivan, D.T. (2010a) Evidence-based practice (EBP) project guidelines and grading criteria. Retrieved September 15, 2015, from http://qsen.org/evidence-based-practice-ebp-project-guidelines-and-grading-criteria/.

Sullivan, D.T. (2010b) Staff RN perspective on evidence supporting practice. Retrieved September 15, 2015, from http://qsen.org/staff-rn-perspective-on-evidence-supporting-practice/.

Sullivan, D.T., Hirst, D., and Cronenwett, L. (2009) Assessing quality and safety competencies of graduating prelicensure nursing students. *Nursing Outlook, 57*, 323–331.

Tetroe, J., Graham, I., Foy, R., Robinson, Eccles, M. P., Wensing, M., et al. (2008). Health research funding agencies' support and promotion of knowledge translation: An international study. *Milbank Quarterly, 86*(1), 125–155.

Titler, M.G., Kleiber, C., Steelman, V.J., Rakel, B.A., Budreau, G., Everett, L. Q., *et al.* (2001) The Iowa model of evidence-based practice to promote quality care. *Critical Care Nursing Clinics of North America, 13*(4), 497–509.

University of South Australia International Centre for Allied Health Evidence. (2014) Critical appraisal tools. Retrieved September 24, 2015 from http://www.unisa.edu.au/research/sansom-institute-for-health-research/research-at-the-sansom/research-concentrations/allied-health-evidence/resources/cat/#Qualitative.

Williamson, K.M., Fineout-Overholt, E., Kent, B., and Hutchinson, A.M. (2011) Teaching evidence-based practice: Integrating technology into academic curricula to facilitate evidence-based decision making. *Worldviews on Evidence-Based Nursing, 8*(4), 247–251.

Winters, C.A., and Echeverri, R. (2012) Teaching strategies to support evidence-based practice. *Critical Care Nurse, 32*(3), 49–54.

Yoder, L.H., Kirkley, D., McFall, D.D., Kirksey, K.M., StalBaum, A.L., and Sellers, D. (2014) Staff nurses' use of research to facilitate evidencee based practice. *American Journal of Nursing, 114*(9), 26–37.

Resources

American Association of Colleges of Nursing. www.aacn.nche.edu
Cochrane Library. www.cochranelibrary.org
EBM Librarian. https://sites.google.com/site/ebmlibrarian
Joanna Briggs Institute. www.joannabriggs.org
PRISMA Group. http://www.prisma-statement.org/2.1.2%20-%20PRISMA%202009%20Checklist.pdf

8

Safety

Jane Barnsteiner, PhD, RN, FAAN

> *John, a new-to-practice nurse, was orienting to his position in the perioperative area. He was assigned to shadow the circulating nurse for a hip replacement surgery for Michael James, a 67-year-old man. During the timeout procedure, the surgeon stated the surgery was to be on the right hip. John spoke up and said no it was the left hip. He had been talking with the patient in the hallway when he arrived in the perioperative area, and he was sure the patient had stated he was having his left hip replaced. The procedure was stopped, Mr. James was awakened, and he and his wife clarified the surgery was indeed to be on his left hip. Confusion had arisen as both hips would eventually need to be replaced, but it was the left one being done first. John was commended for speaking up, and a root cause analysis identified a number of areas that needed tightened up around site marking and documentation for all orthopedic surgical patients.*

The Institute of Medicine (IOM) (1999) defined patient safety as freedom from accidental injury. On March 15, 2016, the IOM was renamed the Health and Medicine Division (HMD) of the National Academies of Science, Engineering and Medicine. In this chapter, publications and citations prior to the change will be noted using IOM and after the change as HMD.

Estimates originally projected that upward of 98,000 people die each year as a result of preventable harm from health care that is supposed to help them, however, more recent estimates put the number much higher: between 251,000 (Makary and Daniel, 2016) and 440,000 (James, 2014), and is the third leading cause of death in the United States. Indeed, the issue of health care safety is so serious, the IOM has produced numerous reports devoted to identifying the issues and recommending how to solve them (http://www.nationalacademies.org/hmd/Global/News%20Announcements/Crossing-the-Quality-Chasm-The-IOM-Health-Care-Quality-Initiative.aspx).

Nurses in executive positions and at the frontlines of care are instrumental in preventing harm to patients and improving patient outcomes. To do this, nurses need to 1) have the necessary Knowledge, Skills and Attitudes (KSAs) about safety science and how it improves the quality of care for patients, and 2) be knowledgeable about system vulnerabilities and how to address them.

Learning about patient safety as a fundamental quality of patient care needs to begin in prelicensure programs and be an integral part of learning in all phases of nursing education and practice (Cronenwett *et al.*, 2007; Cronenwett *et al.*, 2009; Finkelman and Kenner, 2009). Although a health care culture of safety has been a practice priority in nursing for many years, there has been insufficient attention to incorporating the specific content related to the science of safety into the education of health care professionals in both the clinical and academic settings.

Quality and Safety in Nursing: A Competency Approach to Improving Outcomes, Second Edition.
Edited by Gwen Sherwood and Jane Barnsteiner.
© 2017 John Wiley & Sons, Inc. Published 2017 by John Wiley & Sons, Inc.

This chapter will discuss the mechanism of developing a culture of safety in learning organizations, and how understanding the principles of safety science improves a nurse's ability to deliver, high quality, safe nursing care.

A National Mandate

The work of the IOM has been to move the emphasis to widespread system change to promote safety. The message in IOM's *To Err Is Human* was to prevent, recognize, and mitigate harm from error. Errors are defined as the "failure of a planned action to be completed as intended or the use of a wrong plan to achieve an aim" (IOM, 1999). There are multiple places where errors can take place. The medication prescribing-dispensing-administration cycle, wrong site surgery, equipment designs and failure, and handoffs at change of shift reporting are but a few examples (Mitchell, 2008).

In addition to the Institute of Medicine, many organizations have become involved in working to make health care safer. These include the Institute for Healthcare Improvement, the Joint Commission, the American Association of Colleges of Nursing, the National League for Nursing, the American Nurses Association, and the National Patient Safety Foundation, among many others. Some strides have been made. According to a CMS report released in 2015, from 2011 to 2014 Hospital Acquired Conditions (HACs) across the country dropped by 17 percent. It was estimated that this reduction saved 87,000 lives and $20 billion in costs. The CDC (2016) also reported reductions of most health care associated infections when compared with the 2008 baseline.

Yet much work remains to be done, and nurses play a key role in assuring safe patient care. Although delivery of health care is extremely complex and there are tremendous system challenges, nurses often have been held accountable for harm to patients, even while they have not had input into system designs and have little understanding of how complex systems leave them vulnerable to making errors. Key aspects of complex systems involving safety science include the fact that nurses must better understand that errors come in many forms and that cultures of safety, high reliability organizations and human factors are integral components of safe health care systems.

Categories of Errors

Students and clinicians need to understand that errors can take place across the health care system and occur in many forms. *Latent failures*, sometimes called the "blunt" end, arise from decisions that affect organizational policies, procedures, and allocation of resources. For example, the decisions made by the purchasing department regarding the types of monitoring equipment to buy without input from frontline clinicians may result in equipment that does not work seamlessly in the daily work at the frontlines of care. *Active failures* occur at the interface of contact with the patient. For example, a nurse being interrupted during medication administration loses her concentration and pulls the wrong syringe from the medication drawer. This is sometimes referred to as the "sharp" end. Organizational system failures, or *indirect failures*, are related to management, organizational culture, policies/processes, transfer of knowledge, and external factors, for example, how decisions are made regarding staffing and scheduling. *Technical failures* are the indirect failure of facilities or resources, such as when a backup generator does not function during an electrical blackout that would then result in nonfunctioning monitor alarms and ventilators.

Figure 8.1 Reason's Swiss cheese model.
Source: Reason 2000. Reproduced with
permission of BMJ Publishing Group Ltd.

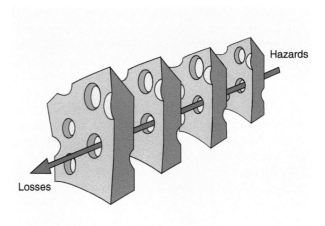

Figure 8.1 Reason's Swiss cheese model. Source: Reason 2000. Reproduced with permission of BMJ Publishing Group Ltd.

A commonly used framework for considering the components related to patient safety is Reason's Adverse Event Trajectory, often referred to as the Swiss cheese model (Reason, 2000). See Figure 8.1.

When a system fails, the immediate question should be *why* it failed rather than *who* caused the failure, for example, which safeguards failed. Reason created the Swiss cheese model to explain how faults in the different layers of the system can lead to errors. The Swiss cheese framework describes the numerous triggers that can set up a sequence of events that may cause an error to occur. These include institution triggers such as incomplete or overly complicated procedures and policies; organization triggers such as patient flow pressures; professional triggers such as delegation authority; team triggers such as inadequate communication training; individual triggers such as distractions; and technical triggers such as the use of universal connections. Multiple defenses that have been set up to prevent errors from occurring occasionally line up so that gaps in each of the multiple triggers align to allow an accident to occur. Hence, the name Swiss cheese model: the holes are aligned.

Sammer *et al.*, (2010) identified seven subcultures of patient safety from the research on safety culture; these form a framework that answer the question "What is a patient safety culture?" The seven subcultures identified are leadership, teamwork, evidence-based, communication, learning, just, and patient-centered. They align closely with the QSEN competencies.

Culture of Safety

The goal of a culture of safety is to "minimize the risk of harm to patients and providers through both system effectiveness and individual performance" (Cronenwett *et al.*, 2007). This acknowledges the influence of complex systems and human factors within the health care delivery system in general and within nursing practice specifically. There are numerous threats to patient safety and errors that can occur at all interfaces of care delivery. Common situations that are obstacles to a safe system include an extremely complex and inherently risk-prone system that can produce unintended consequences; lack of comprehensive verbal, written, and electronic communication systems; tolerance of individualistic practices and lack of standardization; fear of retribution inhibiting reporting; and organizational lack of ownership for patient safety.

Elements of a culture of safety in an organization are the establishment of safety as an organizational priority, shared core values and goals, teamwork, patient involvement, openness/transparency, and accountability (Hershey, 2015). A balance needs to be achieved between recognizing system and process design flaws and not blaming individuals for errors while at the same time not tolerating reckless and egregious behavior. This is currently referred to as a "fair and just culture" (Barnsteiner and Disch, 2012).

Culture is not necessarily uniform within a single organization. Within a health care setting, each discipline may have a different culture as may each patient care area. Although differences may benefit the work of the practice group or organization, more frequently it can result in communication difficulties, particularly around patient handoffs (Berger, Sten, and Stockwell, 2012). In a culture of safety, the focus is on effective teamwork to accomplish the goal of safe, high-quality patient care. Within a culture of safety, when an adverse event occurs, the focus is on *what* went wrong, not *who* is the problem.

In health care, a culture of blame has been pervasive. The focus has often been to try to determine who has been at fault and, all too often, to mete out discipline. This approach leads to hiding rather than reporting errors and is the antithesis of a culture of safety. More recent efforts have been directed to changing this approach and to develop environments that encourage people to report problems so they can be addressed (Barnsteiner and Disch, 2012).

A patient safety culture is nonpunitive and emphasizes accountability, excellence, honesty, integrity, and mutual respect. It incorporates safety principles such as designing jobs and working conditions for safety; standardizing and simplifying equipment, supplies, and processes; and avoiding reliance on memory (Oster and Braaten, 2016). A safety culture requires strong, committed leadership, and engagement and empowerment of all employees. It entails periodic assessment of the culture by employees about the relationship between the organization's culture and the quality and safety within the organization (Wachter and Pronovost, 2009). Numerous tools are available for measuring the health care safety culture within an organization. The most widely used is the Hospital Survey of Patient Safety Culture developed by the AHRQ (2004). See Table 8.1.

High-reliability Organizations

Although individual health care providers are the critical link to safe practice, safety science posits that safety is dependent on the health care systems and organizations in which they work. In addition, patients should be safe from injury caused by interactions with these systems and organizations of care (Shortell *et al.*, 2005). Health care is exceedingly complex and dynamic with a potential for great benefit and risk. Yet there are organizations that are high risk, dynamic, and potentially hazardous yet operate nearly error free. These organizations are called HROs (Oster and Braaten, 2016).

Organizations that have cultures of safety, foster a learning environment and evidence-based care, promote positive working environments for nurses, and are committed to improving the safety and quality of care are considered to have high reliability. Examples include organizations within the nuclear and aviation industries. Characteristics of these organizations include having a safety- and quality-centered culture, direct involvement of top and middle leadership, safety and quality efforts aligned with the strategic plan, an established infrastructure for safety, and continuous improvement and active engagement of staff across the organization (Oster and Braaten, 2016). They exhibit characteristics of having all employees fully engaged in the process of detecting high-risk situations, there are resources dedicated to bringing about the changes suggested, everyone is empowered to act in dangerous situations, and there is a work environment that is fair to employees (Page, 2004). The safety and quality of care can be improved by holding administration accountable, redesigning systems and

Table 8.1 Safety culture assessment tools.

Tool	Web Site
Agency for Healthcare Research and Quality (AHRQ)	http://www.ahrq.gov/professionals/quality-patient-safety/patientsafetyculture/index.html
Five surveys on patient safety culture: • Nursing Home Survey on Patient Safety Culture • Medical Office Survey on Patient Safety Culture • Hospital Survey on Patient Safety Culture • Community Pharmacy Survey on Patient Safety Culture • Ambulatory Surgery Center Survey on Patient Safety Culture Health care organizations can use these survey assessment tools to: • Assess their patient safety culture • Track changes in patient safety over time • Evaluate the impact of patient safety interventions • Compare their findings with national benchmarks	
Patient Safety Culture Improvement Tool (PSCIT) to assess the patient safety culture maturity level (Fleming and Wentzell, 2008)	http://www.longwoods.com/product.php?productid=19604

processes to mitigate the effects of human factors, and using strategic improvements to move toward zero harm (Chassin, 2015). Health care organizations are moving toward becoming high reliability but, given the extent of errors still occurring, have not yet consistently achieved that level of performance.

Human Factors

Human factors is the science of the interrelationship among humans, the technology they use, and the environment in which they work (IOM, 1999). It is identifying and applying what we know about human capabilities and limitations so we can design products, processes, systems, and environments to achieve more effective and safer health outcomes. Thinking is automatic, rapid, and effortless. Actions often are a result of mental models that are based on recurrent aspects of our lives, such as the way one drives to work or the routine for admitting a postoperative heart transplant patient. Fatigue, distraction, and interruptions affect cognitive abilities and problem solving. Errors result when one is tired, distracted, or interrupted and consequently deviates from safe operating procedures, standards, and policies, which can be routine and necessary (Reason, 2000).

Human factors considers the "human condition," or our inability to focus on multiple things at once and perform accurately (National Research Council, 2010). Everyone, regardless of the role he or she plays in a health care system, needs to be mindful of the interdependent system factors and their importance in shaping safe care. Studies indicate that nurses were interrupted on average almost 12 times per hour and 22% of the time while administering medications, as well as frequently while performing safety-critical tasks (Brixey, 2010; Trbovich *et al.*, 2010). Understanding the complex and demanding clinical environment helps us be aware of the components and relationships that influence the safety of care. Systems need to be designed to protect against human errors; hence, the focus needs to be on system failures, not human failures, and on meeting the needs of clinicians within the health care system.

What Students and Clinicians Need to Know About Safety

The IOM outlined the components of quality care as being safe, timely, effective, efficient, equitable, and patient centered. STEEEP is a useful acronym to remember the components (Acronym Finder, 2009). The QSEN definition of safety is adapted from the IOM and is defined as "minimiz[ing] risk of harm to patients and providers through both system effectiveness and individual performance" (Cronenwett *et al.*, 2007).

The QSEN project (Cronenwett *et al.*, 2007, 2009) was developed to identify the competencies prelicensure and graduate students need for safe practice. With funding from the RWJF, a group of experts, with consultation and input from multiple accrediting and professional groups, developed the competencies and disseminated them in publications (Cronenwett, 2012; Cronenwett *et al.*, 2007; Cronenwett *et al.*, 2009;); a web site (www.qsen.org); through an annual national forum; and in "train the trainer" workshops for nurse educators across the United States. Didactic, simulation laboratory and clinical fieldwork teaching strategies have been developed to assist clinicians and educators to incorporate a culture of safety into the curriculum and into practice. This chapter describes the components of the safety competency that need to be embedded into nursing curricula and strategies for doing so.

The QSEN definition of safety incorporates the need for students to understand that "safe, effective delivery of patient care requires understanding of the complexity of care delivery, the limits of human factors, safety design principles, characteristics of high reliability organizations, and patient safety resources" (Cronenwett *et al.*, 2007). Our traditional focus of education for nursing students and clinicians has been steeped in the care of individual patients and families with understanding of the complexity of care delivery systems being notably absent.

To teach the safety competency requires teaching of all the QSEN competencies (Barnsteiner, 2011). *Patient-centered care* (Walton and Barnsteiner, 2017) ensures that the patient and family are at the center of the decision-making process and understands the plan of care that can prevent errors from occurring. *Evidence-based practice* (Tracey and Barnsteiner, 2017) ensures clinicians are using up-to-date science in addition to considering clinical expertise and patient values in designing a plan of care. *Teamwork and collabora*tion (Disch, 2017) ensures that the health care team is communicating and working together effectively with shared decisions among professionals to achieve safe, high-quality care. *Quality improvement* (Johnson, 2017) addresses trending and analysis of data to be able to benchmark with comparable organizations and identify vulnerabilities in the system needing correction. *Informatics* (Clancy and Warren, 2017) enables clinicians to use information and technology to communicate, access knowledge, and support decision making to promote safe care. The QSEN project separated quality improvement and safety into two separate competencies to more comprehensively address the science underlying each of the two and to better describe the KSAs necessary for effective nursing practice. Previously the IOM had listed them as one competency (Sherwood, 2011; 2017).

Appendices A and B list the KSAs of the safety competency that students and clinicians need to know to practice safely. Content includes the elements of a culture of safety, types of health care errors and why they occur, and how to make care safer.

Safety Challenges in All Settings

Most of the work on patient safety has focused on acute care. There is increasing attention on ambulatory care particularly with emphasis on improving the diagnostic process. The latest evidence indicates that at least 5% of ambulatory care visits will result in a diagnostic error (Balogh, Miller, and Ball, 2015).

Human factors challenges have been identified in home care. Care in the home can range from simple tasks such as feeding and bathing to complex issues including home dialysis and caring for a person on a ventilator. Household safety checklists to assess hazards in the household and Internet access for data transfer and remote monitoring enable high quality safe care (National Research Council, 2010).

Skilled nursing facilities (SNF) have not had the same focus on patient safety as other sites of care. In 2014, the US Department of Health and Human Services Office of Inspector General (OIG) reported that an estimated 33 percent of Medicare beneficiaries admitted to SNFs following a hospital stay experienced an adverse event during their SNF stays, with 59 percent of the identified harm events deemed preventable (OIG, 2014).

The Joint Commission established the National Patient Safety Goals to promote specific improvements in patient safety. The requirements highlight problematic areas in health care and describe evidence and expert-based solutions to these problems. The goals that are reviewed and updated annually focus generally on systemwide solutions for hospitals, behavioral health settings, ambulatory settings, home care, and other health care settings (Joint Commission, 2016).

Making Care Safer

It is clear that system thinking and design are necessary to mitigate risk. Students and clinicians need to understand how nurses may contribute to making care safer. The IOM (2001) described nine categories that provide opportunities to improve patient safety by incorporating these into organizations that have a culture of safety:

1) **User-centered design**. A user-centered design makes it easier for the clinician to perform the right action. Approaches include making things visible so the user is able to see actions possible at any time, affordance, constraints, and forcing functions. For example, making something visible would be a sign outside a patient door alerting providers that the patient is at risk for falls so clinicians passing by the room would look in more frequently to check on the patient. Affordance indicates how something is to be used, such as marking the correct limb before surgery or a sign on a door indicating which way to open it. A constraint makes it hard to do the wrong thing, and a forcing function makes it impossible to do the wrong thing, such as connecting equipment to a patient improperly.

2) **Avoid reliance on memory**. Standardizing and simplifying procedures and tasks decreases the demand on memory, planning, and problem solving. The use of protocols and checklists reduces reliance on memory and serves as a reminder for the steps to be followed. Simplifying processes minimizes problem solving. Simplification of processes include having the usual dose of a medication as the default in an electronic order entry, or having an easy-to-use checklist in the procedure tray for central line placement that outlines correct steps.

3) **Attend to work safety**. Work hours, workloads, staffing ratios, distractions, and interruptions all affect patient safety. In many health care settings, realizing that interruptions are a major cause of medication administration errors, nurses have chosen to wear something visually apparent such as a vest to indicate they should not be interrupted when they are preparing or administering medications. Standardizing practice with implementation of "red rules," safe zones, and sacred spaces are all practices that attend to a safe working environment. Having policies and processes in place that require that staff take lunch breaks to recharge promotes patient safety.

4) **Avoid reliance on vigilance**. Checklists, well-designed alarms, rotating staff, and breaks decrease the need for remaining vigilant for long periods. Well-designed alarms that differentiate a potential emergency from a non-pressing situation decrease the need for continuous vigilance.

For example, one alarm may signal a disconnected ventilator needing immediate response, while another may notify of an intravenous pump needing adjustment. Rotating staff assignments and staff taking scheduled breaks and meals also decreases the need for remaining vigilant for long periods.

5) **Training concepts for teams**. The literature is replete with more than 20 years of evidence outlining the importance of teamwork and collaboration. Training programs for effective intra- and interprofessional communication and collaboration include standardizing transitions in care and handoffs, and implementation of crew resource management skill. Many organizations are implementing TeamSTEPPS to provide a framework for interprofessional collaboration and communication and instill a skill set consistent with a safety climate (www.ahrq.gov).

6) **Involve patients in their care**. Patients and families should be in the center of the care process. This includes clinicians obtaining accurate information and including patients and families in decisions about treatments and comprehensive discharge planning and education. Knowing the plan of care, holding rounds in patient rooms, and having patients/families participate promote the concept of patients being at the center and source of control. It allows patients to become knowledgeable about their care and to correct any misinformation. This also means clinicians have a responsibility to assist patients and families to become health literate.

7) **Anticipate the unexpected**. Reorganization and organization-wide changes result in new patterns and processes of care. Introduction of new processes and technologies depends on a chain of involvement of frontline users and the need for pilot testing before widespread implementation to identify vulnerabilities that may affect patient safety. When implementing changes, such as the implementation of an electronic health care record, that call for new ways to deliver care, it would be important to increase organizational vigilance with additional staffing. Additional information system resources during implementation of a new electronic health care record system promotes safe care by anticipating unexpected breakdowns that may happen when putting in a large-scale change.

8) **Design for recovery**. Errors will occur despite the existence of a culture of safety. Designing and planning for recovery will allow reversal or make it hard to carry out irreversible critical functions. Simulation training promotes the practice of processes and rescues using models and virtual reality. Having backup generators in place in the event of an electrical failure, and disaster management programs in place and practiced on a regular basis, help to promote a smooth recovery with minimal harm to patients.

9) **Improve access to accurate, timely information**. Information for decision making needs to be available at the point of care. This includes easy access to drug formularies, evidence-based practice protocols, patient records, laboratory reports, and medication administration records.

Nurses are in a central position to improve the quality and safety of care through patient safety activities because nurses are in the position to coordinate and integrate the multiple aspects of care, monitoring, and identifying hazards and changes in patient conditions before errors and adverse events can occur. Nursing is also in a position to positively affect high-quality, safe care with strong leadership, adequate staffing, and strong interprofessional communication and collaboration.

Work Environment

The IOM report *Keeping Patients Safe: Transforming the Work Environment of Nurses* (2004) emphasized the importance of the work environment in which nurses provide care. Recommendations from the report included the need for the following:

1) The chief nurse executive to have a leadership role in the organization, which provides a voice for nursing and safe patient care at the top levels of the organization.

2) Evidence-based staffing models, which decrease stress and workload and positively impact patient outcomes.
3) Evidence-based scheduling, which modulates the effect of fatigue.
4) Safe work environments such as safe patient handling programs, which minimize injury and disability and promote healthy work environments.

The Joint Commission identified the pervasive effect on patient safety related to disruptive behavior among health care clinicians. Disruptive behavior is psychological and physical intimidation as well as overt and passive activities meant to intimidate or disrupt care. Disruptive behavior/bullying/abuse has a negative effect on quality of care, patient safety, and nurse retention and job satisfaction (Barnsteiner, 2012; Clarke and Donaldson, 2008). The Joint Commission (2009) identified that disruptive behaviors undermine a culture of safety and has instituted two leadership standards for accreditation that will facilitate civility in the workplace and give staff a mechanism for reporting disruptive behavior:

- EP 4: The hospital/organization has a code of conduct that defines acceptable and disruptive and inappropriate behaviors.
- EP 5: Leaders create and implement a process for managing disruptive and inappropriate behaviors.

In addition to disruptive behavior, components in the design of the physical environment can produce vulnerabilities to patient safety and clinician safety as well. Having "no lift" policies and sufficient patient lifting equipment prevents patient and clinician injuries. Limiting work hours and adequate staffing prevents fatigue. Workspace design that promotes flow of patient care and fewer interruptions decreases the chance of errors.

Work-arounds may present patient safety hazards. Clinicians regularly encounter problems or impediments in delivering care and invent a quick work-around to solve those problems. This first-order change occurs because clinicians are really busy and need to get the problem solved. Examples include using equipment for purposes it was not intended or bypassing the procedure for barcoding medication administration because the process has too many steps. Many organizations do not provide a way to report problems and develop solutions in a timely or effective fashion. This frequently used approach to problem solving leaves systemic problems untreated, and this risk-taking behavior is potentially a cause of error that may result in patient harm.

Transitions in Care and Handoffs

The Joint Commission International Center for Patient Safety (2005) defines handoff communication as "the realtime process of passing patient specific information from one caregiver to another or from one team of caregivers to another for the purpose of ensuring continuity and safety of the patient/client/resident's care." Handoff of patient care from one nurse to another is an integral part of nursing practice (Berger, Sten, and Stockwell, 2012; Riesenberg *et al.*, 2010). The term handover rather than handoff is increasingly being used in practice to indicate the process is not one-sided. Handoff is used in this chapter as it is the more commonly used term.

Transitions in care and handoffs create vulnerabilities in health care that require special attention. Central to effective handoffs is effective communication. Ineffective communication and inadequate handoffs have negative consequences for patients. Standardization in the processes of handoffs with face-to-face communication remains key to addressing patient safety concerns (Dayton and Henricksen, 2007; Friesen, White, and Byers, 2008; Saint *et al.*, 2005; Welsh, Flanagan, and Ebright, 2010).

Handoffs may be facilitated through the use of standardized change of shift reporting checklists. SBAR has become a frequently used approach both for interprofessional communication and nurse to nurse communication (Berger, Sten, and Stockwell, 2012; Riesenberg *et al.*, 2010). At the direct work group/team level, the use of safety huddles has been demonstrated to engage frontline staff in improving patient safety (Gerke, Uffelman, and Chandler, 2010). Increasingly, handoffs are taking place in the presence of the patient with the patient participating. This enables the patient to contribute, ask questions, and verify the information being passed among clinicians (Walton and Barnsteiner, 2017).

Processes for Examining Safety Threats

Root cause analysis (RCA) and failure mode and effects analysis (FMEA) are two methods for examining the factors leading to an adverse event or a close call (Johnson, 2017). There are numerous resources for RCAs and FMEAs on the AHRQ web site (www.patientsafety.gov). The Joint Commission recommends an RCA after all sentinel events to outline the sequence of events that led up to the event, identifying causal factors and root causes. It is followed by defining a course of action to eliminate risks.

FMEA is an evaluation technique used to identify and eliminate known and/or potential failures, problems, and errors from a system, design, process, and/or service before they actually occur (NPSF, 2016). The goal of an FMEA is to prevent errors by attempting to identify all the ways a process could fail, estimate the probability and consequences of each failure, and then take action to prevent the potential failures from occurring. Simulating equipment failures has been shown to be useful to hone provider skills and identify equipment vulnerabilities and to evaluate alternative approaches or procedures (Waldrop *et al.*, 2009).

Transparency

Transparency is the free flow of information open to examination by others. There has been increasing movement toward transparency at all levels of the heath care system. Results have been better than anyone expected both in terms of improved performance and fewer issues. Hospital performance on core measures has improved since CMS began public reporting. Rapid disclosure and honest explanations to patients/families have been demonstrated to increase satisfaction with care and lead to lower malpractice settlements (Kachalia, *et al.*, 2010). Yet in a survey of health professionals only 15% reported they were satisfied with the degree of transparency in their organization (NPSF, 2015a).

Transparency and accountability to patients and families is a hallmark of a culture of safety. Disclosure of errors to patients is linked to patient safety efforts and is mandated by many state patient safety requirements. Transparency with patients and families includes promptly providing patients and families with full information about any harm from treatment and an apology, and offering a fair resolution (NPSF, 2015a). It involves both communicating information as well as addressing the patient's emotions. High-reliability organizations have in place policies, processes, and training directed toward disclosing health care errors and significant near misses to patients and their families. Students and clinicians need to understand the disclosure process for the health care organization and develop disclosure communication skills related to how to deliver difficult news.

Transparency among clinicians can lead to system change and create a safe supportive environment. Interprofessional processes for reporting, analyzing, sharing, and using safety data for improvement promotes transparency, teamwork, and collaboration leading to safer care. Institutional processes to address challenges to accountability such as disruptive behavior, violation of safe practices, and inadequate supervision of performance also help to promote transparency.

Transparency among health care organizations, through sharing of information, can facilitate the more rapid adoption of best safety practices. Participation in improvement collaboratives, such as through the IHI, is one way to accelerate improvement.

Increasingly we are seeing transparency of clinicians and health care organizations (HCO) with the public through the reporting of data about performance. Publicly displayed measures, such as scorecards and dashboards used for monitoring quality and safety, make data usable by patients. These include HCAHPS data about patient satisfaction and CMS measures about quality indicators such as hospital-acquired conditions.

Voluntary Versus Mandatory Error Reporting Systems

The IOM (2001) differentiated between mandatory and voluntary reporting of health care errors. Voluntary reports may encourage practitioners to report near misses and errors, thus producing important information that might reduce future errors. However, there is concern that with voluntary reporting, the true error frequency may be many times greater than what is actually reported. Mandatory reporting systems, usually enacted under state law, generally require reporting of sentinel events, adverse events causing patient harm, and unanticipated outcomes such as serious patient injury or death (Schumann, 2017).

The IOM (2001) has called for a nationwide reporting system that would provide funds for state governments to organize systems for reporting errors. The goal is to have a national patient safety center that would receive state reports and aggregate data for intensive analysis. To date, this legislation has not been passed, but 27 states and the District of Columbia currently have mandatory reporting and have designed databases to aggregate and report statewide data.

Processes such as regulation, legislation, accreditation, linking payment with performance, commitment of professional organizations, and public engagement can impact the safety and quality of nursing care and health care (Schumann, 2017). Numerous states such as Pennsylvania and Texas now have error reporting laws. Accrediting organizations such as the Joint Commission influence patient safety with explicit standards such as the National Patient Safety Goals and handoff communications. The Centers for Medicare and Medicaid Services are linking reporting performance on quality indicators such as pressure ulcer prevalence and central line infections with hospital payment. An initiative of the National Council of State Boards of Nursing, the Practice Breakdown Advisory Panel, was established to study nursing practice breakdown and identify common themes related to events and recommend strategies to correct unsafe practices (NCSBN, 2010). It is expected that this work will shift the focus of state boards of nursing from punishment to prevention and correction. The ANA has widely publicized standards related to prevention of workplace injuries from needle sticks and patient lifting. The American Association of Critical-Care Nurses (2016) recently updated their standards for establishing and sustaining healthy work environments. All of these efforts are initiating positive changes in the work environment for nurses (Flynn *et al.*, 2012; Kupperschmidt, *et al.*, 2010; Schumann, 2017).

Openness is a critical factor in a culture of safety. It indicates there is acceptance of human elements in error and a means of reporting any error or near miss or identified potential for error. Many errors go unreported by health care workers. A major concern clinicians have is that self-reporting may result in repercussions. Lack of reporting of errors and near misses have consequences for individual clinicians as well as for the organizations in which they work. Unreported errors remove the opportunity of analyzing to improve patient safety, thereby limiting improvements because there is no understanding of what works to prevent the errors. Openness is important so that errors and potential problems are exposed and solved before they endanger others. Within a culture of open-ness, there is a "fair and just culture" where discipline is limited to reckless or egregious behavior (Barnsteiner and Disch, 2012).

Near misses are more common than adverse events and provide valuable information regarding weaknesses in systems that predispose to adverse events (Bagian *et al.*, 2001). Aggregate data from near-miss analyses are used to direct attention to critical safety issues. Discussions of near misses usually do not generate the defensive reaction often associated with discussion of adverse events. Institutional reporting systems should be nonpunitive and should keep reported information confi-dential and nondiscoverable. Information should be used for system improvements. The reporting process should be uncomplicated and preferably electronic to lead to rapid analysis. The opportunity for anonymous reporting is thought to lead to greater willingness to report errors. Traditional reporting mechanisms have utilized verbal reports and paper-based incident reports to detect and document clinically significant medical errors, yet the correlation with actual errors has been low. CMS reported that in a review of a large number of Medicare records 86% of errors with harm had not been reported (OIG, 2012). Reporting errors and near misses through established systems pro-vides opportunities to prevent future similar, and perhaps even more serious, errors. Several factors are necessary to increase error reporting: having leadership committed to patient safety; eliminating a punitive culture and institutionalizing a culture of safety; increasing reporting of near misses; pro-viding timely feedback and follow-up actions and improvements to avert future errors; and having a multidisciplinary approach to reporting (Barnsteiner and Disch, 2012; NPSF, 2015b).

Second Victim

Health care professionals report feeling worried, guilty, and depressed following serious errors, as well as being concerned for patient safety and fearful of disciplinary actions (Conway *et al.*, 2010; Rassin, Kanti, and Silner, 2005; Rossheim, 2009; Scott *et al.*, 2010; Wolf, 2005). They also are aware of their direct responsibility for errors. Many nurses accept responsibility and blame themselves for serious-outcome errors. Wu (2000) coined the phrase *second victim* to describe the impact of errors on profes-sionals. The use of the term is controversial. Consumer advocates challenge the use of the term *second victim* on the basis that it takes attention away from the patient who suffered because of an error. However, health care professionals practice the art and science of health care delivery within very com-plex environments. Rather than allow clinicians to suffer alone after an adverse event, it is imperative that systems be developed to help them understand the event, to stimulate healing, and to improve the health care system (Denham, 2007; Institute for Safe Medication Practices, 2011; White *et al.*, 2008).

Even though it has been recognized for some time that clinicians experienced significant personal and professional emotional distress in the aftermath of unanticipated patient safety events, recent research has also demonstrated that having a support system in place positively influences the overall culture of patient safety in an organization (Scott, 2015).

Integrating a Culture of Safety into the Curriculum and into the Ongoing Education of Clinicians

Sherwood (2011) described initiatives taking place worldwide for integrating quality and safety science in nursing education and practice. These include curriculum mapping for spreading the competencies across the curriculum, educational standards for incorporating the competencies into accrediting organizations, curriculum essentials documents, and regional institutes held across the country that use a train-the-trainer development model to help educators transform curricula. Barton *et al.* (2009) used a developmental approach—beginning, intermediate, and advanced stages of the curriculum—in a Delphi study to identify where in the curriculum the 162 QSEN competencies should be introduced and where they should be emphasized (see Appendix C). Early introduction was recommended for the safety competency and indeed should be integrated in all phases of an educational program. The NCSBN in their Transition to Practice model recommends the QSEN competencies be incorporated into nurse residency programs for new-to-practice nurses (Spector, Ulrich, and Barnsteiner, 2017). Content related to safety should be a component of all health professional education and a part of ongoing professional development programs across all health care agencies (Health and Medicine Division of the National Academies of Science, Engineering and Medicine, 2016).

Teaching the Safety Competency

Students and clinicians alike need to understand that safe, effective delivery of patient care requires understanding of the following: the complexity of health care systems, the limits of human factors, safety design principles, characteristics of high-reliability organizations, and patient safety resources. There needs to be a rebalance of the curricular equation with a balance between teaching patient care and creating a culture of system responsibility. Safety education needs to move from the "background" of implicit learning to the "foreground" of established curriculum. For educators to teach safety, whether in the academic or clinical setting, they must be knowledgeable and current about the components of a safe culture. Activities that may facilitate up-to-date learning follow: 1) becoming members of a clinical agency committee such as Quality Improvement, Patient Safety, pharmacy, and other quality and safety committees, 2) advancing an academic/clinical partnership between schools of nursing and clinical agencies holding quarterly or twice yearly meetings of nursing executives and clinical leaders with deans/directors and key educators, and 3) gaining familiarity with resources to use when teaching, such as on the QSEN web site (www.qsen.org). The IHI Open School has courses on quality and safety that are free for clinicians, faculty, and students.

Most nurses, including nurse educators, have not been educated in error prevention or trained as patient safety coaches (Reid and Catchpole, 2011). When a teaching moment presents itself, as with a medication administration near miss by a student, a nurse will typically base educational outcomes on success or failure, automatically designating errors or near misses as failures without analyzing the circumstances surrounding the incident. Teaching strategies should stress the complexity of patient safety, using near misses as well as sentinel events as educational tools to improve delivery of care. A case-based curriculum provides opportunities for role-play in "ideal" models as well as "real" situations. Scenarios should stress truth telling, responsible behavior, error reporting, and follow-up to error reporting. Finally, a comprehensive curriculum should prepare nurses to anticipate the potential for error. Multiple strategies may be employed to teach a culture of safety. These are usually divided into classroom, simulation laboratory, and clinical activities. See Textboxes 8.1–8.3).

Summary

Making progress on a culture of safety begins with learning how to learn about safety. Change, however, will occur at different stages and speed. Cultural transitions can take 10 years or more. Educators and clinicians need to be proactive and remain persistent in the commitment to help develop the

---

Textbox 8.1 Classroom Education Activities to Teach Safety Competency

- Demonstrate prescribing, dispensing, and medication error vulnerabilities and solutions during pharmacy classes.
- Evaluate the research on work hours and fatigue and have discussion of how these affect quality of care and risk of errors.
- Discuss sentinel event and serious reportable event–"never event"–statistics.
- Discuss the Joint Commission videos such as *Speak Up: Prevent Errors in Your Care*, which may be accessed on YouTube, retrieved from: http://www.youtube.com/watch?v=EccuE-_2_2E
- Use unfolding case studies incorporating multiple QSEN competencies within cases appropriate for the course content. See www.qsen.org web site for examples.
- Invite patients and/or their families to tell their stories and what they want from health care providers.
- Incorporate problem-based learning with clinical scenarios in classroom with participants working in teams.
- Develop pocket guides–brief self-contained learning modules on the components of safety–for clinicians and students to use.

Textbox 8.2 Simulation Education Activities to Teach Safety Competency

- Use a patient model to simulate safety breaches.
- Simulate equipment failures with scenarios to detect and correct equipment problems.
- Set up a clinical room with opportunities to identify and correct multiple hazards and errors.
- Demonstrate how a near miss or error is documented.
- Practice SBAR for effective handoffs and communication between and among clinicians.
- Use high-fidelity clinical simulations to assess ability to deliver safe care in the clinical setting.
- Read and interpret medication labels, some of which are correct and some of which contain errors. Have participants rewrite labels for clearer understanding.
- Use a complex set of discharge medication orders and set up a schedule of medications. Have participants set up a mediset using small candies.

Textbox 8.3 Clinical Education Activities to Teach Safety Competency

- Observe and evaluate teamwork communication and collaboration while attending patients.
- Design a checklist for a common procedure, e.g., insertion of foley catheter.
- Serve as "secret shoppers" and observe staff and other students' technique, such as hand hygiene or interruptions. Track findings and report the data.
- Discuss near misses and adverse events with staff nurses during clinical experiences.
- Attend an RCA and/or FMEA.
- Observe and evaluate teamwork, communication, and collaboration on patient/walk rounds.
- Develop QI projects, and engage an interprofessional team to implement the project. Share project results with students, educators, and agency members.
- Attend patient safety rounds.
- Incorporate reflective exercises on patient safety in clinical postconferences.
- Complete TeamSTEPPS and assess communication and collaboration on interprofessional patient rounds.

- Develop a safety rounds checklist and have teams make unit rounds to complete the checklist. Have participants share results with staff and initiate a discussion of the findings.
- Perform peer review of documentation to assess for any errors in documentation.
- Set up error/near miss reporting system to trend student errors/near misses.
- Complete an environmental safety scan of a clinical area and evaluate the lighting, space, and accessibility for patients, families, and staff. Assess traffic and noise, and accessibility of supplies and equipment, including space for medication preparation.
- Working in teams, have nursing, medical, and pharmacy students examine a complex patient health record and complete a medication reconciliation analysis from admission through discharge.
- Design approaches to reduce interruptions, such as wearing vests during medication administration and establishing no-interruption zones such as the medication preparation area.

knowledge, skills, and attitudes necessary to reshape the education and practice environment. Reducing health care errors is complex business. Safe, effective delivery of patient care requires understanding of the complexity of health care systems, the limits of human factors, safety design principles, characteristics of high reliability organizations, and patient safety resources. These components are critical to the preparation of safe clinicians and essential for twenty-first century health care delivery.

References

Acronym Finder. (2009) Retrieved on June 29, 2011, from http://www.acronym-finder.com/Safe%2c-Timely%2c-Effective%2c-Efficient%2c-Equitable%2c-Patient_Centered-(Care%3b-Baylor-Health-Care-System)-(STEEEP).html.

American Association of Critical-Care Nurses. (2016) *AACN standards for establishing and sustaining healthy work environments: A journey to excellence.* 2nd Ed. Retrieved from: www.aacn.org.

Bagian, J.P., Lee, C., Gosbee, J., DeRosier, J., Stalhandske, E., Eldridge, N., *et al.* (2001) Developing and deploying a patient safety program in a large health care delivery system: You can't fix what you don't know about. *Joint Commission Journal on Quality Improvement, 27*(10), 522–532.

Balogh, E.P., Miller B.T., and Ball, J. (2015). *Improving diagnosis in health care.* Washington DC: National Academies Press.

Barnsteiner, J., and Disch, J. (2012). A just culture for nurses and nursing students. *Nursing Clinics of North America. 47*(3):407–16.

Barnsteiner, J. (2012) Workplace abuse in nursing. In D. Mason, J. Leavitt, and M. Chafee (Eds.), *Politics and policy in nursing and healthcare*, 6th Ed. London: Elsevier.

Barnsteiner, J. (2011) Teaching the culture of safety. *Online Journal of Issues in Nursing, 16*(3), Ms. 5.

Barton, A., Armstrong, G., Preheim, G., Gelmon S., and Andrus L. (2009) A national Delphi to determine developmental progression of quality and safety competencies in nursing education. *Nursing Outlook, 57*, 331–332.

Berger, J.T., Sten, M.B., and Stockwell, D.C. (2012) Patient handoffs: Delivering content efficiently and effectively is not enough. *International Journal of Risk and Safety Medicine. 24*(4):201–205.

Brixey, J. (2010) Interruptions in workflow for RNs in a level one trauma center. March/April, *Patient Safety and Quality Healthcare*, 25–30.

Clarke, S., and Donaldson, N. (2008) Nurse staffing and patient care quality and safety. In Hughes, R.G., (Ed.), *Patient safety and quality: An evidence-based handbook for nurses* (pp. 2-111–2-136). Rockville, MD: Agency for Healthcare Research and Quality, Publication No. 08-0043.

CDC. (2016) *National and State Healthcare Associated Infections Progress Report.* http://www.cdc.gov/HAI/pdfs/progress-report/hai-progress-report.pdf.

Chassin, M.R. *(2015) High reliability in healthcare: Working toward zero harm.* http://www.arabhealthmagazine.com/press-releases/2015/issue-4/high-reliability-in-healthcare-working-toward-zero-harm/.

Center for Medicare and Medicaid Services. (2015) *Hospital-acquired conditions update: Interim data from national efforts to make healthcare safer, 2010–2014.* http://www.ahrq.gov/sites/default/files/publications/files/interimhacrate2014_2.pdf.

Conway, J., Federico, F., Stewart, K., and Campbell, M.J. (2010) Respectful management of serious clinical adverse events. IHI Innovation Series white paper. Cambridge, MA: Institute for Healthcare Improvement.

Cronenwett, L. (2012) A national initiative: Quality and Safety Education for Nurses (QSEN), In G. Sherwood and J. Barnsteiner (Eds.), *Quality and safety in nursing: A competency approach to improving outcomes.* Hoboken, NJ: Wiley-Blackwell.

Cronenwett, L., Sherwood, G., Barnsteiner, J., Disch J., Johnson, J., Mitchell, P., *et al.* (2007) Quality and safety education for nurses. *Nursing Outlook, 55,* 122–131.

Cronenwett, L., Sherwood, G., Pohl, J., Barnsteiner, J. Moore, S., Sullivan, D. T., *et al.* (2009) Quality and safety education for advanced practice nurses. *Nursing Outlook, 57,* 338–348.

Dayton, E., and Henriksen, K. (2007) Communication failure: Basic components, contributing factors, and the call for structure. *Joint Commission Journal on Quality and Patient Safety/Joint Commission Resources, 33*(1), 34–47.

Denham, C.R. (2007) Trust: The 5 rights of the second victim. *Journal of Patient Safety, 3,* 107–119.

Disch, J. (2017) Teamwork and collaboration. In G. Sherwood and J. Barnsteiner (Eds.), *Quality and safety in nursing: A competency approach to improving outcomes.* 2nd Ed. Hoboken, NJ: Wiley-Blackwell.

Finkelman, A. and Kenner, C. (2009) *Teaching IOM: Implications of the Institute of Medicine reports for nursing,* 2nd Ed. Silver Springs, MD: Nursebooks.org.

Flynn, L., Liang, Y., Dickson, G.L., Xie, M., and Suh, D. (2012) Nurses' practice environments, error interception practices, and inpatient medication errors. *Journal of Nursing Scholarship. 44*(2):180–186.

Friesen, M.A., White, S.V., and Byers, J. (2008) Handoffs: Implications for nurses. In R.G. Hughes (Ed.), *Patient safety and quality: An evidence-based handbook for nurses* (pp. 2-285–2-333). Rockville, MD: Agency for Healthcare Research and Quality. Publication No. 08-0043. 34.

Gerke, M., Uffelman, C., and Chandler K. (2010) Safety huddles for a culture of safety, May/June. *Patient Safety and Quality Healthcare,* 24–28.

Health and Medicine Division, National Academies of Sciences, Engineering, and Medicine. (2016). *Envisioning the future of health professional education: Workshop summary.* Washington, DC: The National Academies Press.

Hershey, K. (2015) Culture of Safety. *Nursing Clinics Of North America. 50*(1):139–152.

Institute of Medicine. (1999) *To err is human: Building a safer health system.* Washington, DC: National Academies Press.

Institute of Medicine. (2001) *Crossing the quality chasm: A new health system for the 21st century.* Washington, DC: National Academies Press.

Institute of Medicine. (2004) *Keeping patients safe: Transforming the work environment of nurses.* Washington, DC: National Academies Press.

Institute for Safe Medication Practices. (2011) Too many abandon the "second victims" of medical errors. *ISMP Safety Alert*, *16*(14), 1–3.

James, J.T. (2014) A new, evidence-based estimate of patient harms associated with hospital care. *Journal of Patient Safety*, *9*(3)122–128.

Johnson, J. (2017) Quality improvement. In G. Sherwood and J. Barnsteiner (Eds.), *Quality and safety in nursing: A competency approach to improving outcomes*. 2nd Ed. Hoboken, NJ: Wiley-Blackwell.

Joint Commission. (2009) Leadership committed to safety. Sentinel Event #43, Retrieved from http://www.jointcommission.org/assets/1/18/SEA_43.pdf.

Joint Commission. (2016) *2016 National Patient Safety Goals*. Retrieved from https://www.jointcommission.org/standards_information/npsgs.aspx.

Joint Commission International Center for Patient Safety. (2005). *Strategies to improve hand-off communication: Implementing a process to resolve questions*. Retrieved June 29, 2011, from http://www.jcipatientsafety.org/15274/.

Kachalia, A., Kaufman, S.R., Boothman, R., Anderson, S., Welch, K., Saint, S., Rogers, M.A. (2010) Liability claims and costs before and after implementation of a medical error disclosure program. *Annals of Internal Medicine 153*(4):213–21.

Kupperschmidt, B., Kientz, E., Ward, J., and Reinholz, B. (2010) A healthy work environment: it begins with you. *Online Journal of Issues in Nursing*. 1D.

Makary, M. and Daniel, M. (2016) Medical error—the third leading cause of death in the US. *British Medical Journal*. May 3. British Medical Journal 2016;353;i2139.

Mitchell, P. (2008) Defining patient safety and quality care. In R.G. Hughes (Ed.), *Patient safety and quality: An evidence-based handbook for nurses* (pp. 1–1–1–6). Rockville, MD: Agency for Healthcare Research and Quality. Publication No. 08-0043.

National Council of State Boards of Nursing. (2010) *Nursing pathways for patient safety*. Mosby St. Louis, MO: Mosby.

National Patient Safety Foundation. (2016) RCA^2: Improving Root Cause Analyses and Actions to Prevent Harm Retrieved from: http://www.npsf.org/?page=RCA2.

National Patient Safety Foundation. Lucien Leape Institute. (2015a) *Shining a light: Safer healthcare through transparency*. Boston, MA: National Patient Safety Foundation. Retrieved from: http://npsf.org/transparency.

National Patient Safety Foundation. (2015b) *Free from harm: Accelerating Patient Safety Improvement 15 years after To Err is Human*. Retrieved from: www.npsf.org/free-from-harm.

National Research Council. (2010) The Role of Human Factors in Home Health Care: Workshop Summary. Steve Olson, Rapporteur. Committee on the Role of Human Factors in Home Health Care, Committee on HumanSystems Integration. Division of Behavioral and Social Sciences and Education. Washington, DC: The National Academies Press.

Office of Inspector General. (2014) Adverse Events in Skilled Nursing Facilities: National incidence among Medicare beneficiaries. Retrieved from: http://oig.hhs.gov/oei/reports/oei-06-11-00370.pdf.

Office of Inspector General. (2012) Hospital incident reporting systems do not capture most patient harm. Retrieved from: http://oig.hhs.gov/oei/reports/oei-06-09-00091.pdf.

Oster, C., and Braaten, J. (2016) *High Reliability Organizations: A Healthcare Handbook for Patient and Safety Quality*. Indianapolis, IN: Sigma Theta Tau International.

Page, A. (2004) *Keeping patients safe: Transforming the work environment of nurses*. Committee on the Work Environment for Nurses and Patient Safety, Board on Health Care Services. Washington, DC: National Academies Press.

Rassin, M., Kanti, T., and Silner, D. (2005) Chronology of medication errors by nurses: Accumulation of stresses and PTSD symptoms. *Issues in Mental Health Nursing*, *26*(8), 873–886.

Reason, J. (2000) Human error: Models and management. *British Medical Journal, 320*, 768–770.

Reid, J., and Catchpole, K. (2011) Patient safety: A core value of nursing—So why is achieving it so difficult? *Journal of Research in Nursing, 16*, 209–223.

Riensenberg, L.A., Leitsch, J., and Cunningham, J.M. (2010) Nursing handoffs: A systematic review of the literature. *American Journal of Nursing, 110*(4), 24–34.

Saint, S., Kaufman, S.R., Thompson, M., Rogers, M., and Chenowith, C. (2005) A reminder reduces urinary catheterizations in hospitalized patients. *Joint Commission Journal on Quality and Patient Safety, 31*(8), 455–462.

Sammer, C., Lykens, K., Singh, K., Mains, D., and Lackan, N. (2010) What is patient safety culture? A review of the literature. *Journal of Nursing Scholarship, 42*, 156–165.

Schumann, M.J., (2017) Policy implications driving national quality and safety initiatives. In G. Sherwood and J. Barnsteiner (Eds.), *Quality and safety in nursing: A competency approach to improving outcomes.* 2nd Ed. Hoboken, NJ: Wiley-Blackwell.

Scott, S.D. (2015) Second Victim Support: Implications for patient safety attitudes and perceptions. *Patient Safety and Quality Healthcare. 12*(5):26–31.

Sherwood, G. (2011) Integrating quality and safety in nursing education and practice. *Journal of Research in Nursing, 16*, 226–239.

Sherwood, G. (2017) Driving forces for quality and safety: Changing mindsets to improve health care. In G. Sherwood and J. Barnsteiner (Eds.), *Quality and safety in nursing: A competency approach to improving outcomes.* 2nd Ed. Hoboken, NJ: Wiley-Blackwell.

Shortell, S.M., Schmittdiel, J., Wang, M.C., Li, R., Gillies, R., Casalino, L., *et al.* (2005) An empirical assessment of high-performing medical groups: Results from a national study. *Medical Care Research and Review, 62*(4), 407–434.

Spector, N., Ulrich, B., and Barnsteiner, J. (2017) New graduate transition into practice: Improving quality and safety. In G. Sherwood and J. Barnsteiner (Eds.), *Quality and safety in nursing: A competency approach to improving outcomes.* 2nd Ed. Hoboken, NJ: Wiley-Blackwell.

Tracey, M.F., and Barnsteiner, J. (2012). Evidence-based practice. In G. Sherwood and J. Barnsteiner (Eds.), *Quality and safety in nursing: A competency approach to improving outcomes.* Hoboken, NJ: Wiley-Blackwell.

Trbovich, P., Prakash, V., Stewart, J., Trip, K., and Savage, P. (2010) Interruptions during the delivery of high-risk medications. *Journal of Nursing Administration, 40*, 211–218.

Wachter, R.M., and Pronovost, P.J. (2009) Balancing "no blame" with accountability in patient safety. *New England Journal of Medicine, 361*(14), 1401–1406.

Waldrup, W., Murray, D.J., Boulet, J.R., and Kraus J.F. (2009) Management of equipment anesthesia failure: A simulation-based resident skill assessment. *Anesthesia and Analgesia, 109*, 426–433.

Walton, M.K. and Barnsteiner, J. (2017) Patient-centered care. In G. Sherwood and J. Barnsteiner (Eds.), *Quality and safety in nursing: A competency approach to improving outcomes.* 2nd Ed. Hoboken, NJ: Wiley-Blackwell.

Warren, J. and Clancy, T. (2017) Informatics. In G. Sherwood and J. Barnsteiner (Eds.), *Quality and safety in nursing: A competency approach to improving outcomes.* 2nd Ed. Hoboken, NJ: Wiley-Blackwell.

Welsh, C., Flanagan, M., and Ebright, P. (2010) Barriers and facilitators to nursing handoffs: Recommendations for redesign, *Nursing Outlook, 58*, 148–154.

White, A.A., Waterman, A., McCotter, P., Boyle, D., and Gallagher, T.H. (2008) Supporting health care workers after medical error: Considerations for healthcare leaders. *Journal of Clinical Outcomes Management, 15*, 240–247.

Wolf, Z.R. (2005) Stress management in response to practice errors: Critical events in professional practice. *PA-PSRS Patient Safety Advisory*, 2(4), 1–4.

Wu, A.W. (2000) Medical error: The second victim. The doctor who makes mistakes needs help too. *British Medical Journal*, 320(7237), 726–727.

Resources

Agency for Healthcare Research and Quality (AHRQ). www.ahrq.gov

AHRQ SBAR (situation-background-assessment-recommendation). http://www.innovations.ahrq.gov/disclaimer.aspx?redirect=http%3a%2f%2fwww.ihi.org%2fIHI%2fTopics%2fPatientSafety%2fSafetyGeneral%2fTools%2fSBARTechniqueforCommunicationASituationalBriefingModel.htm

American Hospital Association. http://www.aha.org/

American Nurses Association. http://nursingworld.org/

American Society of Health System Pharmacists. http://www.ashp.org/

AORN Information for Surgical Patients. http://www.aorn.org/aboutaorn/whoweare/informationforsurgicalpatients/

Centers for Disease Control and Prevention. www.cdc.gov

Center for Medicare and Medicaid Services. http://www.cms.hhs.gov/center/quality.asp

Consumers Advancing Patient Safety. www.patientsafety.org

Emergency Care Research Institute. www.mdsr.ecri.org

Food and Drug Administration. www.fda.gov

Institute for Healthcare Improvement. http://www.ihi.org/ihi

Institute for Healthcare Improvement Open School for Health Professions. www.ihi.org/OpenSchool

Institute for Healthcare Improvement. Skilled Nursing Facility Trigger Tool for Measuring Adverse Events. Retrieved from: http://www.ihi.org/resources/Pages/Tools/SkilledNursingFacilityTriggerTool.aspx

IHI SBAR Tool Kit retrieved from: http://www.ihi.org/resources/Pages/Tools/SBARToolkit.aspx

Institute for Safe Medication Practices. www.ismp.org

Institute of Medicine. http://www.iom.edu/

The Joint Commission (formerly known at JCAHO). http://www.jointcommission.org/

The Joint Commission International Center for Patient Safety. http://www.jcipatientsafety.org/

The LeapFrog Group. http://www.leapfroggroup.org/about_us

Massachusetts Coalition for the Prevention of Medical Errors. http://www.macoalition.org/

Medical Error and Patient Safety Learning. www.medicalerrorreduction.com

Medwatch. http://www.fda.gov/medwatch/index.html

National Coordinating Council for Medication Error Reporting and Prevention. http://www.nccmerp.org/

National Center for Patient Safety. http://www.patientsafety.gov/

National Family Caregivers Association. http://www.thefamilycaregiver.org

National Patient Safety Foundation. http://www.npsf.org/

National Quality Forum. http://www.qualityforum.org/

Partnership for Patient Safety. www.p4ps.org

P.U.L.S.E. (Persons United Limiting Substandards and Errors in Healthcare).www.pulseamerica.org

Quality and Safety Education for Nurses. www.qsen.org

VA National Center for Patient Safety—Patient Safety Resources. www.va.gov/NCPS/resources.html

Voice4Patients.com. http://www.voice4patients.com/

World Health Organization—International Alliance for Patient Safety. http://www.who.int/en/

9

Informatics

Thomas R. Clancy, MBA, PhD, RN, FAAN and Judith J. Warren, PhD, RN, BC, FAAN, FACMI

As a care coordinator for a large health system, Hannah was responsible for managing the health needs of the systems diabetic population. Her typical day started by accessing the health systems EHR and running a report on all newly diagnosed diabetics seen in the systems' hospitals and or clinics. Knowing that all new diabetics were given access to the health systems portal, Hannah sent an email to each patient's home address to inform them that she would be contacting them in the next day to set up a virtual visit by computer. During the visit Hannah would show each patient how to track their Hba1c in their personal health record (PHR) as well as how to input their daily glucose readings. Hannah also enrolled each patient in the hospitals online support group and patient diabetic education center. Finally, Hannah oriented patients on the mobile application that alerted patients when their medications and blood sampling was due.

Hannah then turned to the existing population of diabetics in the health system and reviewed the clinical outcomes dashboard displayed in the EHR. By drilling down on key indicators in the dashboard, Hannah was able to determine opportunities to improve care. Using advanced clinical decision support systems, Hannah was able to predict which patients were at the highest risk of suffering an event that would result in a hospital admission. She then reviewed the most current data on these patients, which included vital signs from sensors in home monitoring devices and wearable technology, lab results from implanted pumps, nutrition, exercise and sleep logs from the PHR, medication compliance from the mobile app, and participation in online support groups and education. Finally, Hannah contacted those patients at highest risk and set up an intervention plan to get them back on track.

If you think this is a glimpse of the future, think again. This is the world of nursing informatics today!

> In attempting to arrive at the truth, I have applied everywhere for information, but in scarcely an instance have I been able to obtain hospital records fit for any purposes of comparison. If they could be obtained they would enable us to decide many other questions besides the ones alluded to. They would show the subscribers how their money was being spent, what amount of good was really being done with it, or whether the money was not doing mischief rather than good. Florence Nightingale (1863,)

Florence Nightingale, an informatics nurse at heart, demonstrated what could be done with data and information to improve patient care. In her quote above, she alludes to the uses of organized patient records that would reveal the contributions of nursing to cost effective, safe, quality patient care. As information and computer technologies have evolved, they have been identified as strategies

Quality and Safety in Nursing: A Competency Approach to Improving Outcomes, Second Edition.
Edited by Gwen Sherwood and Jane Barnsteiner.
© 2017 John Wiley & Sons, Inc. Published 2017 by John Wiley & Sons, Inc.

to ensure safe patient care (IOM, 2001). The patient safety series of books commissioned by IOM have consistently identified informatics as a major infrastructure component of patient safety, including presenting patient information as a structure that supports clinical decision making, as are providing alerts, reminders, and clinical decision support; serving as a communications tool for the health care team; and supporting quality improvement and clinical research. As information and computer sciences have matured, the vision of health information technology and electronic health records is being achieved. Now the challenge is to educate our educators, students, and clinicians on how to take advantage of these new clinical tools in caring for patients.

Nursing informatics is emerging into the forefront of patient care issues as a result of three major innovations: the maturing of health information technology, national legislation requiring the transformation of health care through the use of health information technology, and nursing education initiatives responding to the technology and legislative trends. HIT has evolved and produced EHRs that are able to store and organize the information captured during clinical work flows and return that information in views designed to support clinical design making. As work has progressed on sharing patient information within an organization, health information exchange between organizations has become important. This ensures that a patient's information follows them wherever they need care. For health information exchange to work in a safe, secure manner, the importance of harmonizing health information through evidence-based protocols, quality measures, health informatics standards, and standardized health and nursing terminologies has emerged as major efforts in the delivery of patient care. Social networking is another powerful information technology being used in patient care. Health care providers are using Facebook, LinkedIn, Twitter, RSS feeds, Listservs, virtual worlds, and dynamic web pages to interact with patients, providing services, information, and education (Mayo Clinic, 2011). Being competent in the use of these technologies is becoming essential for the nursing and the health care team.

Health care reform has been the initiator of transformations in the use of HIT in recent years, creating an intense focus on the implementation and use of information in patient care through use of EHRs and health information exchange (HIE). The Health Insurance Portability and Accountability Act (HIPAA) of 1996 was the first major legislation to influence the use of standards and terminology in patient records, as well as ensuring the privacy and confidentiality of those records (HIPAA, 1996). These regulations have come to be known as administrative simplification. The American Recovery and Reinvestment Act of 2009 included provisions for the infusion of resources and funding for HIT in health care. The section of the act that focused on HIT has become known as the HITECH Act (HITECH, 2010). HITECH provided funds for education and research in informatics and financial incentives for the "Meaningful Use" of electronic health records (Office of the National Coordinator for Health IT, 2011). Providers must demonstrate meaningful use of EHRs between 2011 and 2015 to qualify for the financial incentives. Features of this demonstration include a patient problem list and quality measures, among other requirements. In 2010, the Patient Protection and Affordable Care Act was passed with additional requirements for the use of HIT in patient care, mainly in the form of administrative simplification aimed at reducing health care costs (Affordable Care Act, 2010). These three landmark pieces of legislation, and their resultant regulations, have created a demand for health care professionals who are competent in meaningfully using HIT, including EHRs.

The final innovation is education's response to the maturing of technology and the legalization demand for meaningful use of that technology (Warren and Connors, 2007). IOM, as part of their patient safety series of reports, issued a call to the health profession's educators to transform professional education to include patient-centered care, teamwork and collaboration, evidence-based practice, quality improvement, and informatics (Greiner and Knebel, 2003). They saw these five areas of competency as essential to providing safe patient care. The QSEN project was a major nursing response to this call (Cronenwett *et al.*, 2007; Cronenwett *et al.*, 2009). As a result of the QSEN work, both the AACN and the NLN have integrated the work in their accreditation criteria for schools of nursing. Until these criteria were published, nursing informatics was viewed as a nursing specialty taught in graduate programs, and only a few of those existed.

Development of the QSEN Informatics Competencies

The first step in developing competencies is to define the domain for the work. The ANA defines the specialty of nursing informatics as the facilitation of the integration of data, information, knowledge, and wisdom to support patients, nurses, and other providers in decision making. This is accomplished through the use of information structures and information technology. Nursing informatics is the study and implementation of structures and algorithms to improve communication, understanding, and management of nursing information. Informatics nurses develop symbolic representations of nursing information that can be processed in information systems, regardless of the type of technology used. Structures and algorithms are essential and distinguish nursing informatics from other nursing specialties where the information context is the distinguishing feature. The core phenomena of nursing informatics are 1) all data, information, and knowledge involved in nursing; and 2) the symbolic representation of nursing phenomena (American Nurses Association, 2008). The challenge now is to determine the informatics competencies needed in general and in advanced nursing practice and how to educate our workforce.

Informatics Competencies

Early work on defining informatics competencies was conducted by Staggers, Gassert, and Curran (2001; 2002) as they studied competencies for four levels of practice: staff nurses, administrative nurses, informatics nurses, and informatics researchers. This Delphi study was composed of a panel drawn from informatics experts and informatics educators. Subsequent work on informatics competencies is based on this foundational study. Curran expanded the competencies by identifying those for nurse practitioners (2003). As this work was being completed in the United States, Australia (Smedley, 2005) and Canada (Booth, 2006) were developing informatics competencies using the work of Staggers and colleagues. Most of the competencies identified were basic computer competencies, literacy competencies, and information management (informatics) competencies.

The TIGER Summit was convened to create a nursing profession-wide consortium to promote informatics and technology competencies (Ball *et al.*, 2011). Again the work of Staggers was used to begin the work of identifying informatics competencies. The QSEN informatics competencies were then added to the analysis (Cronenwett *et al.*, 2007; Cronenwett *et al.*, 2009). Computer competencies, though not part of QSEN, were added to the TIGER work. The work of Hobbs (2002) was consulted for adding these competencies. Other competency work being conducted in education and staff development was used to refine the list of informatics competencies (Barton, 2005; Desjardins *et al.*, 2005; McNeil *et al.*, 2003; McNeil *et al.*, 2005; Sackett, Jones, and Erdley, 2005; Simpson, 2005). Finally, information literacy was included in the competencies. The information literacy competencies are based on the work of the National Forum on Information Literacy (n.d.).

The development of the QSEN informatics competencies also was based on the Staggers work. However, the decision was made not to include computer literacy and basic computer skills. The IOM report (Greiner and Knebel, 2003) concerning informatics was clear that computer skills were not included; the focus was on the information management and representation portion of the informatics domain. Information literacy was included as that is essential not only for informatics competencies but also the evidence-based practice competencies. The competencies were then leveled for prelicensure students and advanced nursing practice students (Cronenwett *et al.*, 2007; Cronenwett *et al.*, 2009). The final competencies are listed in Appendices A and B. The informatics competency threads through all six QSEN competencies. Managing patient history, data, and preferences in the EHR enables patient-centered care (Walton and Barnsteiner, 2017). The tools and strategies utilized in developing evidence-based standards of care are based on informatics application (Tracey and Barnsteiner, 2017). Quality improvement can only happen through technology-based tools and decision support software (Johnson, 2017). Safety alerts, error reporting systems and management, and system improvements use informatics application (Barnsteiner, 2017). Interprofessional teams communicate and manage collaborative relationships via technology (Disch, 2017). Informatics is integrated to some degree throughout quality and safety.

Educational Strategies for Teaching Informatics

Educating Nurse Educators

A significant percentage of nurse educators lack education or experience in informatics, as this area of expertise has only recently evolved. As nursing students require more informatics knowledge, skills, and attitudes, it is imperative that nurse educators master the QSEN advanced nursing practice informatics competencies so that they may create curricula and learning strategies to help students become competent in this area. Academic administrators must encourage and support nursing educators to get involved in lifelong learning activities concerning informatics (Bakken *et al.*, 2004; Booth, 2006). Bakken and colleagues (2004) recommend three strategies to achieve nurse educator competence: seminars and small workshops related to informatics, consultation with informatics nurses on developing assignments to ensure informatics content, and having informatics nurses as guest lecturers or as part of the course team. A fourth strategy is to partner with a clinical agency that has an EHR and have educators spend time at the agency learning how the EHR is designed, built, implemented, and used on a daily basis. Talk with them about the impact of federal legislation and reimbursement policies on the demand for electronic information. Other strategies would be to work with QSEN consultants (http://www.qsen.org/consultants.php) and to attend QSEN conferences.

Creating Curricula

There are two tools that may help educators integrate informatics knowledge, skills, and attitudes into their courses: curriculum/course maps and course sequencing guides. A curriculum map lays out the content and its relationships so that educators can ensure that essential content and requirements are taught. As educators plot the content in a curriculum map and propose learning activities, they should investigate the way students are taught to manage patient data, not only the documentation of care but the retrieval of information about the patient for care and quality purposes. It is the representation and manipulation of data and information that is informatics, regardless of technology used. The content reveals the discipline of nursing. Second, a national Delphi study was conducted to provide guidance on sequencing QSEN competencies in the undergraduate curriculum (Barton *et al.*, 2009). The results of this survey will assist in knowing where and when in the curriculum to introduce and reinforce informatics content and competencies.

A second approach to curriculum and course design is mind mapping. Mind mapping provides an opportunity to look at related concepts that can be combined to teach a variety of competencies. See Figures 9.1 and 9.2 for examples of mind maps using the QSEN prelicensure and advanced nursing practice informatics competencies as source material. When the material is presented as a map with relationships, new ideas of working with the competencies or placing them in courses may emerge.

A helpful resource used in creating an informatics curricula is to develop a crosswalk that aligns those competencies created by professional organizations such as AACN, ANA, TIGER, QSEN, and others with examples. Table 9.1 provides one illustration of a crosswalk between the AACN

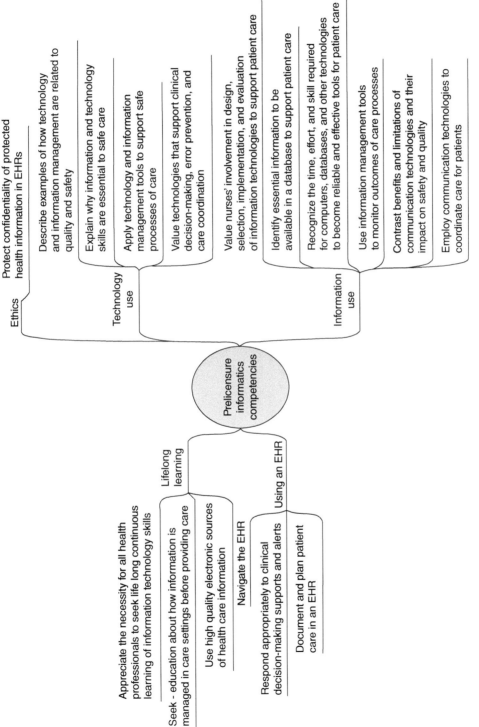

Figure 9.1 Mind map of the pre-licensure informatics competencies group by conceptual categories using FreeMind, a mind mapping tool, available at http://freemind.sourceforge.net/wiki/index.php/Download

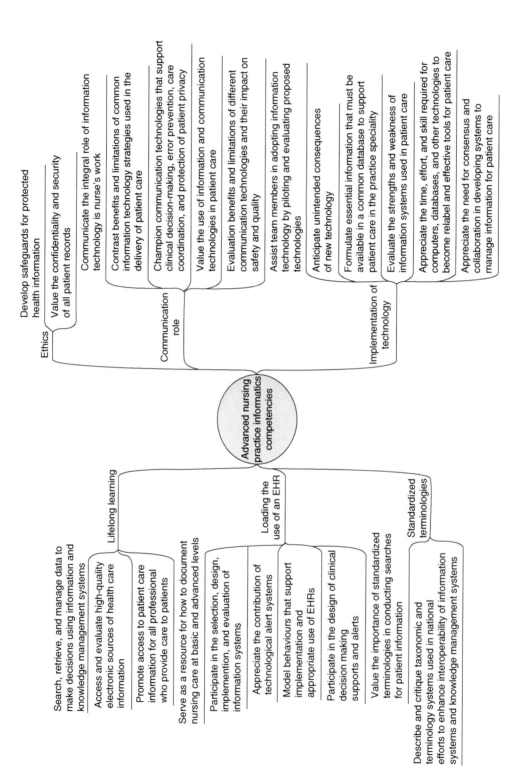

Figure 9.2 Mind map of the advanced nursing practice informatics competencies group by conceptual categories, using FreeMind. Source: using FreeMind, a mind mapping tool, available at http://freemind.sourceforge.net/wiki/index.php/Download

Table 9.1 Crosswalk for AACN BSN Essentials, TIGER Competencies, and QSEN KSAs for Informatics.

#	AACN[1]	Definitions of Terms	AACN Sample Content	TIGER[2] Competencies	QSEN[3] Knowledge	QSEN Skills	QSEN Attitudes
1	Demonstrate skills in using **patient care technologies**, **information systems**, and **communication devices** that support safe nursing practice.	**Patient Care Technologies** • Computers, printers • IV smart pumps • Bar coded medication management systems • Pulse oximeters • Automated blood pressure and pulse • Monitoring equipment (ECG, arterial blood pressure, respirations) • Automated temperature • Defibrillators **Communication Devices** • Smart phones, hands-free mobile communication devices (Vocera), tablets (iPads)	Computer skills that may include basic software, spreadsheet, and health care databases Use of patient care technologies (e.g., monitors, pumps, computer-assisted devices)	**Basic Computer Competencies** 1.1 Hardware 1.2 Software 1.3 Networks 1.4 Information and communication technology 2.1 Operating systems 2.2 File management 2.3 Utilities 2.4 Print management 3.1 Applications 7.1 The Intranet 7.2 Browser 7.3 Using the web 7.4 Web outputs	Explain why information and technology skills are essential for safe patient care.	Seek education about how information is managed in care settings before providing care.	Appreciate the necessity for all health professionals to seek lifelong, continuous learning of information technology skills.
2	Understand the use of **CIS (clinical information systems)** to document interventions related to achieving nurse sensitive outcomes.	**Clinical Information Systems** Electronic health records in: • Acute care • Ambulatory care • Skilled nursing care • Home and community health systems • Public health systems	Electronic health records/physician order entry	**Information Management Competencies** 1.0 Demographics 2.0 Consents 3.0 Medicationmanagement 4.0 Planning care 5.0 Order results 6.0 Care documentation		Document and plan patient care in an electronic health record. Navigate the electronic health record.	

(Continued)

Table 9.1 (Continued)

#	AACN[1]	Definitions of Terms	AACN Sample Content	TIGER[2] Competencies	QSEN[3] Knowledge	QSEN Skills	QSEN Attitudes
		Applications to manage care: • Provider order entry • Clinical documentation (assessment, care planning, other) • Results reporting • Bar coded medication administration (BCMA) • Electronic medication administration record (eMar) • Ancillary systems (pharmacy, lab, radiology)					
3	Advocate for the use of new patient care technologies for safe, quality care	New Patient Technologies: • Emobile health • Telehealth • Patient engagement/ personal health records • Social media • Predictive analytics and "Big Data" • Robotics • Nano-technology and 3D computing • 3D Printing • Wearable technology					

#	Competency		Knowledge	Competencies			
4	Use **telecommunication technologies** to assist in effective communication in a variety of healthcare settings.	**Telecommunications technologies:** Email Telehealth: • Patient monitoring technologies (virtual assessments, ICUs) • Home sensing devices (weight scale, blood pressure (BP) monitor, bed chair, glucose meter, implant monitors, baby monitors, spirometer, medication monitoring, pedometer) Patient engagement: • Personal health records • Health literacy web sites • Social networking	Technology for virtual care delivery and monitoring Information literacy Interstate practice regulations (e.g., licensure, telehealth)	**Basic Computer Competencies** 1.9 Information and communication technology 7.5 Electronic communication 7.6 Using e-mail 7.7 E-mail management Information Management Competencies: 9.0 Facilitating communications	Contrast benefits and limitations of different communication technologies and their impact on safety and quality.	Employ communication technologies to coordinate care for patients.	
5	Apply **safeguards** and **decision-making support tools** embedded in patient care technologies and information systems to support a safe practice environment for both patients and health care workers.	**Safeguards and decision-making support (Information Systems)** • *Medication dosing support* (medication pick lists, dosing calculators) • *Order facilitators* (order sets for specific conditions based on evidence based guidelines: pneumonia, adult prosthetic hip replacement, myocardial infarction [MI]) • *Point of care alerts* (drug to drug interactions, duplicate therapy, drug allergies, contraindications to specific conditions)	Use of technology and information systems for clinical decision making Technology and information systems safeguards (e.g., patient monitoring, equipment, patient identifications systems, drug alerts, IV systems, and bar coding)	**Information Management Competencies** 1.0 Decision support 2.0 Notifications	Describe examples of how technology and information management are related to the quality and safety of patient care.	Respond appropriately to clinical decision-making supports and alerts. Apply technology and information management tools to support safe processes of care.	Value technologies that support clinical decision-making, error prevention, and care coordination.

(Continued)

Table 9.1 (Continued)

#	AACN[1]	Definitions of Terms	AACN Sample Content	TIGER[2] Competencies	QSEN[3] Knowledge	QSEN Skills	QSEN Attitudes
6	Recognize the role of information technology in improving patient care outcomes and creating a safe care environment.	*Point of care reminders* (immunizations, cancer screenings, fall prevention, pain management). *Information displays* (dashboards of relevant data)					
7	Use **standardized terminology** in a care environment that reflects nursing's unique contribution to patient outcomes.	**Standardized terminologies** • Multidisciplinary terminologies (SNOMED-CT, LOINC) q1 need to define these? • Nursing terminologies (CCC, ICNP, NANDA, NIC, NOC, OS, PNDS) q1 and these?	Information management for patient safety	**Information Literacy** 2.9 Understand how to use classification systems and their rationale.	Identify essential information that must be available in a common database to support patient care.	Use information management tools to monitor outcomes of care processes.	
8	Evaluate data from all **relevant sources,** including technology, to inform the delivery of care.	Relevant sources • Literature search methods to access, evaluate information, apply to practice and evaluate outcomes	Retrieval information systems, including access, evaluation of data, and application of relevant data to patient care On-ine literature searches Technological resources for evidence-based practice Web-based learning and online literature searches for self and patient use	**Information Literacy Competencies** 1) Knowledge 2) Access 3) Evaluate information 4) Application 5) Evaluate outcomes		Use high quality electronic sources of health care information.	

#					
9	Apply patient-care technologies as appropriate to address the needs of a diverse patient population.	Diverse patient population • Ethnic/racial • Gender • Cultural • Uninsured/under-insured/homeless • Sexual orientation • Elderly/adult/adolescent/pediatric			
10	Recognize that redesign of **work flow and care processes** should precede implementation of care technology to facilitate nursing practice.	**Work Flow and Care Processes** • SDLC–Systems Design Life Cycle • Human computer interaction		Recognize the time, effort, and skill required for computers, databases, and other technologies to become reliable and effective tools for patient care.	Value nurses' involvement in design, selection, implementation, and evaluation of information technologies to support patient care.
11	Participate in evaluation of information systems in practice settings through policy and procedure development.				
12	Uphold ethical standards related to **data security, regulatory requirements, confidentiality,** and **clients' right to privacy.**	**Data Security, regulatory, confidentiality, right to privacy** • HIPAA • Copyright laws • Ethical behavior	Ethical and legal issues related to the use of information technology, including copyright, privacy, and confidentiality issues	**Basic Computer Competency** 1.10 Security 1.11 Law	Protect confidentiality of protected health information in electronic health records.

Source:
[1] American Association of Colleges of Nursing Essentials of Baccalaureate Education for Professional Nursing Practice and Took Kit. (2008) Accessed August 30, 2015 http://www.aacn.nche.edu/education-resources/BaccEssentials08.pdf
[2] TIGER Competencies for Practicing Nurses. (2015) Accessed August 30, 2015 http://www.thetigerinitiative.org/docs/TigerReport_InformaticsCompetencies.pdf
[3] QSEN Institute web site, Frances Payne Bolton School of Nursing, Case Western University. (2015) Accessed August 30, 2015 http://qsen.org/competencies/

Information Management and Technology Essentials for Baccalaureate Education for Professional Nursing Practice, the TIGER Informatics Competencies for Practicing Nurses, and the QSEN competencies for informatics. Creating a crosswalk provides an opportunity to define each competency, illustrate examples, and better understand common themes. This also aids in ensuring each competency is integrated in the curricula and can be readily located during accreditation surveys.

Educating Students

There are many strategies for teaching informatics competencies. The most obvious are lectures with readings, slides, or handouts highlighting the most critical competencies. Attitudes may also be taught in this manner, with the educator serving as role model and mentor. Most professional attitudes are learned through this approach. Online courses present learning material through the use of modules that contain overviews, objectives, readings, resources (videos, software, web pages, podcasts, virtual worlds, and games), and assignments (quizzes, discussion boards, projects, papers, concept maps, mind maps, web site evaluations, etc.) to teach all three types of competencies. The QSEN web page has numerous activities with directions and resources for educators to adapt and use to develop assignments for lectures and modules (http://www.qsen.org/view_strategies.php).

Assignments fostering information literacy are essential for students who must live and work in the information age. Flood, Gasiewicz, and Delpier (2010) have developed a sequence of five assignments to increase a student's ability to recognize the need for knowledge. In the first assignment the students are taught to search and evaluate the literature. The second assignment is the development of a teaching brochure based on a literature review. In the third assignment, the student identifies an organizational policy or procedure, conducts a literature review, compares the policy to the evidence, and then makes recommendations. The fourth assignment is a care plan for a complex patient based on a literature review and evidence evaluation. The final assignment has the student selecting a clinical setting and identifying how informatics and health information are used to make decisions. Planning activities with library literature searches meets one of the informatics competencies. Including information literacy is essential as it is part of the QSEN and TIGER competencies, yet many do not consider this as part of informatics (Dixon and Newlon, 2010).

Another literature evaluation activity is to evaluate a web site that provides health information. Eight questions guide a good critique: What can the URL tell you? Who wrote the page and are they a qualified authority? Is it dated, current, timely? Is the information cited authentic? Does the page have overall integrity and reliability as a source? Are there biases in the presentation of information? Could the page or site be ironic, like a satire or a spoof? If you have questions or reservations, can you ask them? The QSEN web site has other web page evaluation criteria and activities. This activity helps the student learn how to select a good web site to recommend to a patient and family and how to tell a patient and family whether the information they are getting from the web is accurate and safe to use.

Engaging students in evaluating their own competency achievement is a powerful strategy to promote engagement in learning and rich feedback. Although the assessment tool can be used in a variety of ways, the tool that best helps students focus is the completion of the self-assessment at the beginning of a course. Then the student can develop a personal action plan to achieve or enhance their competency attainment. During the semester, they should work on the plan. At the end of the course, students should complete the self-assessment again and evaluate their strategies for attaining competency.

The next strategy is to review current assignments. If the assignment is about patient information management or care planning, is it done on paper? If it is on paper, consider replacing that assignment with managing the patient data electronically using software such as a spreadsheet, a database, or an EHR. Review the patient simulations, both low and high fidelity, and include electronic documentation of the patient information in an EHR optimized for academic uses (the software selection is growing to meet a variety of needs) to increase the fidelity and to add informatics skills. Also, include retrieval of patient information for purposes of gathering information for clinical decision making, quality improvement analysis, administrative reporting, and clinical research.

Every curriculum contains education concerning ethics. HIPAA and the ACA have very strong requirements for safeguarding the confidentiality, privacy, and security of patient records, both paper and electronic. Most hospitals require HIPAA training before students are allowed to care for their patients. Be sure to identify this education as achieving both informatics knowledge and attitude competencies. If the information and practice about managing usernames and passwords is added to the lesson, then a skill competency also is achieved.

Nursing care plans are another teaching strategy. From an informatics perspective, this is the overarching representation structure of nursing knowledge. We teach students about assessment data, nursing problem lists, goals, interventions, and outcomes. Most EHRs have designed and structured nursing information in accordance with this representation. The structure may be displayed similarly to a paper format of a care plan or it may put each of the care plan structures in a different location. Either way, students need to be taught about the components in order to learn how to navigate an EHR to enter and find the patient information they need. An added benefit of teaching the components of a nursing care plan in an EHR is that it provides images to the student of what is being discussed. By adding this teaching strategy, visual learners are supported and nursing process skills are improved (Kennedy, Pallikkathavil, and Warren, 2009). As we move to EHRs, the use of standardized languages becomes imperative. It is only through coded structured data that we can aggregate, summarize, and analyze nursing's contribution to patient care outcomes (Lundberg *et al.*, 2008). The ANA has recognized both nursing-specific and health care-specific terminologies and classifications to represent nursing in a structured way. See their web site at http://nursingworld.org/npii/terminologies.htm. This web site provides links to learn about each terminology and classification and is a good resource for educators. Introducing standardized language representing nursing knowledge is critical. Most often this knowledge is taught during the nursing process learning activities.

Finally, add experiences with EHRs, both real and simulated. Initially, hospitals were reluctant to grant EHR privileges to students. As health care reform has evolved, more hospitals are implementing EHRs and are automating all patient information. They have more resources to manage EHRs and to train users. As this expertise grows, hospitals are beginning to grant EHR privileges to all students. This is another opportunity to partner with clinical agencies to provide opportunities for student to attain informatics skills in working with EHRs. Clinical agencies are beginning to realize they will be educating nurses either before or after graduation. It is better for students to learn a clinical work flow that includes EHRs than to learn one that includes paper only and then have to learn a new work flow involving EHRs. Review the competencies and add clinical activities that foster the mastery of the competencies.

In early 2001, the need for an EHR optimized for academic purposes was identified (Connors *et al.*, 2002). In a pilot project, a production EHR was adapted for use in the classroom and clinical laboratory. An insight was that the design of forms and order sets could facilitate learning by using learning theories concerning the gestalt (field/ground), advance organizers, constructivism, reinforcement, and active engagement. By interacting with the academic EHR, students learn about the data, information, and knowledge of nursing while attaining informatics skill competencies (Connors, Warren, and Weaver, 2007; Warren *et al.*, 2004; Warren *et al.*, 2010). Assignments in the EHR included completing case studies by entering assessment data and planning care, scavenger hunts to learn navigation, graded care plans based on patients from the clinical settings (taking precautions to be HIPAA compliant), and reviewing information on forms and orders as preparation for class. Evidence-based nursing protocols were integrated into the EHR so that students could experience, analyze, and appreciate how these protocols are deconstructed and then implemented into an EHR (Weaver, Warren, and Delaney, 2005). As a result of the success of this pilot, more than 40 schools have adopted this particular learning strategy. Furthermore, simulated EHRs have joined the market to fill the need of having students engage with EHRs.

Combining the EHR with simulations, both low and high fidelity, creates an optimal learning environment. Students can engage in simple and complex scenarios while performing work flows required in clinical practice. The EHR requires point of care documentation. Clinicians depend on the information in the EHR to be accurate and current. Clinicians, once they thoroughly integrate the EHR in their work flows, base their decision on the information available. The information age has taught us that we can go to one electronic source and have all information brought to us—the EHR vendors sell their products based on this fact. Learning to give care and document at the point of care is a necessary skill and must be learned—simulations provide the place to begin this learning. A typical simulation would have the students accessing the EHR to find information about the patient in their simulation. During the simulation they would document the care given, looking up labs, orders, and other tasks done in the clinical setting. Debriefing would explore how the student accessed information and responded in the case. In a low-fidelity simulation, such as a skills check off, documenting the skill in the EHR would be the last step in the check off, as this is the preferred clinical work flow (Warren *et al.*, 2010).

Strategies for Building an Informatics Curriculum

Given the growing specialization of the information technology, it is unrealistic to expect all faculty to acquire the skill and knowledge to teach informatics. Rather, it is important to concentrate informatics expertise among a core group of faculty that has an interest in the field. These members can then teach informatics courses and act as a resource to other faculty for integration of informatics concepts and applications in their courses. This core group can also attend workshops, certification courses, and other professional development events to stay abreast of current technology.

There is a common misperception that informatics is focused, primarily, on gaining proficiency in the use of EHRs. Becoming competent in navigating EHRs is an important skill for clinical nurses; however, nursing informatics is much more than this. It encompasses the management of information surrounding a body of knowledge specific to nursing. Thus, the field includes knowledge representation through standardized nursing languages, information system design, and analysis of nursing work flow, telehealth, consumer informatics and patient engagement, clinical decision support, robotics, mobile technology, information literacy, data science, and a host of other areas. To experience these many areas, it is important for faculty teaching informatics to either obtain an advanced degree in the field or complete a certification course in informatics. A number of universities and professional organizations now offer these resources (American Medical Informatics Association, 2015; University of Minnesota School of Nursing, 2015).

A key strategy in building an informatics program is the development of academic/practice partnerships between nursing schools and health systems. The financial resources required to purchase simulated EHRs, bar coded medication dispensers, telehealth equipment, and other types of information technology can be substantial. Integrating an informatics curriculum into a health system's existing training programs can provide many benefits. Nursing schools can expose students to state of the art information systems without a large, upfront capital investment in EHR software. Faculty members also have the opportunity to jointly develop with health system educators, the training curriculum for both clinical nurses and nursing students. Successful creation of an academic/practice partnership for shared information technology will need to include the EHR vendor currently in use at the health facility. A training "sandbox" can be created with simulated patient medical histories, orders,and nursing documentation flow sheets. The partnership may also include more advanced equipment and applications such as shared telehealth equipment, care coordination software, and patient engagement portals.

An emerging resource for informatics faculty is online training and software applications, many of which are free on the web. For example, Northstar, a non-profit agency, has made available a free online certificate program that focuses on basic computer skills such as email, Intranet browsers, file management, word processing, using spreadsheets and social media (Northstar, 2015). Edith Cowan University has made available free YouTube tutorials on basic computer literacy skills (Edith Cowan, 2015). Open EMR is a free open source electronic health record that is used by many healthcare facilities (Open EMR, 2015). The application can be used to develop use cases for student teaching if faculty members are willing to create simulated patient data. The Healthcare Systems and Management Society (HIMSS) hosts the TIGER Virtual Learning Environment, an interactive online portal for academic professionals, students, adult learners, and clinical educators that contains a host of health information technology (IT) resources (Edith Cowan, 2015). The AACN, the University of Minnesota School of Nursing, and the Gordon and Betty Moore Foundation have supported the development of informatics webinars, workshops, and online resources specifically aimed at nursing school faculty (National Nursing Informatics Deep Dive Program, 2015). The American Medical Informatics Association (AMIA) provides an introductory course and certification course in health care informatics called the AMIA 10x10 (American Medical Informatics Association 10x10 Courses, 2015). The key point is that many of these resources are now available on the web to assist faculty integrate applications into an informatics curricula.

Implications for Nursing Practice

Nurses are expected to provide safe care in an increasingly technical environment. This technology has changed the role of the nurse and significantly altered the interactions between the nurse and patient. Nurses who have not mastered basic informatics competencies will be at a disadvantage as health care moves to achieve 100% EHR adoption by 2014, a presidential goal. To meet this challenge, the TIGER Summit was convened (http://www.tigersummit.com/Competencies_New_B949.html). The membership of the summit was drawn from professional nursing organizations from the areas of practice, education, administration, and research. The goals of the summit were to develop a strategic plan in which all organizations could work collaboratively to achieve the challenge. A team composed of volunteers was established with the summit to develop informatics competencies for the practicing nurse. The competency model consists of basic computer competencies, information literacy, and information management (including use of an EHR; TIGER Summit, n.d.). The work of QSEN was shared with this team. This competency work is foundational to the work of the other teams for staff development, educator development, and leadership development. The work of the TIGER Summit also identified development needs for educators that may be used to help them gain informatics competencies (Hebda and Calderone, 2010).

The HITECH act has ensured that informatics competencies are a high priority for all health care organizations. The legislation provides funds for HIT training, regional EHR support for small practices and hospitals, research on the use of HIT, and state health information exchange initiatives. A second part of the legislation ties Medicare and Medicaid reimbursement at a preferential rate to those providers who can demonstrate "meaningful use." The criteria for this demonstration are the use of patient problem lists, allergy lists, immunization records, discharge summaries, computerized provider order entry, and quality measures. Furthermore, there is a requirement for reimbursement information to be submitted electronically to Medicare and Medicaid. This requirement has created a major stimulus for purchasing and implementing EHRs that are certified for this purpose. Health care organizations are challenged with not only implementing EHRs but also training their workforce to be meaningful users. There is a need for new graduates who are entering the workforce to have informatics competencies.

Kaiser-Permanente provides an exemplar of the challenges in nursing practice when implementing EHRs. The nursing department wanted an information system that promoted evidence-based practice, supported a professional practice framework, and enabled point of care documentation (Chow and Fong, 2010). Nurses in leadership and staff positions were involved in the selection, design, and implementation of the EHR—a major informatics competency. The design included a requirement to compare information across their practice sites in order to promote quality patient care and to identify normal variances in practice. Terminology had to be standardized and brand names eliminated from care documentation. They also created standard data definitions for describing common patient observations, for example, pain, falls, and pressure ulcers. Evidence-based scales were selected to ensure data quality and standardization. Assessment forms from multiple sites were harmonized so that core documentation would occur at all Kaiser-Permanente sites. What is described is a new environment for the practice of nursing that is heavily influenced by technology and informatics. Both practice and academia need to retool and partner with each other to ensure the success of nursing practice in this environment.

In 2008, the RWJF and the IOM collaborated on a project to assess and transform the nursing profession: *The Future of Nursing: Leading Change, Advancing Health* (IOM, 2011). Two of the recommendations include informatics initiatives. Recommendation 2 was to "Expand opportunities for nurses to lead and diffuse collaborative improvement efforts." Private and public funders are charged with providing funds to advance research on models of care and innovative solutions, including information technology that will contribute to improved health and health care. Health care organizations must engage nurses to work with developers in the design, development, purchase, implementation, and evaluation of EHRs. Recommendation 6 was to "Ensure that nurses engage in lifelong learning." The recommendation encouraged educators to partner with health care organizations to develop and prioritize competencies so curricula can be updated regularly to ensure that graduates at all levels are prepared to meet the current and future health needs of the population.

Emerging Informatics Trends and Implications for Nurse Educators

A major challenge faced by nurse educators in the coming years will be staying current in the face of explosive growth of new information technology. The convergence of four key technology trends today will dramatically change how and where clinical nurses practice. These trends include exponential growth in computer processing power, the ongoing digitization of new forms of data, the relentless buildout of the Intranet, and the transition to mobile technology.

Since first being observed by Gordon Moore in 1965, computer processing power has been doubling every year (Intel, 2015). Much of this has been related to better design of microprocessors, improved computer storage capacity, and the efficiencies gained moving from analog to digital signal processing. As a result, future technology will continue to be faster, smaller, and less costly than today's. This has enabled enormous improvements in micro-sensors that are now embedded in just about everything (including humans through implanted and wearable technology). Today's sensors collect multiple types of data that include physical activity, physiological data, geo-spacial location, sleep patterns, and other data through the quantified self-movement. Social media and patient engagement sites provide a rich source of data on human behavior and social patterns. Add to this the growth of data processed through EHRs and the emerging field of human genomics and the opportunities for creating knowledge value from large scale data sets or "big data" is enormous. And connecting all these devices and systems is the relentless buildout of the Intranet and growth in mobile technology.

It is estimated that the Intranet contributes to the creation of 2.5 quintillion bytes of data daily and that 90% of the stored data in the world was created in just the last two years alone (Marcia Conner Website, 2015). For example, in health care, the number of biomedical and research journal articles has grown from 200,000 in the year 2000 to 750,000 in 2010 (Smith, Stuckhardt, and McGinnis, 2012). The build-out of the Intranet has enabled the flow of information, once accessed only in hospitals, to providers and patients anywhere. Of note is the key device emerging to facilitate this data flow: the smart phone. Of the approximately 7 billion people in the world today, it is estimated that 6 billion own a cellphone, more than the number of those with access to a bathroom (Time, 2013).

The exponential growth in new sources of data as described has provided researchers opportunities to discover patterns that can be used to describe and predict disease conditions and health care events. For example, patterns in the data or "knowledge value" can be used to predict patients at high risk for falls, pressure ulcers, central line infections, sepsis, readmission, and a host of other applications (Canton, 2015). These patterns can be represented by algorithms and then programmed as clinical decision support applications in EHRs and smart phones. Thus, nurses will have access to sophisticated clinical decision support embedded in smart phones such as symptom checkers, point of care lab testing and ultrasound capability, electrocardiogram and lung function testing, and other point of care applications (Topel, 2015). In other words, nurses and information systems will have a symbiotic relationship that enables augmented cognition and vastly improves decision making. The key point is that the technology no longer needs to reside in a hospital or ambulatory care facility. It is mobile and can be accessed in the home.

The convergence of sensor technology and new mobile applications as described is also driving, in part, the so-called "Intranet of Things" (IoT). The IoT represents a global network where devices have the capacity to transfer data without requiring human-to-human or human-to-computer interaction (Canton, 2015).

Although the IoT is in its infancy, the potential to design smart homes for seniors and those requiring close monitoring is enormous. We are already seeing homes that automatically adjust temperature, lighting, and security to appropriate levels. Fall prevention carpets (Aud *et al.*, 2010), electronic medication administration reminders (Glowcap, 2015) and bed alarms are being integrated into homes along with activity monitors and cameras.

Information technology will be a key driver in how and where nurses practice in the next 10 years. The hospital centric model is rapidly transforming to a patient centric one where the shift of care to ambulatory centers and patients homes is accelerating. The Intranet has democratized health care information, and patients are now more engaged in their health care decisions and share information readily through networked support web sites. Information technology, in part, is driving the later phases of the HITECH Act and the meaningful use of EHRs. For example, Phase 3 and 4 of meaningful use focus on care coordination, patient self-management, registries to manage specific patient populations, and patient-engaged communities (HealthIT.gov, 2015). These skills will require nurses to have knowledge of home monitoring devices, wearable technology, and population management and care coordination software.

It is imperative that clinical nurses of the future are competent in the use of information technology. Electronic health records, mobile devices, and the Intranet will be woven into the fabric of everything nurses do. For illustration, the following is a list of emerging roles for nurses and the technology that is enabling them:

Care Coordination (patient-centered medical homes)

- Advanced implantable monitoring devices (diabetic pumps, pace-makers)
- Health maintenance (smart scales, home monitoring devices)
- Population management (descriptive and predictive analytics)

Telemedicine

Virtual ambulatory care (protocol-driven virtual home visits)
Telehealth (patient assessment via telemonitoring equipment)
Remote nursing units (virtual ICUs)

Health Coaching

- Patient engagement (personal health records and health literacy)
- Self-care management through the quantified self movement (wearable technology and the IoT)
- Self and family support through social networks (self and family caregiver online support groups)

Nurse Data Scientist

- Knowledge value creation using advanced computational methodologies (big data, clinical decision support embedded in EHRs and mobile devices)
- Clinical and administrative performance improvement through descriptive and predictive analytics (dashboards)

Just as computer processing speed is growing exponentially, so too are the competencies required of new graduates and clinical nurses for information management and patient care technologies. The AACN Essentials for Informatics and Healthcare Technologies created for masters level programs are rapidly becoming those of generalists. At the masters level, these competencies include the following (AACN, 2015):

1) Analyze current and emerging technologies to support safe practice environments, and to optimize patient safety, cost-effectiveness, and health outcomes.
2) Evaluate outcome data using current communication technologies, information systems, and statistical principles to develop strategies to reduce risks and improve health outcomes.
3) Promote policies that incorporate ethical principles and standards for the use of health and information technologies.
4) Provide oversight and guidance in the integration of technologies to document patient care and improve patient outcomes.
5) Use information and communication technologies, resources, and principles of learning to teach patients and others.
6) Use current and emerging technologies in the care environment to support lifelong learning for self and others.

These essentials align well with those informatics trends described earlier and will become expected competencies for generalists in the future. For example, Table 9.2 presents an illustration of

Table 9.2 Matriculation Crosswalk: AACN Essentials for Patient Technologies and Information Management.

BSN Essentials	Masters Essentials	DNP Essentials
Demonstrate skills in using patient care technologies, information systems, and communication devices that support safe nursing practice.		**Analyze and communicate** critical elements necessary to the selection, use, and evaluation of health care information systems and patient care technology.
Understand the use of CIS systems to document interventions related to achieving nurse-sensitive outcomes.	**Provide oversight and guidance** in the integration of technologies to document patient care and improve patient outcomes.	
Apply safeguards and decision-making support tools embedded in patient care technologies and information systems to support a safe practice environment for both patients and health care workers.		
Use telecommunication technologies to assist in effective communication in a variety of health care settings.	Use information and communication technologies, resources, and **principles of learning to teach patients and others.**	
Advocate for the use of new patient care technologies for safe, quality care.	**Analyze current and emerging technologies** to support safe practice environments, and to optimize patient safety, cost-effectiveness, and health outcomes. **Use current and emerging technologies** in the care environment to support lifelong learning for self and others.	
Evaluate data from all relevant sources, including technology, to inform the delivery of care.		Evaluate consumer health information sources for accuracy, timeliness, and appropriateness.
Use standardized terminology in a care environment that reflects nursing's unique contribution to patient outcomes.		
Participate in evaluation of information systems in practice settings through policy and procedure development.		Demonstrate the conceptual ability and technical skills **to develop and execute an evaluation plan** involving data extraction from practice information systems and databases.
Recognize the role of information technology in improving patient care outcomes and creating a safe care environment.	**Evaluate outcome data** using current communication technologies, information systems, and statistical principles to develop strategies to reduce risks and improve health outcomes.	**Design, select, use, and evaluate programs** that evaluate and monitor outcomes of care, care systems, and quality improvement including consumer use of health care information systems.

(Continued)

Table 9.2 (Continued)

BSN Essentials	Masters Essentials	DNP Essentials
Apply patient-care technologies as appropriate to address the needs of a diverse patient population.		
Recognize that redesign of work flow and care processes should precede implementation of care technology to facilitate nursing practice.		
Uphold ethical standards related to data security, regulatory requirements, confidentiality, and clients' right to privacy.	**Promote policies** that incorporate ethical principles and standards for the use of health and information technologies.	**Provide leadership in the evaluation and resolution** of ethical and legal issues within health care systems relating to the use of information, information technology, communication networks, and patient care technology.

American Association of Colleges of Nursing Essentials Series. (2015) Retrieved on August 30, 2015 at http://www.aacn.nche.edu/education-resources/essential-series

how the AACN Essentials for Information Management and Patient Care Technologies matriculate across bachelor of science in nursing (BSN), masters and doctor of nursing programs and progressively advance the scope of practice for clinical nurses.

Conclusion

Transforming health care requires the integration and mastery of the QSEN competencies to achieve safe, quality, cost-effective care. This chapter focused on informatics, however, all of the competencies must work together to produce this outcome. Collaboration and partnerships between academia and practice are critical to ensure a competent nursing workforce that must use health information technology and EHRs in daily practice.

References

Affordable Care Act. (2010) Retrieved from http://frwebgate.access.gpo.gov/cgibin/getdoc.cgi?dbname=111_cong_bills&docid=f:h3590enr.txt.pdf.

American Association of Colleges of Nursing Essentials Series. (2015) Retrieved from http://www.aacn.nche.edu/education-resources/essential-series.

American Medical Informatics Association. (2015) Retrieved from https://www.amia.org/.

American Medical Informatics Association 10x10 courses. (2015) Retrieved from https://www.amia.org/education/10x10-courses.

American Nurses Association. (2008) *Scope and standards of nursing informatics practice.* Washington, DC: American Nurses Publishing.

American Recovery and Reinvestment Act. (2009) Retrieved from http://frwebgate.access.gpo.gov/cgi-bin/getdoc.cgi?dbname=111_cong_bills&docid=f:h1enr.pdf.

Aud, M.A., Abbott, C.C., Tyrer, H.W., Neelgund, R.V., Shriniwar, U.G., Mohammed, A., and Devarakonda, K.K. (2010) Smart Carpet: Developing a sensor system to detect falls and summon assistance. *J Gerontol Nurs.* 2010 Jul; *36*(7), 8–12.

Bakken, S., Cook, S.S., Curtis, L., Desjardins, K., Hyun, S., Jenkins, M., *et al.* (2004) Promoting patient safety through informatics-based nursing education. *International Journal of Medical Informatics, 73,* 581–589.

Ball, M.J., DuLong, D., Newbold, S.K., Sensmeier, J.E., Skiba, D.J., Troseth, M.R., *et al.* (2011) *Nursing informatics: Where technology and caring meet.* New York: Springer.

Barnsteiner, J. (2017) Safety. In G. Sherwood and J. Barnsteiner (Eds.), *Quality and safety in nursing: A competency approach to improving outcomes.* 2nd Ed. Hoboken, NJ: Wiley-Blackwell.

Barton, A.J. (2005) Cultivating informatics competencies in a Community of Practice. *Nursing Administration Quarterly, 29*(4), 323–328.

Barton, A.J., Armstrong, G., Preheim, G., Gelmon, S.B., and Andrus, L.C. (2009) A national Delphi to determine developmental progression of quality and safety competencies in nursing education. *Nursing Outlook, 57*(6), 313–322.

Booth, R.G. (2006) Educating the future eHealth professional nurse. *International Journal of Nursing Education Scholarship, 3*(1), Article 13. Retrieved from http://www.bepress.com/ijnes/vol3/iss1/art13.

Canton, J. (2015) *Future smart: Managing the game-changing trends that will transform your world.* Philadelphia: De Capo Press, 93–112, 23.

Chow, M.P., and Fong, V. (2010) Nursing leadership and impact. In L.L. Liang and D.M. Berwick (Eds.), *Connected for health: Using electronic health records to transform care delivery* (pp. 69–81). San Francisco: Jossey-Bass.

Connors, H.R., Weaver, C., Warren, J.J., and Miller, K. (2002) An academic-business partnership for advancing clinical informatics. *Nursing Education Perspectives, 23*(5), 228–233.

Connors, H., Warren, J.J., and Weaver, C. (2007) HIT plants SEEDS in healthcare education. *Nursing Administration Quarterly, 31*(2), 129–133.

Curran, C.R. (2003) Informatics competencies for nurse practitioners. *AACN Clinical Issues: Advanced Practice in Acute and Critical Care, 14*(3), 320–330.

Cronenwett, L., Sherwood, G., Barnsteiner, J., Disch, J., Johnson, J., Mitchell, P., *et al.* (2007) Quality and safety education for nurses, *Nursing Outlook, 55*(3), 122–131.

Cronenwett, L., Sherwood, G., Pohl, J., Barnsteiner, J., Moore, S., Sullivan, D.T., *et al.* (2009) Quality and safety education for advance nursing practice. *Nursing Outlook, 57*(6), 338–348.

Desjardins, K.S., Cook, S.S., Jenkins, M., and Bakken, S. (2005) Effect of an informatics evidence-based practice curriculum on nursing informatics competence. *International Journal of Medical Informatics, 74,* 1012–1020.

Disch, J. (2017) Teamwork and collaboration. In G. Sherwood and J. Barnsteiner (Eds.), *Quality and safety in nursing: A competency approach to improving outcomes.* 2nd Ed. Hoboken, NJ: Wiley-Blackwell.

Dixon, B., and Newlon, C.M. (2010) How do future nursing educators perceive informatics? Advancing the nursing informatics agenda through dialogue. *Journal of Professional Nursing, 26*(2), 82–89.

Edit Cowan University Basic Computer Skills Orientation. (2015) Retrieved at https://www.youtube.com/watch?v=DwsKeoXOa9I.

Flood, L.S., Gasiewicz, N., and Delpeir, T. (2010) Integrating information literacy across a BSN curriculum. *Journal of Nursing Education, 49*(2), 101–104.

FreeMind. Retrieved from http://freemind.sourceforge.net/wiki/index.php/Download.

Greiner, A.C., and Knebel, E. (Eds.) (2003) Institute of Medicine Committee on the Health Professions Education Summit. *Health professions education: A bridge to quality.* Washington, DC: National Academies Press.

Glowcap. (2015) Retrieved at http://www.glowcaps.com/.

Health Information Technology for Economic and Clinical Health (HITECH) Act. (2010) Retrieved from http://www.hipaasurvivalguide.com/hitech-act-text.php.

HealthIT.gov. (2015) Retrieved from http://healthit.gov/providers-professionals/meaningful-use-definition-objectives.

Health Insurance Portability and Accountability Act. (1996) Retrieved from https://www.cms.gov/hipaageninfo.

Hebda, T., and Calderone, T.L. (2010) What nurse educators need to know about the TIGER initiative. *Nurse Educator, 35*(2), 56–60.

Hobbs, S.D. (2002) Measuring nurses' computer competency: An analysis of published instruments. *CIN: Computer, Informatics, Nursing, 20*(2), 63–73.

Institute of Medicine. (2001) *Crossing the quality chasm: A new health system for the 21st century.* Washington, DC: National Academies Press.

Institute of Medicine. (2011) *The future of nursing: leading change, advancing health.* Washington, DC: National Academies Press.

Intel. (2015) Retrieved from http://www.intel.com/content/www/us/en/silicon-innovations/moores-law-technology.html.

Johnson, J. (2017) Quality improvement. In G. Sherwood and J. Barnsteiner (Eds.), *Quality and safety in nursing: A competency approach to improving outcomes.* 2nd Ed. Hoboken, NJ: Wiley-Blackwell.

Kennedy, D., Pallikkathavil, L., and Warren, J.J. (2009) Using a modified electronic health record to develop nursing process skills. *Journal of Nursing Education, 2,* 96–100.

Lundberg, C., Warren, J., Brokel, J., Bulechek, G., Butcher, H., Dochterman, J.M., *et al.* (2008) Selecting a standardized terminology for the electronic health record that reveals the impact of nursing on patient care. June. *Online Journal of Nursing Informatics, 12*(2). Retrieved from http://www.ojni.org/12_2/lundberg.pdf.

Marcia Conner Big Data Web Page. (2015) Retrieved from http://marciaconner.com/blog/data-on-big-data/.

Mayo Clinic Center for Social Media. http://socialmedia.mayoclinic.org.

McNeil, B.J., Elfrink, V.L., Bickford, C.J., Pierce, S.T., Beyea, S.C., Averill, C., and Klappenbach, C. (2003) Nursing information technology knowledge, skills, and preparation of student nurses, nursing faculty, and clinicians: A U.S. survey. *Journal of Nursing Education, 42*(8), 341–349.

McNeil, B.J., Elfrink, V.L., Pierce, S.T., Beyea, S.C., Bickford, C.J., and Averill, C. (2005) Nursing informatics knowledge and competencies: A national survey of nursing education programs in the United States. *International Journal of Medical Informatics, 74,* 1021–1030.

National Forum on Information Literacy. (n.d.) *Information literacy competency standards for higher education.* Retrieved from www.infolit.org.

National Nursing Informatics Deep Dive Program. (2015) Retrieved at http://www.nursing.umn.edu/continuing-professional-development/index.htm.

Nightingale, F. (1863) *Notes on hospitals.* London: Longman, Green, Longman, Roberts and Green, p. 176.

Northstar Basic Computer Skills Certificate. (2015) Retrieved at https://www.digitalliteracyassessment.org/.

Office of the National Coordinator for Health IT. (2011) Retrieved from http://healthit.hhs.gov/portal/server.pt/community/healthit_hhs_gov__meaningful_use_announcement/2996.

Open EMR Project. (2015) Retrieved at http://www.open-emr.org/.

Sackett, K., Jones, J., and Erdley, W.S. (2005) Incorporating healthcare informatics into the strategic planning process in nursing education. *Nursing Leadership Forum*, *9*(9), 98–104.

Simpson, R.L. (2005) Practice to evidence to practice: Closing the loop with IT. *Nursing Management*, *36*(9), 12–17.

Smedley, A. (2005) The importance of informatics competencies in nursing: An Australian perspective. *CIN: Computers, Informatics, Nursing*, *23*(2), 106–110.

Smith, M., Saunders, R., Stuckhardt, L., and McGinnis, M. (2012) Best Care at Lower Cost: The Path to Continuously Learning Health Care in America. Institute of Medicine, National Academies Press.

Staggers, N., Gassert, C.A., and Curran, C. (2001) Informatics competencies for nurses at four levels of practice. *Journal of Nursing Education*, *40*(7), 303–316.

Staggers, N., Gassert, C.A., and Curran, C. (2002) A Delphi study to determine informatics competencies for nurses at four levels of practice. *Nursing Research*, *51*(6), 383–390.

TIGER Summit, Informatics Competencies. (n.d.) Retrieved from http://www.tigersummit.com/Competencies_New_B949.html.

TIGER Virtual Learning Environment. (2015) Retrieved at http://www.himss.org/ResourceLibrary/ResourceDetail.aspx?ItemNumber=12325.

Time. (2013) Retrieved from http://newsfeed.time.com/2013/03/25/more-people-have-cell-phones-than-toilets-u-n-study-shows/.

Tracey, M. F., and Barnsteiner, J. (2017) Evidence-based practice. In G. Sherwood and J. Barnsteiner (Eds.), *Quality and safety in nursing: A competency approach to improving outcomes*, 2nd Ed. Hoboken, NJ: Wiley-Blackwell.

Topel, E. (2015) *The patient will see you now: The future of medicine is in your hands.* New York: Basic Books.

University of Minnesota School of Nursing retrieved from http://www.nursing.umn.edu/future-students/index.htm.

Walton, M.K., and Barnsteiner, J. (2017) Patient-centered care. In G. Sherwood and J. Barnsteiner (Eds.), *Quality and safety in nursing: A competency approach to improving outcomes*, 2nd Ed. Hoboken, NJ: Wiley-Blackwell.

Warren, J.J., and Connors, H.R. (2007). Health information technology can and will transform nursing education. *Nursing Outlook*, *55*(1), 58–60.

Warren, J.J., Fletcher, K.A., Connors, H.R., Ground, A., and Weaver, C. (2004) The SEEDS Project: From health care information system to innovative educational strategy. In P. Whitten and D. Cook (Eds.), *Understanding health communication technologies* (pp. 225–231). San Francisco, CA: Jossey-Bass.

Warren, J.J., Meyer, M.N., Thompson, T., and Roche, A. (2010) Transforming nursing education: Integrating informatics and simulations. In Weaver, Delaney, Weber, and Carr (Eds.), *Nursing and informatics for the 21st century: An international look at practice, trends and the future* (pp. 145–161). Chicago: HIMSS Press.

Weaver, C.A., Warren, J.J., and Delaney, C. (2005) Bedside, classroom and bench: Collaborative strategies to generate evidence-based knowledge for nursing practice. *International Journal of Medical Informatics*, *74*, 989–999.

Section 3

Strategies to Build a Culture of Quality and Safety

10

Transforming Education to Transform Practice

Integrating Quality and Safety in Subject-centered
Classrooms using Unfolding Case Studies

Lisa Day, PhD, RN, CNE and Gwen Sherwood, PhD, RN, FAAN, ANEF

Keesha called the School of Nursing Curriculum Committee's monthly meeting to order. Each month, the Committee's first agenda item was The Safety Huddle. Since the faculty had redesigned the curriculum to integrate the QSEN project's six competencies, the Curriculum Committee members had begun sharing what each faculty member was observing and learning in classroom, lab, and clinical settings. In each month's Safety Huddle, the School's Patient Safety Officer highlighted one of the Joint Commission's National Patient Safety Goals (NPSG) with a brief theory burst and crosswalk with the QSEN competencies. The faculty discussed learning experiences already in place and ideas for new experiences to ensure learners would achieve the QSEN competencies and be able to address the NPSGs in practice. As they explored the implications of the QSEN competencies, several broader questions emerged to guide their continued curriculum development:

- *What are the best educational approaches to facilitate learners in achieving the QSEN competencies?*
- *How can teachers create clinically focused interactive classrooms where learners are engaged in clinical reasoning?*
- *What are the best assessment strategies to determine a learner has achieved the QSEN competencies?*

The IOM (2003) recognized education as the bridge to health care quality and proposed six competencies for all health professionals that will enable them to lead and work in systems focused on safety and quality outcomes: patient-centered care, teamwork and collaboration, quality improvement, evidence-based practice, safety, and informatics. Ensuring systems deliver only high quality and safe care requires transforming health professions education so that all health professionals acquire – and are also able to use – KSAs to assess scientific evidence to determine what constitutes best practice; identify gaps between evidence-based best practice and actual practice in different care settings; and to take action to lead change. The six IOM competencies have been endorsed by major professional organizations and credentialing agencies in health care and recommended for inclusion in curricula (Bataldan, Leach, and Ogrinc, 2009), and form the basis for competencies developed for nursing education by the QSEN project. The AACN included the QSEN competencies in the curriculum essentials documents

Quality and Safety in Nursing: A Competency Approach to Improving Outcomes, Second Edition.
Edited by Gwen Sherwood and Jane Barnsteiner.
© 2017 John Wiley & Sons, Inc. Published 2017 by John Wiley & Sons, Inc.

for undergraduate, masters, and DNP programs (AACN, 2008; AACN, 2009; AACN, 2011). The NLN (2010) also recommends the QSEN competencies model for all levels of nursing education.

To achieve the ambitious goals identified in the QSEN project, nurse educators must focus as much on *how* they teach as *what* they teach. In addition to learning experiences that focus on providing care to an individual, nurse educators are also developing strategies that will help learners orient to health care systems and better understand how individual patients live in, and are cared for within, those systems. This chapter opens with a description of the changing health care systems that demand nurses engage in patient safety and quality improvement and that challenge nurse educators to take up interactive, clinically focused instructional methods in classrooms, labs, and clinical settings. It goes on to describe ideas for best practice in professional education and a model – situated coaching with unfolding case studies – that demonstrates how to implement these ideas in the classroom. The final sections provide a guide for teachers in developing unfolding case studies to use in classrooms and ideas for facilitating classroom discussion.

QSEN: Integrating Quality and Safety Competencies in Nursing

Nurses as Leaders in Quality and Safety: The New Reality

Regardless of whether they enter practice with a diploma, an associates, bachelors, masters, or doctoral degree, all registered nurses (RN) are accountable for delivering evidence-based, safe, high-quality, patient-centered care across all settings. The gap increasingly evident between pre-RN education and practice expectations contributes to longer and more costly orientation programs for new nurses (Sherwood and Drenkard, 2007) and to the high turnover rate of new graduates during the first year of employment (Spector, Ulrich, and Barnsteiner, 2012). New role responsibilities create a new clinical reality for nurses and demand changes in both prelicensure and postlicensure nursing education; education and practice exist as mirrors of each other – what happens in one affects the other. Nurses need to recognize clinical questions, describe processes for changing current practice, and evaluate the outcomes of improvement initiatives. Staff development efforts must address the learning needs of practicing professionals whose education did not include quality improvement and safety science. Nurses manage complex processes that require them to balance competing priorities in patient care management. These priorities include understanding the underlying disease processes and medical treatments and how these impact individuals, families, and communities; coordinating care among the entire health care team; using informatics and other technologies safely and efficiently; understanding how to access and use institution-specific policies and procedures; and knowing when and how to use outside resources (Hughes, 2008).

Nurses are expected to coordinate care and collaborate with a wide variety of health professionals across a variety of care settings. Nurses participate in and may lead quality improvement teams, which require coordinating input from the multiple disciplines involved in improving a particular aspect of care. Nurses gather data used to help develop and implement protocols required to meet outside regulatory standards and economic incentives. Nurses use data derived from patients, providers, and systems to monitor the outcomes of care and design, and apply and test improvement methods (Johnson, 2012). Nurses participate in building a culture of patient safety by applying new approaches to error prevention and management like safety checks to ensure that clinicians take certain actions and precautions to protect patients during care delivery (Sammer *et al.*, 2010). Nurses participate in recognizing and reporting errors and near misses, RCA and FMEA, and work with risk management, and patients and their families in responding to adverse events (Barnsteiner, 2017). Rather than ignoring system dysfunction such as breakdowns in communication, workarounds that have become the norm, and ineffective care processes, nurses have a responsibility to speak up when they observe actions that jeopardize patient safety or care that falls short of evidence-based care standards. Working with inter-disciplinary teams, nurses can create new care protocols, design care pathways to set standards of care, use safety reporting systems and analyze risks, examine benchmark data for areas of improvement, and design system changes based on outcomes (Sherwood and Jones, 2010).

Development of the Quality and Safety Education in Nursing Competencies

The goal of the national QSEN project (Cronenwett *et al.*, 2007; Cronenwett, 2012; Sherwood, 2011) was to integrate the six IOM (2003) competencies into nursing practice. The QSEN National Expert Panel defined the six competencies (patient-centered care, teamwork and collaboration, evidence-based practice, quality improvement, safety, and informatics) and used an iterative process to identify KSA objectives for each of the six competencies (Cronenwett *et al.*, 2007; Appendix A). Definitions remain the same across all nursing practices, but graduate-level competencies were further developed with higher-level KSA objectives appropriate for advanced practice nurses (Cronenwett *et al.*, 2009; Appendix B).

A 15-school pilot learning collaborative demonstrated ways to integrate the six QSEN competencies in multiple educational entry programs (Cronenwett, Sherwood, and Gelmon, 2009). Schools mapped ways to integrate the competencies, led faculty development for understanding the competencies, and worked with a clinical partner to implement demonstration projects for transforming their curricula. The QSEN web site (www.QSEN.org/pilot) reports curricular strategies developed by the schools with their practice partners to model integration of the competencies (Cronenwett, Sherwood, and Gelmon, 2009). Barton *et al.* (2009) report a Delphi study for placement of the 162 KSAs defining the six quality and safety competencies for beginning, intermediate, and advanced learners (Appendix C). Cronenwett *et al.* (2009) and Pohl *et al.* (2009) discuss graduate placement.

Results of the Pilot School Learning Collaborative demonstrated the need for educator development in both clinical and academic settings as well as new pedagogical approaches to advance quality and safety (Armstrong, Sherwood, and Tagliarini, 2009; Brown, Feller, and Benedict, 2010; Cronenwett, Sherwood, and Gelmon, 2009). Faculty development was further implemented nationally as the AACN hosted 11 QSEN regional workshops and the QSEN Institute has continued the annual QSEN National Forums (Cronenwett, 2012; Barnsteiner *et al.*, 2013).

Changing Education Paradigms in Academic and Clinical Settings

Whether in clinical or academic settings, it is a challenge to know how to begin to integrate the QSEN competencies into educational programs that are already overloaded with content. Benner *et al.* (2010) pointed out that to prepare nurses for their roles in these complex systems, including key roles in improving patient care quality and safety, curricular redesign must be paired with new pedagogies that engage learners in active, authentic clinical reasoning and focus on achieving deep learning rather than simple memorization.

Infusing quality and safety competencies into nursing education further shifts the focus from con-tent-centered teaching to contextualized learning centered on the main subject of nursing: patient- and family-centered care. The central subject of nursing practice – the patient and family – should be central in the classroom so learning is contextualized and learners are motivated to both acquire and use knowledge. Shifting from passive knowledge acquisition to active knowledge use in the classroom shifts learning from emphasizing what learners should know to what learners should be able to do with the knowledge. Barton and colleagues (2009) completed a Delphi study to assist nurse educators in determining beginner, intermediate, and advanced placement of the QSEN competencies and KSAs (Appendix C). Rather than adding more content, nurse educators can integrate the QSEN

KSAs across a curriculum by threading them through existing courses, clinical experiences, simulations, and learning assignments, and by using quality and safety to form the structure for case studies. The same is true for educational units in practice settings; the QSEN KSAs can be used as the foundation for unit-based simulations, staff development, or more formal education offerings.

The QSEN Pilot Learning Collaborative (Cronenwett, Sherwood, and Gelmon, 2009; Armstrong, Sherwood, and Tagliareni, 2009) found that the most effective instructional methods were those that engaged learners in interactive experiential learning. Theory bursts replaced traditional length lectures; questions were embedded in unfolding case studies; clinical learning experiences included safety and quality discussions; debriefings after clinical or simulation helped learners apply abstract concepts to real clinical situations; learners were mentored in quality improvement initiatives; and learners applied the competencies in simulated clinical situations. The Collaborative demonstrated the essential partnership between academic and clinical settings and how the QSEN competencies can be used in each environment. Clinical nurse educators have also sought new educational models to further develop practicing nurses whose formal academic education did not prepare them for new roles in ensuring patient care quality and safety.

Bold and innovative new pedagogical approaches are necessary for nurses to learn to integrate patient safety and quality improvement into their clinical thinking. Ironside and Cerbie (2012) explored narrative pedagogies to help learners explore multiple concepts from a patient-centered perspective. Both high- and low-fidelity simulation exercises (Durham and Alden, 2017) offer learners a way to develop the QSEN KSAs by practicing medication administration safety, communicate with health care team members including the patient and family, and enter and retrieve data from the electronic health record.

With new educational paradigms, nurse educators are rethinking nursing fundamentals labs that teach discrete skills to one nurse, one patient at a time (Preheim, Armstrong, and Barton, 2009). Schools of nursing skills labs traditionally have been organized around student competence in individual psychomotor skills such as sterile technique, IV insertion, and provision of bed baths and other hygiene needs. In newer models, highly orchestrated clinical learning labs may organize learning around physiologic systems, such as the cardiac-compromised patient; skills may be emphasized in bundled sets via high-fidelity simulation to more closely resemble an actual nursing situation, in some cases creating a virtual hospital (Durham and Alden, 2012).

To prepare nurses for new practice realities that include their key roles in improving patient care quality and safety, more changes are needed in nursing education, especially in classrooms. To improve patient outcomes, well-equipped professional nurses must understand the complexity of the health care system and have skills to seek out best practices and implement change. Shifting from passive knowledge acquisition to interactive experiential learning in the classroom shifts learning from emphasizing what learners should *know* to what learners should *be able to do* with the knowledge, that is, it assists learners in translating their knowledge into actions. The next section of this chapter examines one such pedagogical shift: from content delivery to situated coaching in the classroom.

Situated Coaching to Promote Interactive Knowledge Use

Benner *et al.* (2010) identified situated coaching as a signature pedagogy in nursing education. Signature pedagogies are pervasive teaching methods that define how knowledge is used and that facilitate professional formation within a discipline (Shulman, 2005). Shulman describes signature pedagogies as, "...important precisely because they are pervasive. They implicitly define what counts as knowledge in a field and how things become known. They define how knowledge is analyzed, criticized, accepted or discarded (Shulman, 2005)." For example, medical teaching rounds, where a medical student presents a patient's diagnosis and medical treatment plan to the attending physician on a service, is a signature pedagogy of medical education that emphasizes the knowledge and culture of the discipline. The medical student is expected to gather information and draw conclusions about the patient's medical condition and status independently, then present these findings and ask for guidance in the form of consultation with the attending physician who is also the clinical teacher (Cooke, Irby, and O'Brien, 2010).

Shulman (2005) goes on to outline three dimensions of signature pedagogies:

1) Surface structure: the part of teaching that is visible in the world; what outsiders hear and see happen between a student and teacher.
2) Deep structure: the teacher's assumptions about the knowledge, skills, and ethics of the discipline and about how best to convey these to students.
3) Implicit structure: the values embedded in the discipline that are evident in the teaching.

A signature pedagogy in nursing education, that is, situated coaching, is one that is pervasive across all types of nursing programs and among a diverse array of teachers. The following example of a clinical learning encounter illustrates this signature pedagogy, which involves a teacher coaching a learner while both are immersed in a patient care situation as shown below.

It's 8:30 in the morning and the student nurse is in the hospital medication room preparing to give a subcutaneous injection to a patient for the first time. The clinical instructor is by her side.

Student (checking a pre-filled syringe against the patient's medication administration record): Enoxaparin...that's due at nine a.m., 40 mg subQ. That's the right dose. It's to prevent deep vein thrombosis (DVT), which makes sense because the patient just had a hip replacement.

INSTRUCTOR:	Excellent! Did you review SubQ injection in your skills book?
STUDENT:	Yes.
INSTRUCTOR:	Good. (opens a drawer filled with different size needles) What size needle do you want for that?
STUDENT:	Ummm...(pause)...what are my choices?
INSTRUCTOR:	Any of these (indicates the needles in the drawer).
STUDENT:	Let's see...(picks up two needles and hesitates).
INSTRUCTOR:	What does "subQ" mean?
STUDENT:	Subcutaneous. And the patient is thin so I need a small needle (holds up a 25 gauge, 5/8 inch needle).
INSTRUCTOR:	Excellent choice. How do you think the patient will respond to this needle? Is it going to hurt? Is he anxious about needles?
STUDENT:	I don't know. This is the first time I've given him a shot. But he doesn't seem anxious at all; he's pretty calm. I can ask him before I give it.
INSTRUCTOR:	Good idea (takes a towel off the linen cart and hands the student an empty syringe, the needle the student chose, and an alcohol wipe). Now, show me the proper technique for giving the injection. Pretend this is the patient's skin (indicates the rolled towel).
STUDENT:	Well, I'll give it in the abdomen. I'll pinch the skin up (pinches the towel and wipes the area with the alcohol wipe), and use a 90-degree angle (holds the syringe like a dart with the needle perpendicular to the towel, hesitates)...or should it be 45 degrees?
INSTRUCTOR:	It could be either. How will you decide?

|STUDENT:|The book said it depends on how thick the fat layer is. I'll go with 45 because he's pretty skinny, and I don't want to hit the muscle.|
|INSTRUCTOR:|Very good thinking! So show me.|

(The student completes the injection.)

STUDENT:	And I don't want to rub the site because of the bruising risk. (She moves to recap the needle; the instructor stops her.)
INSTRUCTOR:	That was perfect, but what do you know about needle safety?
STUDENT:	Oh! Never recap. (She activates the safety device on the needle.)

In the illustration above, the student presents information about the medication, and the instructor asks questions to determine the student's readiness to proceed. When the student is puzzled or does not know how to proceed, she asks questions and seeks assistance from the instructor. The instructor responds not with a direct answer, but with a choice or question of his/her own. The discussion revolves around the student's readiness to complete a subcutaneous injection, taking into account the patient's safety and comfort.

The deep structure reflects the true purpose of the situated coaching encounter: to teach the student how to think like a nurse. The instructor coaches the student by offering choices and asking questions in order to help him/her internalize a nursing identity. These are the kinds of things nurses ask themselves, and this is the kind of thinking nurses engage in when making a clinical choice or decision. By talking the student through the thinking process, the instructor invites the student to notice certain things and respond in certain ways and thus to begin thinking like a nurse.

The implicit structure of a signature pedagogy has to do with tacit assumptions and values. In the example of situated coaching, the questions the instructor asks and the guidance she/he gives to the student prioritize the patient and safety. Ensuring the effectiveness of care and keeping the patient and nurse safe are the principal concerns behind the questions. The tacit selection of a private setting away from the patient and the openness with which the instructor engages the student's questions and responds to his/her hesitations reflect the importance of open, undistracted dialogue that is focused on the task at hand. The teacher's choice of coaching as a way to facilitate the student's discovery and use of knowledge she/he already has, rather than direct instruction or giving the student a step-by-step account of what she/he should know and do, reflects the expectation that the student will be prepared to engage in the practice.

This approach is a familiar part of the teaching and learning that takes place in clinical and lab settings. Bringing situated coaching to classroom teaching and learning provides an excellent platform for teachers and learners to engage with the QSEN competencies while moving nursing education toward needed pedagogical transformation. The following example illustrates how situated coaching can be used in the classroom with an unfolding clinical narrative. See Textbox 10.1 for a report from the Emergency Department RN.

TEACHER:	You have heard the report from the RN in the ED. Tell me about Mr. Prince. What concerns do you have based on what you know?
STUDENT #1:	His breathing.
STUDENT #2:	Yes, he's not breathing very well.
TEACHER:	What do you mean? What data do you have that make you think breathing is a problem?
STUDENT #3:	His oxygen saturation is low.
TEACHER:	Okay, his sat is low. What else?
STUDENT #2:	His respiratory rate is 28, and he has crackles in his lungs.

STUDENT #3:   And he's confused.

TEACHER: Good, so, he's breathing fast, is not getting enough oxygen, and he's confused. Why?

STUDENT #4:   It's the pulmonary edema.

STUDENT #5:   And heart failure.

TEACHER: Okay, now think about the pathophysiology and medical treatments. How can you best help Mr. Prince? What are the risks and what are he and his son experiencing? This will help you figure out your priorities of care for Mr. Prince.

(A discussion of the pathophysiology of heart failure, pulmonary edema, dyspnea, and confusion follows with the teacher guiding learners to use appropriate online resources for pieces they do not remember and always connecting the knowledge back to Mr. Prince and what he and his son are experiencing.)

Textbox 10.1 Hand-off Report from the Emergency Department RN

Mr. Prince is a 75-year-old male with a history of hypertension, coronary artery disease (CAD), coronary artery bypass graft (CABG), who was brought in by ambulance when his son found him short of breath and confused and called 911. He arrived short of breath and diaphoretic, and a chest X-ray showed pulmonary edema; there was nothing acute on the ECG, but he's being ruled out for MI. We gave him a dose of furosemide IV and placed a urinary catheter. Right now he's alert, oriented to self and place, moving all extremities with equal strength. Heart rate 100, sinus tachycardia with Premature Atrial Complexes (PAC); Blood pressure 110/70; Respiratory rate 28; oxygen saturation by pulse oximetry 93% on 2 liters nasal cannula oxygen; oral temperature 37 degrees centigrade; denies pain. He says his breathing is a little better. He has a 22 gauge IV in his left forearm running 5% dextrose and water at 30 mL/hour and a 22 gauge saline lock IV in his right hand. The cardiologist thinks he just needs diuresis but might want to start some dobutamine depending how he does in the next couple of hours. He'll need telemetry monitoring. His adult son is here with him.

This exchange, which took place in a classroom with one teacher and 75 learners present, illustrates how a teacher can use a brief client narrative to frame a discussion of content – pathophysiology, physical exam findings, and priorities of care – while keeping the discussion centered on concern for the client. The teacher coaches the learners to use their existing knowledge and to acquire new knowledge to identify and address nursing concerns for a particular client. The discussion illustrates one way to integrate QSEN competencies, patient-centered care, evidence-based practice, safety, and informatics, while moving toward important pedagogical transformation in the following three ways: integrating three high-level apprenticeships of professional education and practice described by Sullivan (2005); creating a subject-centered classroom as described by Palmer (1998); and addressing the four paradigm shifts called for by Benner *et al.* (2010). These ideas will be more fully explored in next section.

Integrating Innovative Ideas into the Nursing Classroom

Three Apprenticeships of Professional Education

Sullivan described three high-level apprenticeships: a cognitive apprenticeship to the profession's unique body of knowledge; a skills-based apprenticeship to the unique skills required for the practice, including psychomotor skills and also ways of thinking and problem-solving; and an apprenticeship of ethical comportment in which learners take up values and ways of relating to others that are embedded in their chosen professional practice community (Sullivan, 2005). All three of these apprenticeships are present in every teaching-learning experience, whether in the classroom, lab, or clinical setting. The word apprenticeship used here is a departure from early nursing models when learners in hospital-based schools of nursing provided low-cost labor. Sullivan's (2005) apprenticeships require a learner to have direct coaching from an experienced professional; this is the kind of discipline-specific learning and values inculcation required to become a professional in any field. The QSEN KSAs, or any traditional formulation of learning objectives, can be mapped to the three apprenticeships. What is unique about Sullivan's model is that it emphasizes the importance of coaching learners to integrate all three apprenticeships and to understand that the knowledge and skills of a profession are always in service to the ethics embedded in the practice community.

Traditionally in nursing education, these three apprenticeships have been separated with the cognitive apprenticeship taught in the classroom, and the skills-based apprenticeship taught in skills labs and clinical settings. Learners most often took up the values-based apprenticeship of ethical comportment by attending to the role modeling of their teachers and preceptors. Sullivan's ideas translate to innovative teaching practices when nurse educators make conscious and planned efforts to integrate all three apprenticeships in all classroom, lab, and clinical settings (Day & Sherwood, 2017).

Subject-centered Teaching and Learning

Based on what we know about learning for a practice, learning involves much more than acquiring information and content. The ways nurses use knowledge in practice as they gather data and problem-solve in changing situations that often are underdetermined, which is the kind of active knowledge-use all nurses must learn how to do, speaks to the inadequacy of static lecture as a main pedagogy in teaching this dynamic practice. When teachers actively engage in guiding learners as they apprentice to the whole of integrated nursing practice, the responsibility as teacher/coach becomes more than presenting content in a well-constructed set of slides.

Palmer (1998) describes an effective way to integrate learning and create a collaborative learning environment by bringing teacher and learners, the two things that are consistently present in the classroom, together with a "third thing," which is the big idea or central subject of the discipline. Bringing the third thing to the center of learning creates what Palmer describes as a subject-centered classroom (Palmer, 1998). In traditional models of schooling, teachers and learners are present in the classroom as two groups ready to engage in teaching and learning, respectively. In teacher-centered instructivist models, teaching is central and is usually equated with imparting information or telling learners things they need to know. Learner-centered models shift the focus from instruction to construction and recognize learners are in control of their own learning. Teachers put learning first in designing classroom environments. Departing from both teacher- and learner-centered models, Palmer makes the *subject* the center of classroom learning. In a subject-centered classroom, teachers and learners are always aware that something is present other than themselves.

In the subject-centered classroom, in addition to learner and teacher, there is a third thing present. The third thing is the subject, the big idea with which learner and teacher will struggle in order to understand the truth. Palmer describes the presence of the third thing or *subject* as palpable, real. It is the teacher's job to conjure the subject in such a way that it cannot be ignored. The subject takes different forms depending on the discipline under study. It is easy to think of the subject as the topic of a traditional nursing class, for example, diseases such as diabetes, heart disease, or peptic ulcer disease, or concepts such as patient safety, perfusion, anxiety, or pain, or skills such as physical exam techniques, teamwork behaviors, or safe medication administration. The nurse will need to learn some content including the physiologic processes that can explain disease and disease progression. The nurse will also need to know how to do certain things like report near misses or errors, obtain a patient-centered health history and place an intravenous line safely. Palmer's idea of the subject goes beyond the content and skills that are the focus of much of nursing education. The big idea or third thing that should be present in the nursing classroom is the whole practice of nursing that integrates Sullivan's (2005) three professional education apprenticeships and grows out of the nurse's relationship with the client, engagement in service in addressing the client's health-related concerns, and integration of the QSEN competencies.

Four Paradigm Shifts

The authors of the landmark Carnegie National Study of Nursing Education (Benner *et al.*, 2010) recommended four paradigm shifts that are consistent with Sullivan's three apprenticeships and with Palmer's subject-centered classroom:

1) Shifting from delivering decontextualized content to teaching for situated cognition, a sense of salience, and action in particular situations.
2) Shifting from separating clinical and classroom to connecting and integrating classroom and clinical learning means that instead of teaching content in the classroom and expecting learners to then apply this in clinical, nurse educators will create learning environments in all settings that make current, and sometimes just-in-time, knowledge *use* central. This recognizes that learners acquire a great deal of cutting-edge content knowledge in clinical settings and that classroom settings where teachers structure lectures based on textbook content may be out of touch with real world practice.
3) Shifting from an emphasis on critical thinking to an emphasis on clinical reasoning that includes the varied modes of thinking nurses use in practice. The Critical Thinking Community defines critical thinking as "the art of thinking about your thinking while you are thinking in order to make your thinking better: more clear, more accurate, or more defensible" (The Critical Thinking Community, 2014). Critical thinking is a vital part of all learning and of nursing practice, but thinking critically is a disengaged, objective, critiquing or puzzle-solving approach. Thinking like a nurse is more than critical thinking as captured in the term clinical reasoning, a larger conceptual umbrella that includes, but is not limited to, critical thinking (Benner *et al.*, 2010; Tanner, 2006). Asking learners to think through an unfolding case study in which the patient situation changes over time and information may be lacking allows learners to develop many aspects of clinical reasoning including critical thinking.
4) Shifting from socialization, the demonstration of externally imposed behaviors, to formation allows the internal growth and development of a commitment to the values that sustain nursing practice (Benner *et al.*, 2010). Student nurses often think being a nurse means knowing certain things and having certain psychomotor and time management skills, an impression reinforced when teachers use classroom time only to deliver content, telling learners what they need to know, showing them how to complete step-by-step tasks, and enforcing rules for classroom and clinical conduct, all methods of socialization that help learners develop the external manifestations of the practice. Learners memorize the content and steps of the procedures and abide by the rules in order to pass their courses and graduate but may not have accomplished the

transformation necessary to become good nurses. Nurses are professionals who use a unique set of knowledge and skills in order to enact the values of their practice in the world. Shifting from a focus on socialization to formation means bringing values to the center of learning by expecting learners to acquire knowledge and skills for the sake of service. Organizing classroom learning around a clinical narrative creates the expectation that knowledge and skills will be acquired and used for the sake of service to a patient, family, or community, not simply to achieve a particular score on an exam or grade in a course.

These four paradigm shifts transform classroom time from an instructivist model where teachers focus on content, to a collaborative problem-solving environment where teachers and learners think and solve problems together. Centering the learning on a client situates the learners as nurses involved in planning and delivering care to clients. At the same time, the case study situates the teacher as an expert clinical coach who role-models clinical reasoning and what nurses care about, that is, the values embedded in the practice. The narrative gives learners and teachers a puzzle or problem to solve and encourages the teachers to coach learners to think like nurses, i.e., attend to the most salient aspects of the situation by engaging in clinical reasoning.

The exchange between teacher and learners that opened this section is an example of Palmer's third thing or big idea in nursing education. Starting class with the hand-off report on a hospitalized patient given in Textbox 10.1 centers classroom learning on the true subject of nursing and gives learners and teachers something to care about, that is, Mr. Prince, his health and well being, his family, and community.

Shifting from Content-based Instruction to Situated Coaching Using Unfolding Clinical Narratives

By bringing a clinical narrative into the classroom, the teacher introduces learners to a client situation and invites them to join in planning best care. In this learning model, rather than introduce disease categories and lists of signs and symptoms, or nursing diagnoses and possible interventions, the teacher acts as a coach to guide learners toward the resources and information they will need. Learners acquire knowledge and facts and make connections as they use this learning to be of best service in the situation (Day, 2011; Glendon and Ulrich, 2001; Palmer, 1998). This kind of thinking and awareness promotes a culture of safety and illustrates the QSEN competencies in action.

Because it is seen as an efficient way to deliver content to a large number of learners, nurse educators often use the classroom setting to cover cognitive domain learning objectives, the so-called "content to be covered" that students need for nursing practice. Classroom lecture is the most efficient method to transfer the information learners need to know. Transferring information, however, is not the sum and substance of teaching, and learning to use the knowledge required for nursing is not as easy as passively listening to a lecture. In order to learn to think and use knowledge and content, learners need coaching in all three of Sullivan's apprenticeships because content delivery through lecture will be inadequate (Benner *et al.*, 2010). For example, Textbox 10.2 shows a series of slides that deliver context-free content on oxygenation. The slides provide a cataloging of possible medical diagnoses, physical examination findings and nursing interventions that provide an organized method for delivering information similar to that found in a textbook. The teacher might elaborate on each bullet point in her or his lecture and might provide examples from practice to make the content more interesting.

Textbox 10.2 Presenting Patient Using Decontexualized Content Compared with Textbox 10.1 Using Clinical Narrative

---

Slide #1, Left-sided Heart Failure: Signs and Symptoms

- Shortness of breath/dyspnea
- Fatigue
- Altered mental status
- Oliguria
- Weak pulses
- Lung sounds: bilateral crackles at bases
- Cough with frothy white or pink sputum
- Chest Xray: pulmonary edema

Slide #2, Heart Failure: Medical Treatment

- Diuresis: furosemide PO or IV
- Beta blockers and ACE inhibitors
- Inotropic support
  - Lanoxin PO or IV
  - Dobutamine IV infusion

A teacher can use the bullet-point slides in Textbox 10.2 to deliver decontextualized content, lists of facts learners think they must memorize in order to prepare for exams. In contrast, a teacher can use the clinical narrative introduced in Textbox 10.1 to situate learners' thinking, guide them toward identifying the most important aspects of the situation and selecting the most important facts to memorize, and help them decide how to prioritize the action steps they will need to take in response. Textbox 10.1 is an example of how the lecture slides in Textbox 10.2 can be transformed so that content becomes secondary to the central subject of nursing practice: the client/family-nurse relationship. Textbox 10.1 captures the content contained in the three parts of Textbox 10.2 but instead of simply cataloging this content, the opening case study narrative gives part of a hand-off report on a patient hospitalized with pneumonia. See Textbox 10.3 for a hand-off report from an ED nurse. Allowing learners to encounter information in a situation similar to practice engages them in problem solving and shifts the focus from content as central while still requiring them to learn content. This model for a subject-centered classroom that integrates Sullivan's three apprenticeships blends ideas from the following sources:

- Problem-based learning in which learners use information and prior knowledge to solve discipline-specific problems.
- Team-based learning in which learners work in teams to discover and construct the information and knowledge they need to solve discipline-specific problems or with learners from multiple disciplines to examine broader care implications.
- Simulation where students participate in mock client-care situations.
- Narrative pedagogy where students and teachers co-construct the knowledge needed to engage in nursing practice.
- Case-based teaching and learning, such as used in law and business school classrooms.

Textbox 10.3 Hand-off Report from the Emergency Department RN (see Textbox 10.1)

Step 1

Mr. Prince arrives from the ED to the cardiac telemetry unit on a gurney accompanied by a middle-aged man he introduces as his son. He is sitting up breathing shallowly at a rate of 20, which increases to 28 when he moves from gurney to bed. Oxygen saturation is 95% on 2 liters nasal cannula oxygen. Heart rate 100, rhythm as below; lungs with crackles at both bases, otherwise clear; heart sounds S1, S2, S3; Pulses palpable bilaterally, radial 2+, pedal 1+. Urinary catheter in place draining clear yellow urine; IV catheters are intact. Mr. Prince's son says his father must be hungry; he hasn't eaten since yesterday. He offers to go to the cafeteria to get his father some soup.

Telemetry rhythm:

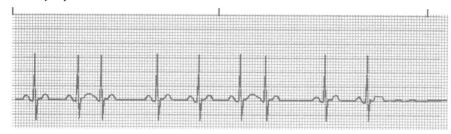

Step 2

The telemetry technician alerts you that Mr. Prince's heart rhythm has changed to this:

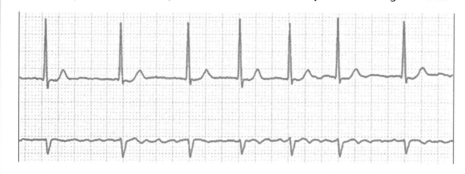

The most important feature of using unfolding clinical narratives in a subject-centered classroom is the learner-teacher relationship, which includes the teacher's engagement and commitment to the following: 1) the subject; 2) guiding students toward the truths that live in the community of nurses and become evident in relationship with the client; and 3) inviting learners to join this community.

When teachers invite learners to join them in nursing practice they remove barriers and create a more level hierarchy, two things that have been shown to improve learning outcomes in higher education (Palmer, 1998; Greer *et al.*, 2010). Authentic exchange of ideas and true dialogue between teachers and learners as they construct, deconstruct, and reconstruct knowledge and truth shift the power balance in the classroom from teacher-controlled learning to learner-centered teaching. Yet learners do need to receive new information and acquire new knowledge, and educators do need to cover some content. Some teachers fear a loss of control of the classroom environment, and some learners are most comfortable with a familiar teaching format, for example, a lecture, where they get what they think they need: answers to questions on the next exam. A teacher guiding learners through projected slides to deliver content and information meets these needs but presents few opportunities to exchange ideas or engage in dialogue. In this teaching model learner-teacher contact is limited to question-answer where learners ask questions, the teacher provides answers; the teacher asks questions, the learners provide answers. Without dialogue, teachers do not know the reasons behind a learner's incorrect answer and cannot see how learners are thinking or how they will use the knowledge they acquire to improve their practice.

To create a classroom environment that is a collaborative space where teacher and learners together engage in best nursing practice, the teacher will have to surrender some control and focus on promoting and coaching learners' thinking. By bringing a client narrative into the classroom the teacher introduces learners to a client situation and invites them to join in planning best care. Teachers do not introduce disease categories and lists of signs and symptoms, or nursing diagnoses and possible interventions; they do not insist that learners remember certain facts and connections. Rather, the teacher as coach guides learners toward the resources and content they will need in order to be of best service in the client situation. This kind of thinking and awareness promotes a culture of safety; it is the QSEN competencies in action.

A Method for Constructing an Unfolding Case Study

There are different ways to center learning on the client. For example, problem-based learning experiences in nursing education are centered on a client and the client's health-related concerns. The client may be presented on paper as a case study or may be presented in the simulation lab or on video with an actor playing the part. In all of these methods, the client's situation takes a narrative form and changes over time as learners receive results of diagnostic tests and new information from the client and other sources, thus the case unfolds. The teacher's choice of a narrative and decisions about how the story will unfold are crucial to the learning experience. The first step in crafting an effective unfolding case study or narrative for use in a subject-centered classroom that incorporates the QSEN competencies is to examine five specific questions relative to objectives, content/concepts, context and narrative.

Objectives

When a teacher plans a course that will use case studies or narrative, she or he begins with course objectives and the objectives for the given class period (Glendon and Ulrich, 2001). These can include the QSEN KSAs specifically or embed these into other objectives. Either way, the objectives, whether addressing KSAs, should answer the question "What do I want learners to be able to do with the knowledge and skills they acquire during this class period?" (Michaelsen and Sweet, 2008). By shifting the approach to course design from knowledge *acquisition* to an emphasis on knowledge *use*, the teacher takes a step toward integrating classroom and clinical learning. For example, in designing a class on cardiac diseases, fluid balance, or symptom management, the teacher might start with the following QSEN-based knowledge objectives: "Describe reliable sources for locating evidence reports and clinical practice guidelines," and "Locate evidence reports related to clinical practice topics and guidelines." Then the teacher might restate these as a knowledge use objective, such as learners will be able to use knowledge of best evidence to assist a client with heart failure to maintain sodium restriction as a symptom management and health promotion strategy. With this restatement of the classroom learning objectives, the classroom becomes a place where learners actively engage with the knowledge of the discipline to be of service to a client, family, or community. Learners are motivated to learn as the teacher/coach helps them acquire the KSAs they will need as nurses to provide best care to the client.

Concepts and Content

The next important question is "What concepts and content should I use as the medium to facilitate learning?" This question casts the content as the medium rather than the message and further emphasizes knowledge *use* over knowledge acquisition. To transform the classroom into a learning experience situated in nursing practice that puts Palmer's subject or "third thing" in the center, teaching and learning content lies in thinking and responding like a nurse, that is, the purpose of learning the content and concepts is to develop the ability to think and respond like a nurse in situations that demand such a response. The nurse who has acquired evidence-based knowledge that a sodium-restricted diet will improve the health of clients with heart failure will not necessarily know how to use this knowledge effectively to deliver patient-centered care through teamwork and collaboration with other providers. In an encounter with a client or other members of the health care team, the nurse must integrate this knowledge with communication, teaching, and trust-building skills, and with values of compassion, empathy, and understanding to provide high quality, safe care.

Context

The next question speaks to the context that situates the learning in nursing practice: "What client situation will take us there?" For example, if by the end of a class period the teacher wants learners to be able to respond appropriately as nurses to clients who have just returned from a diagnostic procedure, one effective context may be care of a client after diagnostic cardiac catheterization. This procedure offers enough complexity in managing safety and quality, such as intravenous contrast, an arterial puncture, sedation, post-procedure risks, or client and family anxiety, to introduce many QSEN competencies and objectives while encouraging learners to consider seriously the nursing roles and responsibilities in this and similar situations where clients are exposed to the risks of diagnostic procedures or treatments.

 Crafting these types of objectives and using content in this way moves content delivery from a central role to a facilitative role. The teacher will use content in order to help learners acquire certain abilities. These abilities might be very specific and task-oriented safety skills (e.g., be able to follow the proper steps to administer medications safely), be data collection/assessment related (e.g., be able to interpret and respond appropriately to changes in cardiac rhythm), or be more broadly concerned with patient/family-centered care (e.g., be able to elicit and respond appropriately to health-related concerns from an older adult client). The third question, regarding context, brings the client to the center and gives teachers and learners a reason to care about the content, as well as a motive for learning and discovering. These first three questions also shift the teacher's preparation for classroom learning from passive knowledge acquisition with the question "What do I want learners to know?" to active learning and accomplishment, as shown in the question "What do I want learners to be able to do?"

Developing the Narrative

The teacher's answers to the first three questions guide construction of the narrative. The next step delves a bit further in order to situate the learning in a specific nursing care context by asking two more questions:

1) Where and under what circumstances will the nurse/student meet the client and learn of the client's health issues?
2) How will the narrative develop?

Textbox 10.4 Outpatient Clinic Visit

Mr. Prince is a 75-year-old male with a history of hypertension, CAD, CABG, and heart failure His son brought him to clinic today for evaluation of a weight gain of one pound over the past week. Mr. Prince says, "I may have cheated on my salt this week." He lives with his son and daughter-in-law and their two school-age children.

Vital signs	Today	3 months ago
HR	100	90
BP	100/80	110/70
RR	20	18
SaO2	97%	96%
T	36.8 c	37 c
Weight	175 lbs	173 lbs

Many different client narratives will work to accomplish the goals of being able to interpret clinical signs and symptoms and begin to develop comfort in talking with older adult clients about their health concerns. But the client's health condition will differ; the nurse will meet the client, learn of the client's concerns and respond in a variety of ways; and the narrative will unfold differently depending on the situation and setting in which the client is introduced. For example, meeting a client in a primary care clinic inspires different questions and responses from the nurse than does meeting a client in the acute medical unit of the hospital. Textbox 10.4 illustrates a second possible beginning narrative in the context of the outpatient clinic.

To stimulate and develop learners' clinical imaginations, it is important to ensure authenticity in the narrative and include information from believable sources given the context. For instance, in a primary care clinic, the nurse typically first receives information from the client or family directly as a report of what brought them to clinic and/or answers to health history questions. In acute care settings, the nurse typically first meets the client through some form of hand-off report from another nurse who might be giving a report from the previous shift, from the ED where the client was admitted, from the post-anesthesia care unit or critical care unit, or from a long-term care facility. Which narrative a teacher chooses to develop and where she or he chooses to begin the story will depend on what learning she or he wants to emphasize as the narrative develops and changes. By using the acute care narrative introduction shown in Textbox 10.1 and report from the ED nurse, the unfolding narrative can take the client through an entire hospitalization with multiple opportunities for learners to plan and evaluate safety and team collaboration, and to engage with health system informatics as they search for reliable sources to support their choice of interventions. This further promotes an understanding of systems thinking in managing client care so important in quality and safety. If the acute care narrative begins with a report from the previous shift on a more stable client who will be discharged to home that day, or if primary care is the setting, learners and teachers can delve more deeply into QSEN competencies and KSAs related to patient-centered care as they engage in discharge planning.

The two examples of beginning development of unfolding clinical narratives in Textboxes 10.1 and 10.4 illustrate different concerns and a different sense of urgency for the nurse. Ms. Baker's acuity is different in each scenario, and each introduction predicts a different unfolding in step 2. By carefully choosing, combining, and re-combining facts, the teacher can develop a narrative that takes teachers and learners into many different areas of concern and areas of conflicting concern. For example, for the Mr. Prince introduced in Textbox 10.1, the nurse's priority is his breathing, but Mr. Prince or his son might have different concerns that risk pulling the nurse away from this priority. This creates an opportunity to explore the tensions between two QSEN competencies: patient-centered care and safety. The choices the teacher makes about how the narrative will evolve will determine how the priorities of care shift. For example, the Mr. Prince introduced in Textbox 10.1 might stabilize and his narrative unfold to the Mr. Prince in Textbox 10.4 where the priority may be questions and concerns he has about going home. By adding facts that are less relevant to the main priority as the narrative unfolds, like the slight changes in vital signs introduced in step 1 of each, the teacher can coach the learners to attend to the most pressing concerns first and guide them toward developing a sense of salience.

Using clinical narratives in classroom teaching is a way to situate learning for the students and encourage them to begin thinking like nurses. Centering class discussion on a narrative that unfolds over time situates the learners and teachers as nurses with the teacher as coach. The next section of this chapter will discuss how teachers can support students' thinking and coach with carefully constructed questions and reflective practice strategies as they discover the content and concepts embedded in the narrative.

Reflective Practice and Questioning Strategies for Situated Coaching

Reflective practice is also a key component of narrative learning. Through mindful inquiry, learners develop a questioning attitude that guides them to ask relevant questions about practice (Day and Smith, 2007). Nurses and learners who adopt this questioning attitude uncover gaps in their own thinking and care delivery or gaps within the system. Learners can use structured reflection to analyze case studies, narratives, practice events, and other learning experiences to consciously examine how their actions are consistent with their beliefs and attitudes (Ironside, Cerbie, and Wonder, 2017). Reflection is a systematic way of thinking about one's actions and responses in order to change future actions and responses, which is the first step to improvement (Freshwater, Taylor, and Sherwood, 2008). Reflection is asking questions.

The QSEN competencies and situated coaching with unfolding case studies rely on a spirit of inquiry so each nurse, learner, and teacher asks questions both to determine the evidence for why actions are implemented while always exploring better ways to do one's work. Developing reflective practice supports Sullivan's three apprenticeships by helping learners analyze values and beliefs (ethical comportment), identify breakdowns in communication with clients and co-workers (skills), and discover gaps in their knowledge (cognitive).

Reflective practice is a basic skill in developing critical reasoning that examines practice situations and cultivates deep learning. Reflective practices help develop affective or attitudinal skills like emotional intelligence, leadership capacity, and engagement in work activities that promote constant improvement and professional maturity (Horton-Deustch and Sherwood, 2008). Reflective practice guides learning from experience by asking practitioners to consider their knowledge, beliefs, and values within the context of the situation. Reflection during and after clinical events helps nurses make sense of what happened and resolve emotional conflicts and questions of personal and professional effectiveness and satisfaction. Reflective practice is a way to organize group dialogue among novice and more experienced nurses or between disciplines to promote learning from and about each other. Nurses may write narratives of meaningful encounters with patients or co-workers and reflect on the meaning from varied perspectives, such as the patient, family, or other providers, to promote patient-centered care, teamwork, and collaboration.

Reflecting in or on action helps develop greater awareness of behavior, skills, and attitudes to help nurses accept accountability for actions. As part of the classroom learning experience with unfolding narratives, the teacher can coach the student to reflect before, in, and on action. Reflecting before action may include the briefing process in planning and coordinating care, considering what one knows as well as what one needs to deliver safe care. Reflecting in action happens in the moment as learners respond to the client's changing condition as the narrative unfolds, to assess actions, clear their mind, or bring focus to the patient being cared for. It may call for a team huddle where learners work in groups to address complex problems, problem solve to get everyone on the same page, clarify miscommunication, strategize on how to engage the patient or family in care, or learn from a near miss. Reflecting on action can be applied at the end of the class to mine events for lessons learned, or learners may write one-minute reflections on their experiences.

Learners can use the following steps to write about a particular event, in the classroom case study or in their clinical or lab experiences, that stands out in their mind or has unresolved consequences:

- Describe what happened, give objective details of the event.
- Examine feelings that arose in the moment and in the aftermath.
- Think about the event from multiple perspectives to see positive and negative aspects.
- Analyze knowledge and attitudes that influenced what happened to make sense of it.
- Consider alternatives; ask what else could you have done? What gaps in knowledge affected what happened?
- Determine the appropriate response by setting an action plan for future situations.
- Adapted from "The Scholarship of Reflective Practice," by Freshwater *et al.*, 2005, Sigma Theta Tau International Task Force on the Scholarship of Reflective Practice. Available for download at http://www.nursingsociety.org/aboutus/PositionPapers/Pages/position_resource_papers.aspx

Critical reflection based on appreciative inquiry can be applied to evaluate or assess achievement of learning objectives, guide learners in self-assessment, or contribute to a professional portfolio for career development. Changes in attitudes or movement toward professional maturity that may not be revealed in standardized tests, multiple choice questions, or traditional performance evaluations may be visible in reflections. Educators may develop rubrics to respond to reflective learning activities, simulations, or case studies. An appreciative inquiry guide with the following questions may lead the learner to reflect on times of success:

- What were standout events (this semester/this work period) when I felt successful?
- What about the events made me feel effective?
- What roles and responses did others have?
- How was this different from other events?
- What are lessons learned to guide my actions in the future?

When learning is situated with an evolving clinical narrative, the teacher can facilitate the learners' discovery and use of the knowledge they need in order to be of best service to the patient/client/family by guiding their reflection and coaching their thinking. In the role of coach and facilitator, the teacher encourages learners to ask questions and discuss ideas with the teacher and with each other. Opening the class discussion with a clinical narrative orients the learners toward the nurse's work and concerns. Then, with guidance and coaching from the teacher and from each other, learners will adopt and assimilate reflective practices and thinking habits. In this way, learners will become aware of their own thinking patterns and develop these patterns into habits of thought that match what is known as thinking like a nurse (Tanner 2006, Armstrong, Horton-Deutsch & Sherwood, 2012).

One coaching strategy is to give students specific questions to consider when approaching an unfolding narrative. For example, after they receive report on a hospitalized client, the teacher can ask learners what the risks are to the client and how the nurse can reduce the risks. In the example of the client with heart failure, one risk is fluid overload, and the nurse can address this risk by managing fluid intake and monitoring output. Two more questions are then appropriate to help learners organize their thinking and anticipate future events: How will the nurse recognize and respond to the risk if it develops? Then when the narrative unfolds, good questions for learners to contemplate include the following: 1) What questions do you have? 2) What essential data are missing? 3) What concerns do you have? 4) What actions will you take and what will you do first? 5) What do you think the client and family are experiencing?

In the beginning, the teacher asks the questions and gives learners ideas about how to organize their thinking to formulate good nursing-oriented and client-centered answers. Eventually, the learners should be able to ask their own questions and arrive at answers that show they are thinking like nurses.

Summary

Integrating the QSEN competencies calls for rethinking nursing curricula to replace simple content delivery with interactive classroom learning where the teacher coaches learners to use what they know in a situated context that mimics real world application. Nurse educators can transform classroom learning by integrating it with clinical learning; integrating Sullivan's three apprenticeships: cognitive, skill-based, and ethical comportment; and centering learning on the true subject of nursing, that is, the client, family, or community. The method presented in this chapter for constructing unfolding case narratives provides the basis for subject-centered, contextualized learning in the classroom that can accomplish all of this while still providing students with the knowledge and information they need. Starting class by introducing a patient and family and then guiding learners as they think through changes in the situation transforms learning into an active, reflective, situated experience, and transforms the teaching role. The teacher becomes coach in using carefully constructed authentic case study narratives that guide learners toward new concepts and content so they plan and provide best care to a particular patient and family.

References

American Association of Colleges of Nursing. (2008) *The essentials of doctor of nursing practice.* Washington, DC: Author.

American Association of Colleges of Nursing. (2009) *The essentials of baccalaureate education for professional nursing practice.* Washington, DC: Author.

American Association of Colleges of Nursing. (2011) *The essentials of master's education for professional nursing practice.* Washington, DC: Author.

Armstrong, G., Sherwood, G., and Tagliareni, E. (2009) Quality and Safety Education in Nursing (QSEN): Integrating recommendations from IOM into clinical nursing education. In T. Valiga and N. Ard (Eds.), *Clinical nursing education: Critical reflections* (pp. 207–226). New York: National League for Nursing Press.

Armstrong, G., Horton-Deutsch, S., and Sherwood, G. (2017) Reflection in clinical contexts: learning, collaboration, and evaluation. In reflective practice: Transforming education and improving outcomes. In S. Horton-Deutsch and G. Sherwood (Eds.), (2nd Ed). Sigma Theta Tau International Press: Indianapolis.

Barnsteiner, J. (2017) Safety. In G. Sherwood and J. Barnsteiner (Eds.), *Quality and safety in nursing: A competency approach to improving outcomes.* Hoboken, NJ: Wiley-Blackwell.

Barnsteiner, J., Disch, J., Johnson, J, McGuinn, K., Chappell, K. and Swartwout, E. (2013) Diffusing QSEN competencies across schools of nursing: the AACN/RWJF Faculty Development Institutes. *Journal of Professional Nursing, 29*(2), 68–74.

Barton, A., Armstrong, G., Preheim, G., Gelmon, S., and Andrus, L. (2009) A national Delphi to determine developmental progression of quality and safety competencies in nursing education. *Nursing Outlook, 57*(6), 313–322.

Batalden, P.B., Leach, D., and Ogrinc, G. (2009) Knowing is not enough: Executives and educators must act to address challenges and reshape healthcare. *Healthcare Executive, 24*(2), 68–70.

Benner, P. (1984) *From novice to expert: Excellence and power in clinical nursing practice.* Menlo Park, CA: Addison Wesley.

Benner, P., Sutphen, M., Leonard, V., and Day, L. (2010) *Educating nurses: A call for radical transformation.* San Francisco: Jossey-Bass.

Brown, R., Feller, L., and Benedict, L. (2010) Reframing nursing education: the Quality and Safety Education for Nurses initiative. *Teaching and Learning in Nursing, 5*, 115–118. doi:101016/j.teln.2010.02.005.

Cronenwett, L. (2017) A national initiative: Quality and Safety Education for Nurses (QSEN). In G. Sherwood and J. Barnsteiner (Eds.), *Quality and safety in nursing: A competency approach to improving outcomes.* Hoboken, NJ: Wiley-Blackwell.

Cronenwett, L., Sherwood, G., Barnsteiner, J., Disch, J., Johnson, J., Mitchell, P., *et al.* (2007) Quality and safety education for nurses. *Nursing Outlook, 55*(3), 122–131.

Cronenwett, L., Sherwood, G., and Gelmon, S. (2009) Improving quality and safety education: The QSEN learning collaborative. *Nursing Outlook, 57*(6), 304–312.

Cronenwett, L., Sherwood, G., Pohl, J., Barnsteiner, J., Moore, S., Sullivan, D. T., *et al.* (2009) Quality and safety education for advanced practice nursing practice. *Nursing Outlook, 57*(6), 338–348.

Day, L. (2011) Using Unfolding Case Studies in a Subject- Centered Classroom. *Journal of Nursing Education, 50*(8), 447–452. doi: 10.3928/01484834-20110517-03.

Day, L., and Sherwood, G. (2017) Transforming Education to Transform Practice: Integrating Quality and Safety in Unfolding Case Studies. In G. Sherwood and J. Barnsteiner (Eds.), *Quality and safety in nursing: A competency approach to improving outcomes.* (2nd Ed). Hoboken, NJ: Wiley-Blackwell.

Durham, C., and Sherwood, G. (2008) Education to bridge the quality gap: A case study approach. *Journal of Urologic Nursing* [Special issue], *28*(6), 431–438.

Durham, C., and Alden, K. (2012) Integrating Quality and Safety Competencies in Simulation. In G. Sherwood and J. Barnsteiner (Eds.), *Quality and safety in nursing: A competency approach to improving outcomes.* Hoboken, NJ: Wiley-Blackwell.

Finkelman, A., and Kenner, C. (2009) *Teaching IOM: Implications of the Institute of Medicine reports for nursing,* 2nd Ed. Silver Spring, MD: American Nurses Association.

Freshwater, D., Horton-Deutsch, S., Sherwood, G., and Taylor, B. (2005) *The scholarship of reflective practice* [Resource paper]. Available at Sigma Theta Tau International web site: http://www.nursingsociety.org/aboutus/PositionPapers/Pages/position_resource_papers.aspx.

Freshwater, D., Taylor, B., and Sherwood, G. (Eds.). (2008) *International textbook of reflective practice in nursing.* Oxford: Blackwell Publishing and Sigma Theta Tau Press.

Glendon, Kellie J., and Ulrich, Deborah L. (2001). *Unfolding case studies: Experiencing the realities of clinical nursing practice.* New Jersey: Prentice-Hall.

Greer, A.G., Pokorny, M., Clay, M.C., Brown, S., and Steele, L.L. (2010) Learner Centered Characteristics of Nurse Educators. *International Journal of Nursing Education Scholarship, 7*(1): 15p–15p. 1p.

Horton-Deutsch, S., and Sherwood, G. (2008) Reflection: An educational strategy to develop emotionally competent nurse leaders. *Journal of Nursing Management, 8*, 946–954.

Hughes, R.G. (2008) *Patent safety and quality: An evidence-based handbook for nurses* (AHRQ Publication No. 08–0043). Rockville, MD: Agency for Healthcare Research and Quality. http://www.ahrq.gov/qual/nurseshdbk.

Institute of Medicine. (2003) *Health professions education: A bridge to quality*. Washington, DC: National Academies Press.

Institute of Medicine. (2010) *The future of nursing: Leading change, advancing health*. Washington, DC: National Academies Press.

Interprofessional Education Collaborative Expert Panel (IPEC). (2011) *Core competencies for interprofessional collaborative practice: Report of an expert panel* Washington, DC: Interprofessional Education Collaborative.

Ironside, P., and Cerbie, E. (2017) Narrative teaching strategies to foster quality and safety. In G. Sherwood and J. Barnsteiner (Eds.), *Quality and safety in nursing: A competency approach to improving outcomes*. Hoboken, NJ: Wiley-Blackwell.

Johnson, J. (2017) Quality improvement. In G. Sherwood & J. Barnsteiner (Eds.), *Quality and safety in nursing: A competency approach to improving outcomes*. Hoboken, NJ: Wiley-Blackwell.

Joint Commission. (2016) *2016 National Patient Safety Goals*. Retrieved from https://www.jointcommission.org/standards_information/npsgs.aspx.

Michaelsen, L.K. and Sweet, M. (2008) The essential elements of team-based learning. *New Directions for Teaching and Learning, 2008*(116), 7–27. doi: 10.1002/tl.330.

National Council of State Boards of Nursing. *Simulation Study*. Accessed May 10, 2016 at https://www.ncsbn.org/685.htm.

National League for Nursing. (2010) *Outcomes and competencies for graduates of practical/vocational, diploma, associate degree, baccalaureate, masters, doctoral and research doctorate programs in nursing*. New York: National League for Nursing.

National Quality Forum. (2012) Serious Reportable Events. Accessed May 10, 2016 http://www.qualityforum.org/Topics/SREs/Serious_Reportable_Events.aspx.

Page, A. (2004) *Keeping patients safe: Transforming the work environment of nurses*. Committee on the Work Environment for Nurses and Patient Safety, Board on Health Care Services. Washington, DC: National Academies Press.

Palmer, Parker J. (1998) *The courage to teach: Exploring the inner landscape of a teacher's life*. San Francisco: Jossey-Bass.

Pohl, J., Savrin, C., Fiandt, K., Beauchesne, M., Drayton-Brooks, S., Scheibmeir, M., and Brackley, M. (2009) Quality and safety in graduate nursing education: Cross-mapping QSEN graduate competencies with NONPF's NP core and practice doctorate competencies. *Nursing Outlook, 57*(6), 349–354.

Preheim, G.J., Armstrong, G.E., and Barton, A.J. (2009) The new fundamentals in nursing: Introducing beginning quality and safety education for nurses' competencies. *Journal of Nursing Education, 48*(12), 694–697.

Sammer, C.E., Lykens, K., Singh, K.P., Mains, D.A., and Lackan, N.A. (2010) What is patient safety culture? A review of the literature. *Journal of Nursing Scholarship, 42*(2), 156–165.

Sherwood, G. (2006) Appreciative leadership: Building customer driven partnerships. *JONA, 36*(12), 551–557.

Sherwood, G. (2011) Integrating quality and safety science in nursing education and practice. *Journal of Research in Nursing, 16*(3), 226–240. doi: 10:1177/1744987111400960.

Sherwood, G. (2017) Driving forces for quality and safety: Changing mindsets to improve health care. In G. Sherwood and J. Barnsteiner (Eds.), *Quality and safety in nursing: A competency approach to improving outcomes*. Hoboken, NJ: Wiley-Blackwell.

Sherwood, G. and Drenkard, K. (2007) Quality and safety curricula in nursing education: Matching practice realities. *Nursing Outlook*, 55(3), 151–155.

Smith, E.L. and Day, L. (2007) Integrating quality and safety content into clinical teaching in the acute care setting. *Nursing Outlook*, 55(3), 138–143.

Spector, N., Ulrich, B., and Barnsteiner, J. (2017) New graduate transition into practice: Improving quality and safety. In G. Sherwood and J. Barnsteiner (Eds.), *Quality and safety in nursing: A competency approach to improving outcomes*. Hoboken, NJ: Wiley-Blackwell.

Sullivan, W. (2005) *Work and Integrity: The Crisis and Promise of Professionalism in America* 2nd Ed. San Francisco: Jossey-Bass.

Sullivan, D.T., Hirst, D., and Cronenwett, L. (2009) Assessing quality and safety competencies of graduating prelicensure nursing students. *Nursing Outlook*, 57(6), 323–331.

Tanner, C.A. (2006) Thinking like a nurse: a research-based model of clinical judgment in nursing. *Journal of Nursing Education*, 45(6), 204–211.

The Critical Thinking Community. (2014) Defining Critical Thinking. Retrieved July 28, 2014 from http://www.criticalthinking.org/pages/defining-critical-thinking/766.

Thornlow, D. and McGuinn, K. (2010) A necessary sea change for nurse faculty development: Spotlight on quality and safety. *Journal of Professional Nursing*, 26(2), 71–81.

Resources

Agency for Healthcare Research and Quality (AHRQ):
Information and resources, including information on TeamSTEPPS, evidence-based practice, relevant research, patient teaching information, and consumer information around quality and safety. http://www.ahrq.gov/

American Association of Colleges of Nursing: www.aacn.nche.edu
Resources for standards and guidelines for education and practice

American Association of Critical Care Nurses:
Clinical Practice resources for standards and guidelines for education and practice related to critical care and the work environment
www.aacn.org/DM/MainPages/PracticeHome.aspx?lastmenu=divheader_clinical_practice

American Nurses Association. The National Center for Nursing Quality Indicators: www.nursingquality.org
Resources for standards and guidelines for education and practice:

Institute for Healthcare Improvement (IHI)
The IHI has information about programs, links to patient safety information and Open School for learners. http://www.ihi.org/IHI/

Institute of Medicine (IOM)
The IOM is a nonprofit organization that provides science-based information about health and science policy. http://www.iom.edu/

Institute for Safe Medication Practices (ISMP)
Educates healthcare providers and the public about safe medication practices with many resources for safe medication practices. http://www.ismp.org/

International Nursing Association for Clinical Simulation and Learning (INACSL)
Promotes research and disseminate evidence based practice standards for clinical simulation methodologies and learning environments. http://www.inacsl.org

Interprofessional Education Collaborative Expert Panel. (2011). *Core competencies for interprofessional collaborative practice: Report of an expert panel.* Washington, D.C.: Interprofessional Education Collaborative. http://www.aacn.nche.edu/education-resources/IPECReport.pdf

Massachusetts Nurse of the Future Core Curriculum
http://www.mass.edu/currentinit/currentinitNursingNurseFutureComp.asp

National Center for Interprofessional Practice and Education
Resources for integrating health professions education and practice into a transformative Nexus. https://nexusipe.org/

National Council of State Boards of Nursing. https://www.ncsbn.org/685.htm

National League for Nursing: Organization promoting and guiding nursing education programs across all levels of education. www.nln.org

North Carolina Board of Nursing Just Culture
Resources to develop a culture that promotes learning from student practice errors while properly assigning accountability for behaviors and consistently evaluating events.
http://www.ncbon.com/dcp/i/nursing-education-resources-for-program-directors-just-culture-information

Oregon Consortium of Nurse Educators. http://ocne.org/index.html

Quality and Safety Education for Nurses (QSEN)
National project for integrating patient-centered care, teamwork and collaboration, evidenced-based practice, quality improvement, safety, and informatics competencies into nursing education and practice. http://qsen.org/

Robert Wood Johnson Foundation
The Future of Nursing: Leading Change, Advancing Health (2010). http://www.iom.edu/Reports/2010/The-Future-of-Nursing-Leading-Change-Advancing-Health.aspx

Simulation Innovation Resource Center (SIRC) National League for Nursing
e-learning site for nursing educators to learn about simulation http://sirc.nln.org/

TeamSTEPPS© (Team Strategies and Tools to Enhance Performance and Patient Safety) Teamwork and communication curriculum developed by the Department of Defense in collaboration with AHRQ. http://teamstepps.ahrq.gov/

11

Using Narrative Pedagogy to Foster Quality and Safety

*Pamela M. Ironside, PhD, RN, FAAN, ANEF, Elizabeth Cerbie Brown, MSN, RN
and Amy Hagedorn Wonder, PhD, RN*

Initially I didn't even plan on going into the room until as I walked by I noticed my patient had a visitor, so I thought this would be a good opportunity to introduce myself and get some information. (It had really been difficult getting information from him because of his complications with speech and everything.) So I introduced myself and then just tried to strike up a conversation with the patient, you know, like "How are you doing? And how are you related?" and all that, and then he told me this was his son and a little bit more information about himself. And once there was a really, you know, a general rapport, I started to ask questions about what brought him here, about his living conditions, and does he know anything about his medications. But once I started asking about if he's ever had any complications I noticed he started to get a little bit cold and distant. He got really quiet. And that's when I started to kind of back away a little bit, like okay, "Well, I'll let you guys spend some time together and let me know if you need anything." And as I started to walk away I heard him utter something under his breath, which I wanted to address because it didn't sound very, it was something to the effect of 'stay out of my business!' And I said, "Excuse me. I didn't hear you," because it's been difficult to understand him the whole time. And he said, "You heard me!" And I could tell he was angry. So I wanted to kind of smooth it over because this was still in the middle of the shift and I'm still going to be caring for him, and I didn't want any more problems. And I just explained that "I'm sorry if I offended you or if you're angry. I'm just trying to get some more background because I don't have all the information I need. Then he expressed his anger some more, and I apologized left the room. (Kelly, prelicensure student)

The goal of the QSEN initiative is to transform nurses' professional identity in such a way that every nurse has a commitment to improve the quality and safety of health care wherever and whenever it is delivered (Cronenwett *et al.*, 2007). To that end, educators across the country are working diligently to embed the QSEN competencies as well as knowledge, skill, and attitude statements into their courses and curricula. To be successful, however, these efforts must go far beyond merely providing learners with more content knowledge about particular aspects of quality and safety or more skills they can proficiently and habitually perform. Rather, achieving a transformation in nurses' professional identity will require a change in how educators think about nursing practice and how we prepare learners to engage in that practice.

Quality and Safety in Nursing: A Competency Approach to Improving Outcomes, Second Edition.
Edited by Gwen Sherwood and Jane Barnsteiner.
© 2017 John Wiley & Sons, Inc. Published 2017 by John Wiley & Sons, Inc.

Teaching Nursing Practice

The predominant approach to teaching nursing in both academic and practice settings is conventional pedagogy, which focuses heavily on cognitive gain and skill acquisition as the basis of all learning encounters. Two common assumptions of this approach are that 1) content knowledge is best presented beginning with simple aspects and progressing to those that are more complex, and 2) when learners have acquired the prespecified content knowledge, they can then apply it in assigned practice settings in a linear, direct, and corresponding manner to provide evidence of their learning (Ironside, 2001). This approach to teaching is pervasive in the discipline, and educators rarely question the utility or limits of using just one pedagogy to prepare learners to provide safe, quality care. Because of this over-reliance on conventional pedagogy, teachers often mistake the mere adoption of innovative strategies as the means by which the QSEN goal can be met.

It is clearly important for students to obtain knowledge of the field and proficiency in practice skills before they enter the workforce. Yet, knowledge and skills alone are insufficient to prepare students for practice. Indeed, research is increasingly explicating the complexity of nurses' work (e.g., Cline, 2015; Sitterding *et al.*, 2012) and the complex web of interconnected, interdependent, and diverse elements (Lindberg, Nash, and Lindberg, 2008) that make up the systems within which care is delivered. Navigating the complexity of care delivery systems requires that students learn diverse skills, such as managing ambiguity and uncertainty, dealing with interruptions and distractions, making qualitative distinctions between different manifestations of health disruptions or different patients' and families' responses to health and illness, and understanding differing perspectives of practice encounters. For example, Kelly's story at the start of the chapter provides teachers and students with a plethora of opportunities to explore different perspectives, real or potential conflicts in how care is experienced, and the meaning these experiences have for nurses, patients, and families. Teaching these aspects of nursing practice will require new pedagogies.

Narrative Pedagogy

Narrative pedagogy, a research-based, phenomenological pedagogy, was first identified during a longitudinal study of the experiences of teachers, students, and clinicians in nursing education (Diekelmann and Diekelmann, 2009). Consistent with its philosophical underpinnings in hermeneutic phenomenology, educators enacting narrative pedagogy shift their attention from merely delivering or demonstrating specific content and skills to co-creating experiences in which they work *with* students to explore their experiences in nursing education and to challenge their preconceived notions and habitual ways of thinking (Ironside, 2015). As teachers and students think together about the situations they encounter, they challenge their assumptions and reflect on, question, and reinterpret their shared experiences. In so doing, they discover new possibilities for learning and practice that are local, at hand, and context-specific.

Importantly, narrative pedagogy is an inclusive pedagogy in that it also embraces research in higher education, including attention to issues such as power (critical pedagogy), voice (feminist pedagogy), and the meta-narratives that shape nursing education and practice (postmodern pedagogy). These diverse pedagogies (conventional, critical, feminist, phenomenological, and postmodern) are not mutually exclusive but rather extend and enhance one another. Bringing multiple pedagogies to bear on learning and teaching in nursing, teachers enacting narrative pedagogy create learning experiences that invite students and clinicians to think differently and to be open to new understandings and possibilities for improving education and practice (Ironside, 2014). When narrative pedagogy is enacted, teachers, students, and clinicians share their experiences communally, most frequently by writing accounts and reading them aloud (Ironside and Hayden-Miles, 2012) or posting them in discussion forums. Writing the account of an experience involves rethinking the experience and making it intelligible to others by filling in details, concerns, and contextual factors that give the account its meaning and set up the possibility of understanding the experience in new ways. For instance, a graduate student began her account as follows:

> It was colder than I ever remember a January night to be. With the fullest, brightest moon, the deepest wind chill, and our Emergency Department no less busy for the weather. The wind was fierce and unforgiving, and the moon in the clearest night of the year lit the way to our doors. It was a cruel night for lost souls. There were more than the usual feverish, fretful children; tired, despondent single mothers; impatient, irritated youth; the homeless and rejected needy. There were too few of our own nurses, a tired and overworked pair of physicians, and no one had thought to bring "treats." I was in charge of it all *(Ironside et al., 1998).*

Because understanding is always already situated, contextual, and directed toward possibilities (Heidegger, 1927/1962), descriptions such as this draw the listener/reader into the experience as they hear this charge nurse describe her worries and concerns in the context of a bitterly cold night, a busy emergency department, short staffing, and "no treats." The listener/reader is drawn into the experience, not as a distanced observer, but as an engaged participant. The listener is right there in the account (Gadamer, 2001) and, together with the teller, must attend to the context, challenges, and opportunities influencing the possibilities for care (Ironside and Hayden-Miles, 2012). Sharing narrative accounts also reveals preconceived notions, oversights, and misunderstandings brought into the experience, as this prelicensure student shared as he began the story of his experience caring for a patient with end-stage renal disease:

> I got report from the night nurse who said my patient, who had end-stage renal disease, was refusing dialysis. I couldn't believe he would do this! He had been on dialysis for a while and things were going well. Obviously I would need to do some teaching about his disease and reinforce the consequences of refusing treatment. But when I met the patient and his wife, he said he hadn't refused dialysis. I was surprised by this because I was sure the night nurse had said he had refused. So then I started wondering if he was confused or if he was lying or what. I mean, maybe he just didn't want his wife to know he wanted to refuse. Why would I hear this in report if it wasn't true?

Teaching students how to make qualitative distinctions between different patients' responses to health and illness requires the exploration of the assumptions that inform their thinking about particular situations. Narrative accounts of experiences and collaboratively engaging in cycles of interpretation provide opportunities for teachers and students to appreciate multiple perspectives and to think through preconceived notions.

To elicit narrative accounts of experiences, some teachers ask students to write an account of their most memorable experience in a particular clinical setting or to write an account in response to prompts such as, "Today I was worried when...," "I didn't know what to do or say when...," or "I was surprised to find..." (Ironside and Hayden-Miles, 2012). Other teachers have invited beginning students to share an experience that stands out for them in which they cared for, or were cared for by, another person (Ironside, 2003). Similarly, when orienting new nurses, staff educators have asked new nurses to bring narrative accounts of a time during the orientation when they were unsure about what was going on clinically with a patient or about a memorable moment they encountered during the orientation. Patient and family stories are also a rich source of narratives to

---

Textbox 11.1 Interpretive Questions to Examine Story

Please reflect on your experiences today in clinical. What stands out for you in this experience? As you think about this time, write the story of your experience. Your story may be of breakdown when nothing went right *or* of making a difference, when everything "fell into place." Include as much detail as possible and tell your story in first person, rather than stepping back and analyzing or describing "objectively." Consider what was running through your head at the time. What you were seeing and hearing? Any little fact of the story you can recall belongs with your experience. After you have given the details of your story, please describe why this story is important to you and what it means to you.

Interpretive Questioning

• How was your attention shifting as the experience unfolded? What were you watching for? distracted by? worried about? surprised by?
• What is the *relationship* between X and Y? By whose account?
• Whose voice is missing/silent? Whose interests were being served?
• You had certain expectations and goals when you came into this experience. Can you say more about if/how these changed as the situation evolved?
• Have you encountered a situation like this before? How was this situation like (or different from) that one?
• What were you hearing from colleagues, faculty, other team members, and the patient/family during this time? What did it mean to you?

---

engage students in thinking about and questioning practice. In each case, the teacher/educator encourages students or patients/families to describe their experience as it happened, highlighting what was "going through their head" at the time or what they were thinking "while they were in the thick of it," rather than stepping back and giving a general overview or listing of what they did or said during the experience (Textbox 11.1). As experiences are shared, teachers and students engage in cycles of interpretation, exploring the meaning and significance of the experience, the assumptions underlying the ways the experience is understood, and the new insights about and possibilities for improving nursing education and practice revealed by this communal and collaborative thinking. Consider this narrative shared by a nurse educator who faced the limits of evidence-based practice when caring for her daughter.

> I'm not new to healthcare. In addition to working at the school of nursing, I've had far too much experience as a patient and family member! I've been dealing with melanoma now for a few years and have had repeated skin excisions from my back, arms, legs and chest. I was able to deal with that, although scheduling was a nightmare with a heavy academic load! But then last fall I learned my dad had stage 4 cancer. It was a shock for us all, and you know how that goes…as the nurse in the family you are just always on call for everyone's questions, concerns, tears, you name it. It was exhausting! So I'm used to talking with healthcare providers about the latest evidence guiding treatment choices and translating that for my family. I read a lot and always stress evidence-based practice with my students. Its something I believe in!
>
> Then quite unexpectedly my 9-year-old daughter came home from school with sharp abdominal pain. 24 hours later she was in the hospital. Come to find out she had pancreatitis and severe stomach ulcers. She was in a lot of pain and was really frightened by the whole event.

I was scared too, and I needed answers! What was happening to my daughter? What were we going to do about it? I sat by daughter's bedside day and night. Although the room was lit only by monitors, the pain in her face was overwhelming to me. She rolled in the bed and quietly cried, begging me to do something to stop the pain. I had never felt so helpless!

What made this even more difficult is that no one knew why she was experiencing this, or what to do about it despite being at a world-class pediatric facility. The nurses and residents spent little time with us. They were uncomfortable not knowing what to say or do, although I'm sure they looked diligently for some options and some evidence to support them. I asked questions, but they had no answers. As the days drug on they started to avoid me, coming into the room less and less. I searched the literature, I searched the internet, I talked with colleagues. I mean, I TEACH evidence-based practice, this is what I DO…how could I not find anything to help? The specialists that visited, and there were a lot of them, had little to offer. They discussed different approaches for treatment with us but because of the unknown cause the best evidence didn't seem to be "best" at all. But treatment decisions had to be made. How can I make informed decisions for my daughter when there's no good evidence? I tapped down the frantic feelings that kept surfacing. And in the meantime, we waited, hoping against hope for some answers.

Cycles of Interpretation

Teachers enacting narrative pedagogy engage students and clinicians in cycles of interpretation of their shared experiences by listening and co-responding, raising questions that provoke thinking. Together they explore the meaningfulness of the story, holding the understanding each brings to the account open and problematic. Seeking new ways to understand, they together attend to multiple perspectives (scientific, critical, feminist, postmodern, phenomenological, as well as perspectives of other team members, the patient, and the family). They also challenge assumptions, critique prevailing perspectives and the limits of current knowledge, and explore the meaning and significance of their interpretations for the emerging practice of the students and new nurses. Importantly, these efforts are not directed specifically toward identifying which perspective or action among those explored is best, most efficient, or most correct. Rather, consistent with the philosophical underpinnings of narrative pedagogy, all understanding is considered tentative as the complexity, uncertainty, and ambiguity of the encounter, as well as the fallibility of current knowledge and understandings, are preserved by cycles of interpretation. Through these cycles of interpretation, students learn to ask unsettling questions rather than rush to judgment about how to intervene in a particular situation.

Again, enacting narrative pedagogy and engaging in cycles of interpretation begin by hearing shared accounts of practice experiences. Consider this experience. Shelly has been a nurse for two years on a pediatric medical unit at City United Hospital, a large urban, acute care hospital. She shared the following story.

Shelly's Story

It's 3:30 p.m. on a busy pediatric medical unit. Afternoons are always busy because we are sending patients off the floor for tests, many of the medical teams are in seeing their patients, all of the consults are in progress, and we begin to get admissions and process discharges. I am assigned four busy patients and have just discharged my easiest patient (asthma exacerbation) to home. Then the charge nurse tells me there is a patient in the emergency department (ED) who needs to be admitted on our unit and I'm up for the admission. Geez, I think to myself, can't I just have 30 minutes to catch up?

I haven't charted all day and I need to spend time with my family in room 27; they have so many questions about their child's new diabetes diagnosis and they need some support. But I just smile at my charge nurse, and tell her OK. Inside I say a little prayer, hoping they won't bring the patient for a good long while. I check in on my patient in room 31 who doesn't have any family with him, but a child life specialist is in playing with him right now (thank goodness!). I decide the charting can wait – it's waited this long – and I head into room 27. The child's grandparents have now arrived and are taking turns playing with the adorable 5 year old. The mom looks at me, and I can see the raw emotion in her eyes. She is exhausted, confused, and terrified of what this new diagnosis means for her child and their family. Just as I pull up a chair to sit next to them, I get called overhead that I have a phone call. Of course I do. (SIGH!) I take the call in the hall, and it is Theresa from the ED. She is calling to report on my new patient and wants to know if she can bring him up in 10 minutes. I explain that I am with a patient and family right now and need to check on the room before she brings him to the floor, so it will be awhile before we are ready. She gets very impatient and says that she is bringing the patient up in 10 minutes, that should be enough time for the room to be ready, and hangs up the phone. OK, then. I flag the charge nurse down, verify that the room will be ready and go back into room 27. I am able to spend at least a little time with this family, answer some of their questions, assure them that the diabetes educators and dietician will be here shortly to spend some time with them. Then I tell them I have to go but will be back and get ready to take this admission. But Theresa is already rolling onto the floor with Brandon, a 15-year-old boy with cystic fibrosis. I know Brandon; he has been on our unit a lot. He looks pretty good, considering, so I breathe a sigh of relief. Theresa quickly gives me all of the charting that she brought with her, gives quick report, and as she asks me if I have any questions, she starts backing away from Brandon and me; it is pretty clear to me that she isn't interested in my questions. I know Brandon well, but with the unit so busy I'm really worried that I'll overlook or forget something. I try to get Brandon settled in his room, but he can't seem to get comfortable and asks for something to eat. This is going to be a long shift! Times like these are so frustrating! I don't know how I am supposed to keep up. Besides, what's the big rush to get Brandon to the unit and why was Theresa so pushy! Can't she see how busy we are?

By sharing experiences, the teller reveals to the listeners how he or she understands (interprets) the experience. But using narrative pedagogy is not just sharing experiences or responding to the teller's understanding; it is communally and collaboratively questioning the experience. It is a call to thinking deeply about everything present and absent in the experience (Diekelmann and Diekelmann, 2009). In adopting this interpretive stance, teachers, students, and clinicians come to explore in a new way the traditions they inherit, what currently occurs in practice, and what is possible.

After taking a few moments for listeners to consider the shared experience, teachers using narrative pedagogy frequently begin with an open question, such as, "What stands out for you in this story?" Open questions are a call to thinking and reveal what students notice, what catches their attention or piques their interest in the experience. By its very nature, this question is substantively different and sets up a different kind of conversation than asking questions from within conventional pedagogy, such as, "If you were in Shelly's position, what's the first thing you would do?" Importantly, the conversation that ensues as teacher and students engage in cycles of interpretation brings multiple perspectives and experiences, current literature, and further questioning to bear on better understanding this experience and on exploring the meaning and significance it has for nursing practice. For instance, as students comment on the tension between Shelly's desire to spend time with a distraught family and a new admission, the teacher may ask: What does it mean to nurses to face competing demands such as an exhausted, confused, and terrified family on one hand and a new admission with a recurrent exacerbation of his cystic fibrosis on the other? How do nurses decide how to spend their limited time? When the needs of a patient and the system conflict, how do nurses decide what approach to take?

These shared narratives are dynamic tellings/showings of the possibilities for nursing practice as well as the ambiguity, uncertainty, limits, and disruptions inherent in day-to-day practice. They are simultaneously about the individual nurse (teller), others involved in the encounter, the context or system in which the encounter occurred, and the traditions of nursing being learned by the student (for better or worse). Even when a particular experience is written about (e.g., clinical experiences of times students made a difference to a patient), there is always an excess of meaning for teachers, students, and clinicians to explore as matters of concern circulate, stand out, or fade into the background (Diekelmann and Diekelmann, 2009).

Teachers may also engage students in cycles of interpretation across the narratives shared by students and clinicians. In some cases, these narratives tell of experiences around a common theme, whereas in others they may include tellings of a shared experience. For example, Theresa, also a nurse at City United Hospital, is a highly experienced nurse in the emergency department.

Theresa's Story

My shift was supposed to start at 0700 this morning, but my phone rang at 0400 asking me if I'd come in a little early. One of the night shift nurses had a family emergency and had to leave. They often call me when they need help. I've been in this ED for 15 years, love what I do, and I'm pretty good at it. Plus, I am recently divorced and need the extra shifts for the money to pay the medical bills for my son. He is 7 years old and was born with a congenital heart malformation. He is doing well, but the medical bills are extensive, and he'll always require some care. Luckily, my family is extremely supportive, and they help whenever they can. Because I live with my sister and her family, they can watch my son so I can work the extra shifts.

When I arrive this morning, the ED is busy as usual. I take my assignment, three children, two who need some teaching before being discharged home and one who is being admitted. I am also to take over as charge nurse for the day shift. I jump right in so the night nurses can finish their shift and head home. We've been short staffed for days, but after 15 years, I guess you learn how to make anything work. This is less than ideal, but we would manage. As our morning goes on, we are working hard, but everything seems to be moving right along. I keep a close eye on everyone, just to be sure that no one gets overwhelmed. All the rooms are filled with patients and there are a few in the hall; the waiting room is packed. The hospital is full, so it is taking forever to get beds. As ED nurses, we are prepared to quickly diagnose, treat, and transfer, not to give care over a long period of time, so having such a backup of patients waiting to transfer can be really stressful for some long-term ED nurses.

I finish my discharges so I can focus on my other patient. His name is Brandon and he has cystic fibrosis. He seems to be doing fine but is being admitted for a "tune-up." We are just waiting for a bed to open up. I have just started talking with Brandon when the call comes in that we are getting a 7-year-old gunshot wound. What? Did they say a 7 year old? I let the trauma team know and get ready to assist. When the ambulance arrives, team members jump and we all start working quickly.

The victim is a beautiful 7-year-old boy who was outside playing in front of his house. He lived in a bad part of town, probably one of the worst, but it was a beautiful summer morning, probably the first one of the year. Unfortunately, as Isaac was playing outside, a stray bullet from a drive-by gang shooting hit him. In the ED we see too many senseless deaths! This is a hard one on our whole team! We work for almost an hour trying to stabilize him so he can get to surgery, but we lose our battle, and we lose him. The family is being called; only the mom is with him in the ED. She is, of course, devastated! She keeps saying, "I knew I shouldn't have let him play outside. Why did I let him play outside?" As I'm consoling her, I look up from where we are and see Brandon sitting up on his cart, looking across the hall at all of this, his big blue eyes just staring. So now I'm thinking, when is that bed going to be ready? What could be taking so long? He does not need to be down here seeing and hearing all this commotion! I motion to the unit secretary to check on the room for Brandon so we can get him out of here and comfortable in his own room, and give him a wave to let him know we're OK and I'll be over soon. I move the mom down the hall to a grief room. The secretary lets me know the bed is open and that I can give report to Shelly. About then the dad arrives and is just realizing what has happened to his son. I take him to his wife and get them settled into a private visitor's room. But by now I'm really worried that no one is checking in with Brandon. As soon as I can, I call to give report so I can get him into a more comfortable place and away from all this commotion and sadness. When I get the nurse, Shelly, on the phone, she says she knows Brandon (Great, I think, that should speed things up!), but I can tell she doesn't want to take this admission right now; she keeps trying to put me off. I mean, come on! Brandon has already been down here for 4 hours, and this is obviously not a good place for him right now! As I'm trying to get off the phone as quickly as I can, more family members arrive and they are sobbing and yelling in the hall near Brandon's room. I tell Shelly that I'll be bringing him up in 10 minutes and quickly hang up to go support the newest family member who has arrived and learned of their loss.

I go back in to check on mom and dad, and ask them if they want to see Isaac, their little boy, one last time. I can see the fear in their eyes, but I tell them I will be right there with them. They are relieved and say they want to say their goodbyes. I tell them to take some time right now with the chaplain, and I'll get the room ready for them. I don't want them to see Isaac this way, so I need a few minutes to prepare him and the room. I'm moving as fast as I can when another experienced nurse walks in, so I ask him to get Isaac ready for his parents while I take Brandon upstairs. He agrees, and shares that Betsy, one of our newer nurses, is extremely upset by this loss so he has sent her to take a short break. I thank him and say we'll have to do some debriefing after this one. Seeing a 7-year-old victim is hard on everyone! I reassure him I will check on Betsy when I get back. I quickly grab Brandon and his stuff, and we head upstairs. He's really quiet, but when I ask he says he is fine. "It's been a tough morning for you, hasn't it?" I ask. Brandon stays quiet. We roll onto the unit and find Shelly. Since she knows Brandon, I give her a quick report and ask if she has any questions. I tell Brandon goodbye and quickly head back down to the ED. I now have one of the hardest parts of my job – helping parents say goodbye to their baby! This makes me think of my own 7 year old for a moment. I can't imagine what his parents are going through. I take the few seconds in the elevator to gather my thoughts. I take a deep breath. Here I go.

The strength of narrative pedagogy lies in seeking to understand an experience and the possibilities for engaging with it as a nurse. In contrast to conventional pedagogy's focus on the application of knowledge or theories (learned elsewhere and applied in a specific situation), with narrative pedagogy, teachers invite students and clinicians to think about the situations they encounter in new ways and from multiple perspectives, using their knowledge and experience as the background for questioning the meaning and significance of the experience. The background, theories, or specific clinical data may be brought to bear in interpreting an account (e.g., understanding Shelly's and Theresa's experiences draws on knowledge of newly diagnosed diabetes and cystic fibrosis in children, family dynamics, grief, handoffs and communication among team members and across departments), but the focus is on seeking to understand the experience before considering what knowledge to apply, or when and how it might be applied.

Further, hearing the narratives shared and the conversations that ensue as teacher, students, and clinicians collaboratively and communally engage in cycles of interpretation reveals how teachers, students, and clinicians understand the situations they encounter and ascertain what knowledge to use when and how. They also consider the limitations of their knowledge and experience (e.g., what do I know and what do I need to know?), current disciplinary knowledge and evidence to guide practice (e.g., what could be wrong with using best practices in this case?), and inherited, idealized views of nursing practice that do not account for the context in which care is given (e.g., what does it mean to nurses to be unable to provide "good" nursing care because of competing demands for their time?). The shift in using narrative pedagogy is to bring the complexity and the multifaceted, interrelated problems facing nurses on a day-to-day basis into the conversation rather than try to simplify or mitigate the complexity of nursing practice in order to teach isolated skills such as communication, organization, or priority setting. Indeed, phenomenologically, it is only through understanding an experience that decisions about what knowledge/skills to apply as well as when and how to apply them in a particular situation are possible.

Experiences are never straightforward or linear, and it is often the case that cycles of interpretation include "unsettling" an experience by persistently asking questions from multiple perspectives (scientific, critical, feminist, postmodern, and phenomenological). This is in stark contrast to the conventional approach of moving linearly from question to answer without considering questions such as the position of the nurse in the experience and how the particular problem being solved became identified as a problem in the first place. With narrative pedagogy, a shared experience is not simply a description of a discrete event; it brings with it past and current experiences and the available possibilities given the situation. Thus, cycles of interpretation are never acontextual or abstract but are rooted in the pressures and contingencies, the norms and policies, the cultures and traditions, and the values and ethics of the environments in which the experience occurred. As teachers, students, and clinicians communally and collaboratively engage in cycles of interpretation, they bring their background knowledge and experience (i.e., past), their perspective (i.e., present), and their anticipated sense of possibilities (i.e., future) into the conversation. Like the hermeneutic circle, understanding is circular, never ending, and always already situated in the experiences teachers, students, and clinicians bring into conversation.

As teachers participate in cycles of interpretation, they approach each conversation as a learner – seeking to learn more about nursing practice and how students learn nursing in the complex and evolving health care system. They also gain insight into the students' thinking. At times, students' thinking shows great depth and insight, and teachers are amazed at the ways students are thinking about their practice (Ironside, 2006; Ironside and Hayden-Miles, 2012). At other times, students' preconceived notions, oversights, prejudices, and misunderstandings are revealed. For example, after hearing Shelly's story, students frequently want to critique Theresa's practice and to contrast it to an idealized notion of good practice, positing the "right" thing for Shelly to do or say. Yet, when Theresa's narrative is heard, those interpretations quickly become problematic, and students must consider new perspectives and ways of thinking about practice. Teachers using narrative pedagogy pose questions to keep students' emerging understandings in play and, together with the students, to learn more about nursing practice. For instance, they might ask: What are the issues of power, control, and authority embedded in Shelly's and Theresa's accounts? Whose voice is missing from these tellings? What assumptions are we making about what constitutes good practice? How are these assumptions influencing our current understanding? What does this experience mean to you as a new nurse (student nurse)? Relying solely on pedagogies directed toward achieving predetermined outcomes or changes in behavior covers over what is to be learned by questioning how we come to understand experiences, the assumptions we make, and the importance of nurses learning together and keeping their practice open and problematic.

Narrative Pedagogy and Quality and Safety Education for Nurses

The QSEN goal of transforming nurses' professional identity in such a way that every nurse has a commitment to improving the quality and safety of health care wherever and whenever it is delivered presents both a challenge and an opportunity for nursing educators (Cronenwett, 2012). The QSEN competencies and the explication of the KSAs required to achieve those competencies sound deceptively straightforward (Appendices A and B). At first glance, it appears that teaching skills such as *act with integrity, consistency, and respect for differing views*, or *provide patient-centered care with sensitivity and respect for the diversity of human experience* (Cronenwett *et al.*, 2007) requires only that teachers transmit these skills to students in such a way that students recognize and can assimilate and articulate these aspects of practice. Teachers can then evaluate students' acquisition of these skills in subsequent classroom, clinical, or simulation experiences. The prevalence of this approach can be seen in faculties' efforts to map the six competencies and the 162 KSA statements across the curriculum so that faculty members, administrators, and regulators are aware of where each of the competencies and KSAs are taught and learned. Yet, research has shown that relying on this approach is problematic because nursing curricula are already overloaded with content and skills to the point where there is little time for thinking (Ironside, 2004). Loosening our grasp on conventional pedagogy as the only, or even the best, approach to teaching nursing creates opportunities for teachers, students, and clinicians to co-create different kinds of experiences in which prevailing views, extant knowledge, assumptions, and the meaning and significance of practice experiences can be communally and collaboratively explored.

Using narrative pedagogy requires that teachers reconsider how they spend their time with students. Working with students and clinicians to co-create experiences that focus on thinking and extending our understanding of nursing practice, with all the complexities that entails, becomes as important as content knowledge or the demonstration of particular skills. For example, relying solely on conventional pedagogy, a teacher might talk with students about the importance of nurses *acting with integrity, consistency, and respect for differing views* and may create case studies about patients with differing views to see if students are able to identify the best way to proceed in each particular situation. Using narrative pedagogy, teachers invite students to think about the complexity of *respecting different views* and may raise questions such as: As a nurse, how would you know if a patient you were caring for felt respected or not? How do nurses exude respectfulness when encountering patients who are predators or who are racist, violent, inappropriate, nonadherent, or aggressive? Could there be times that despite our best efforts to be respectful, patients experience the opposite?

Such questions are unanswerable. That is, the complexity of these questions keeps our experiences, knowledge, and assumptions in play as teachers, students, and clinicians engage in conversation, exploring differing perspectives and thinking together about these aspects of practice. Importantly, because these questions are situated in (and arise from) narrative accounts of experiences, they also show how interrelated the KSAs are in nursing practice. For instance, as teachers, students, and clinicians explore the question of how nurses can exude respectfulness when encountering patients who are predators or who are racist, violent, inappropriate, nonadherent, or violent, they are simultaneously engaging students in thinking about numerous KSAs (e.g., *act with integrity, consistency, and respect for differing views; provide patient-centered care with sensitivity and respect for the diversity of human experience; seek learning opportunities with patients who represent all aspects of human diversity; recognize personally held attitudes about working with patients from different ethnic, cultural, and social backgrounds; willingly support patient-centered care for individuals and groups whose values differ from their own*, and so forth; Cronenwett *et al.*, 2007). When providing care, the QSEN KSA statements are not isolated or discreet aspects of practice to be learned separately and later synthesized into a competency. They are embedded in practice situations in both positive and negative ways.

Thus, much is to be gained from expanding our pedagogical repertoire by using pedagogies grounded in teachers', students', and clinicians' experiences so that conversations about the competencies and KSA statements occur in ways consistent with and reflective of the complexity of current practice.

Narrative pedagogy is not a strategy teachers employ in the service of teaching quality and safety, but it is a way of persistently thinking about nursing education and practice *with* students and clinicians and of communally and collaboratively exploring new possibilities for improving the quality and safety of care provided. Co-creating experiences that focus on thinking together and understanding experiences in new ways and from multiple perspectives extends conventional pedagogy by developing students' interpretive skills (skills related to thinking in new ways and from multiple perspectives). This means that teachers enacting narrative pedagogy can't plan in advance where the conversation around an experience will go or the understandings that will be uncovered. As participants in the conversation, teachers enacting narrative pedagogy focus on questioning current understanding (e.g., whose interests are being served? What does it mean to patients to have these encounters with nurses?), rather than providing or describing one particular view over others. This questioning cultivates deeper consideration of students', teachers', and clinicians' experiences and holds the possibility of new perspectives and ways to improve nursing education and practice.

Teachers enacting narrative pedagogy reclaim for their teaching practice an emphasis on the importance of always questioning the best practices of nursing care, the strengths and weaknesses of current evidence, and the ways in which nurses listen and respond to those in their care. But more than just critiquing current nursing care (although an important practice), teachers enacting narrative pedagogy foster thinking broadly about the tentativeness of answers in clinical practice and the importance of persistently questioning, holding everything currently assumed to be true open and problematic. This is consistent with the literature that shows how navigating the uncertainty and fallibility embedded in current (and future) practice has become as important for nurses (and other health care providers) as content knowledge and skill mastery and that interpreting (learning to read) situations is as important as intervening (Cook, Ironside, and Ogrinc, 2011).

Summary

The importance of preparing students and new nurses to provide safe, quality care cannot be overestimated. The QSEN delineation of specific competencies and of KSA statements identifies important aspects of practice all nurses entering the workforce should possess (Cronenwett *et al.*, 2007). As nursing faculties and clinical educators strive to embed QSEN competencies into their curricula and programs, it is crucial that the complexity of these competencies and KSAs be appreciated and incorporated into teaching and learning encounters in nursing. Using diverse pedagogies, such as narrative pedagogy, affords teachers the opportunity to create substantively different experiences with students and clinicians, experiences focused on thinking together in new ways and from multiple perspectives about the complexities of practice and the possibilities for improvement.

References

Cline, D.D. (2015) Complexity of care: A concept analysis of older adult health care experiences. *Nursing Education Perspectives*, *36*(2), 108–113.

Cook, M., Ironside, P.M., and Ogrinc, G. (2011) Mainstreaming quality and safety: A reformulation of quality and safety education for health professions students. *Quality and Safety in Health Care*, *20*(Suppl 1), 179–182.

Cronenwett, L. (2012) A national initiative: Quality and Safety Education for Nurses (QSEN). In G. Sherwood and J. Barnsteiner (Eds.), *Quality and safety in nursing: A competency approach to improving outcomes*. Hoboken, NJ: Wiley-Blackwell.

Cronenwett, L., Sherwood, G., Barnsteiner, J., Disch, J., Johnson, J., Mitchell, P., *et al.* (2007) Quality and safety education for nurses. *Nursing Outlook, 55*, 122–131.

Diekelmann, N., and Diekelmann, J. (2009) Schooling learning teaching: Toward narrative pedagogy. Bloomington, IN: iUniverse Press.

Gadamer, H.-G. (2001) *Gadamer in conversation: Reflections and commentary*. (R.E. Palmer, Ed. and Trans.). New Haven, CT: Yale University Press.

Heidegger, M. (1962) *Being and time* (J. Macquarrie and E. Robinson, Trans.). San Francisco: HarperCollins. (Original work published 1927).

Ironside, P.M. (2001) Creating a research base for nursing education: An interpretive review of conventional, critical, feminist, postmodern, and phenomenologic pedagogies. *Advances in Nursing Science, 23*(3), 72–87.

Ironside, P.M. (2003) Trying something new: Implementing and evaluating narrative pedagogy using a multi-method approach. *Nursing Education Perspectives, 24*(3), 122–128.

Ironside, P.M. (2004) "Covering content" and teaching thinking: Deconstructing the additive curriculum. *Journal of Nursing Education, 43*, 5–12.

Ironside, P.M. (2006) Using narrative pedagogy: Learning and practicing interpretive thinking. *Journal of Advanced Nursing, 55*, 478–486.

Ironside, P.M. (2014) Enabling narrative pedagogy: Inviting, waiting and letting be. *Nursing Education Perspectives, 35*(4), 212–218.

Ironside, P.M. (2015) Narrative pedagogy: Transforming nursing education through 15 years of research. *Nursing Education Perspectives, 36*(2), 83–88.

Ironside, P.M., Fuhrman, M., Hogan, D., Kavanaugh, K., Ryan, M., and Voss, S. (1998) *Creating a narrative pedagogy in teaching and learning nursing theory: The voices of teachers and students*. Chicago: Chicago Institute for Nursing Education.

Ironside, P.M., and Hayden-Miles, M. (2012) Narrative pedagogy: Co-creating engaging learning experiences with students. In G. Sherwood and S. Horton-Deutsch (Eds.). *Reflective practice: Transforming education and improving outcomes* (pp. 135–148). Indianapolis, IN: Sigma Theta Tau International.

Lindberg, C., Nash, S., and Lindberg, C. (2008) On the edge: Nursing in the age of complexity. Bordentown, NJ: PlexusPress.

Sitterding, M.C., Broome, M.E., Everett, L.Q., and Ebright, P. Understanding situation awareness in nursing work. *Advances in Nursing Science, 35*(1), 77–92.

12

Integrating Quality and Safety Competencies in Simulation

Kathryn R. Alden, EdD, MSN, RN, IBCLC and Carol F. Durham, EdD, RN, ANEF, FAAN

In recent years, the use of simulation-based learning in nursing education has increased exponentially. A large national survey of prelicensure nursing programs in the United States showed that 87% incorporated medium- and high-fidelity simulation learning activities in nursing courses (Hayden, 2010).

The value of high-quality simulation was acknowledged in a large longitudinal, randomized, controlled study by the NCSBN. Results of the study showed that "substituting high-quality simulation experiences for up to half of traditional clinical hours produces comparable end-of-program educational outcomes and new graduates that are ready for clinical practice" (Hayden *et al.*, 2014). The NCSBN study supports that faculty need to be subject matter experts and have formal training in simulation pedagogy, including debriefing methodology. Additionally, adequate staffing, equipment and supplies to provide clinical realism need to be available to create meaningful simulation experiences (Hayden *et al.*, 2014).

In an effort to improve educational practices, increase patient safety, and reduce variability in clinical learning experiences, standards of practice for simulation were developed by the International Nursing Association for Clinical Simulation and Learning (INACSL, 2011). The INACSL Standards of Best Practice: Simulation[SM] are designed to assist educators in maximizing simulation-based learning experiences and to further the science of simulation (Rutherford-Hemming, Lioce, and Durham, 2015). (See Table 12.1). A description of the standard, rationale, expected outcomes, criteria, and guidelines can be found at INACSL's web site (http://www.inacsl.org/i4a/pages/index.cfm?pageID=3407).

Simulation is an effective instructional strategy to teach concepts and practices related to quality and safety in nursing practice (Berndt, 2014; Shearer, 2013). It is also useful in evaluating patient safety competencies (Henneman *et al.*, 2010). The QSEN competencies (patient-centered care, teamwork and collaboration, evidence-based practice, quality improvement, safety, and informatics [Cronenwett *et al.*, 2007]) can easily be incorporated into simulation learning activities, whether for prelicensure, transition to practice, or clinician education (Berndt, 2014; Durham and Alden, 2012; Ironside, Jeffries, and Martin, 2009; Jarzemsky, McCarthy, and Ellis, 2010). Simulation can contribute to improved learner knowledge, attitudes, and confidence related to quality and safety (Gant and Webb-Corbett, 2010; Piscotty, Grobbel, and Tzeng, 2011; Sears, Goldworthy, and Goodman, 2010; Shearer, 2013).

The value of human patient simulation in promoting safe practice is reflected in the IOM report *To Err is Human: Building a Safer Health Care System*. The IOM recommends simulation

Quality and Safety in Nursing: A Competency Approach to Improving Outcomes, Second Edition.
Edited by Gwen Sherwood and Jane Barnsteiner.
© 2017 John Wiley & Sons, Inc. Published 2017 by John Wiley & Sons, Inc.

Table 12.1 INACSL Standards of Best Practice: Simulation ^{SM}

Standard I:	Terminology (Meakim *et al.*, 2013)
Standard II:	Professional Integrity of Participant(s) (Gloe *et al.*, 2013)
Standard III:	Participant Objectives (Lioce *et al.*, 2013)
Standard IV:	Facilitation (Franklin, Boese *et al.*, 2013)
Standard V:	Facilitator (Boese *et al.*, 2013)
Standard VI:	The Debriefing Process (Decker *et al.*, 2013)
Standard VII:	Participant Assessment and Evaluation (Sando *et al.*, 2013)
Standard VIII:	Simulation Enhanced Interprofessional Education (Sim-IPE) (Decker *et al.*, 2015)
Standard IX:	Simulation Design (Lioce *et al.*, 2015)

as a strategy that can be used to prevent errors in the clinical setting: "Health care organizations and teaching institutions should participate in the development and use of simulation for training novice practitioners, problem solving, and crisis management, especially when new and potentially hazardous procedures and equipment are introduced" (Kohn, Corrigan, and Donaldson, 2000).

This chapter focuses on the use of simulation-based education as an instructional strategy and includes information on how to integrate specific QSEN competencies into simulation-based learning activities. Educators have realized only the tip of the iceberg in terms of the potential use of simulation-based education in teaching students about quality and safety in nursing practice.

Simulation and safety are concepts often aligned with one another as educators consider instructional strategies for various courses and situations. It is important for the educator to select or design simulation-based activities to fit learning objectives, needs of the learners, and the setting. In some cases, a variety of simulated-based education approaches can be used in a single patient care scenario. As a prelude to information about using high-fidelity simulation to teach QSEN competencies, it is helpful to understand the various types of simulation-based activities used in nursing education.

Overview of Simulation-based Learning

Simulation is an activity or event replicating clinical practice using scenarios, simulators, standardized patients, role-playing, task trainers, or virtual reality. Simulations can vary from simple to complex and are intended to engage learners in realistic learning activities that promote development and utilization of cognitive and psychomotor skills.

The believability or realism of a simulation learning experience is known as *fidelity*. *INACSL Standards of Best Practice: Simulation* states:

> The level of fidelity is determined by the environment, the tools and resources used, and many factors associated with the participants. Fidelity can involve a variety of dimensions, including (a) physical factors such as environment, equipment, and related tools; (b) psychological factors such as emotions, beliefs, and self-awareness of participants; (c) social factors such as participant and instructor motivation and goals; (d) culture of the group; and (e) degree of openness and trust, as well as participants' modes of thinking (Meakim *et al.*, 2013).

Benefits of Simulation-based Learning

Simulation is a learner-centered approach to nursing education. The focus is not on the educator as the "sage on the stage" but on the learner. It is an immersive, hands-on, experiential learning activity in which learners can assume an active role in a patient care scenario. Using simulation, educators can provide students with risk-free, controlled learning opportunities that bridge the gap from theory and laboratory knowledge to actual patient care situations. During simulation, students reflect and draw upon their knowledge and previous experiences as they collect and analyze patient data, utilize clinical reasoning skills to decide on appropriate interventions, and evaluate the effectiveness of their actions. They can practice assessment and psychomotor skills. Students are assisted to visualize the physiologic responses of the "patient" to medications and other interventions. Because simulation does not endanger the well being of patients, students can be permitted to make mistakes, correct those mistakes, and learn from them while in a supportive environment. Simulation requires learners to use cognitive, technical, and behavioral skills as they interact with the "patient" and other actors in the scenario, such as family members or health team members. Simulation promotes self-efficacy and increases self-confidence of learners in their ability to perform technical skills, care for actual patients, and handle unexpected situations in the clinical setting (Franklin and Lee, 2014). This enhances their ability to provide safe, quality care to patients.

Uses of Simulation-based Learning in Nursing Education

Simulation-based learning is adaptable and flexible, allowing for a broad range of uses in undergraduate and graduate nursing education, continuing education, staff development, and interprofessional education.

Prelicensure Nursing Education Programs

Prelicensure nursing education programs utilize simulation-based learning in a variety of courses. A conclusion of the landmark study on simulation by the NCSBN is that high-quality simulation experiences can be substituted for up to half of traditional clinical hours with comparable educational outcomes at program end and readiness for practice as professional nurses (Hayden *et al.*, 2014).

Using Benner's (1984) theory of novice to expert as a framework, one can trace the utility of simulation in educating nurses for safe practice. It can be used by novice learners in foundational nursing courses to practice physical assessment, therapeutic communication, and psychomotor skills (Stroup, 2014). Before novice students begin their first clinical practicum, simulation scenarios can help prepare them for what they will encounter with real patients, thus reducing their anxiety and stress (Dearmon *et al.*, 2013). As their anxiety is reduced, they are less likely to make mistakes that can affect patient safety.

As students advance in the nursing curriculum, it is ideal for them to have ongoing opportunities to participate in simulation scenarios that are relevant to each course. For example, students in a maternity course can participate in scenarios using a birthing simulator to focus on high-risk intrapartum care, which they may not experience in the acute care setting but need to know (e.g., prolapsed cord or shoulder dystocia). Integrating content from more than one course into simulation learning activities enhances the learning experiences for students. Faculty in maternity and medical/surgical nursing courses can work together to create and implement scenarios that address relevant concepts across both courses such as a postpartum hemorrhage case that progresses to hypovolemic shock. Pediatric and mental health educators can collaborate on scenarios that address care of a child with a head injury and the associated psychological responses and needs of the parents.

For the student who is approaching graduation, simulation scenarios can be designed as synthesis learning experiences. During capstone nursing courses, students can participate in complex patient care scenarios that require high-level clinical reasoning and decision-making. Key concepts surrounding prioritization, leadership, and management can be incorporated into these scenarios.

Simulation is most commonly used in prelicensure medical/surgical, pediatric, and obstetric courses. Educators are challenged to expand the use of simulation-based learning to include patient care environments such as long-term care, outpatient psychiatric care, or community health.

Graduate Nursing Education

High-fidelity simulation can be used to teach advanced practice skills and concepts to nurse practitioner, clinical nurse specialist, and nurse anesthetist students. Simulation scenarios provide opportunities for these advanced practice nursing students to apply knowledge while using diagnostic reasoning and assessment skills (Bryant, 2013; Campbell and LoGiudice, 2013; Elliott, DeCristofaro, and Carpenter, 2012; Garnett, Weiss, and Winland-Brown, 2015; Haut *et al.*, 2014; Mompoint-Williams *et al.*, 2014; Walton-Moss *et al.*, 2012; Pittman, 2012; Rutherford-Hemming and Jennrich, 2013).

There is great potential for the use of simulation in preparing future nurse educators who will supervise students in the clinical setting. Simulation-based activities provide excellent opportunities for graduate students or new educators to facilitate learning with prelicensure students as though they are in the clinical setting (Hunt, Curtis, and Gore, 2015; Shellenbarger and Edwards, 2012).

Professional Development

Increasingly, simulation is being used in health care agencies as part of orientation programs, continuing education, staff development, and certification courses (Hallenbeck, 2012). Simulation is one means of bridging the gap between education and practice for new graduates, thus easing the transition to practice. Health care agencies can utilize simulation to facilitate the shift from student to professional nurse as the new nurses participate in realistic scenarios that involve policies, procedures, protocols, and equipment that are specific to that particular institution (Kaddoura, 2010; Moughrabi and Wallace, 2015). Simulation can be used in staff development, providing nurses with opportunities to learn and practice skills and procedures (Leigh, 2011). Competency evaluation can be accomplished using simulation. Certification courses such as Advanced Cardiac Life Support (ACLS) and the Neonatal Resuscitation Program (NRP) use simulation for practice and competency evaluation (Hallenbeck, 2012; Lucas, 2014).

Faculty Development

Simulation can be utilized in preparing faculty to teach in the clinical setting. New clinical instructors can benefit from participating in simulation scenarios in which they are responsible for facilitating student learning experiences. Professional development of experienced clinical faculty can be enhanced through simulation-based learning activities (Hunt, Curtis, and Gore, 2015; Shellenbarger and Edwards, 2012).

Interprofessional Simulation

Simulation-based learning activities present an excellent opportunity to teach students about interprofessional or interdisciplinary care and to help them understand the roles of other health care professionals. Through involvement of a variety of health team members, including ancillary personnel, nurses gain an awareness and appreciation of the team approach to providing safe and effective patient care.

Collaboration among professional schools within a college or university is prerequisite to offering interprofessional simulation learning activities (Willhaus, 2010). Within health care institutions, interprofessional team training to promote patient safety can be accomplished using simulation-based education (Engum and Jeffries, 2012; Scolaro *et al.*, 2015; Strouse, 2010).

QSEN Competencies and Simulation

Research evidence supports simulation as an effective educational strategy to teach patient safety competencies (Berndt, 2014; Gant and Webb-Corbett, 2010; Henneman *et al.*, 2010; Ironside *et al.*, 2009). The competencies identified by the QSEN project (patient-centered care, teamwork and collaboration, evidence-based practice, quality improvement, safety, and informatics [Cronenwett *et al.*, 2007]) are inherent to most high-fidelity simulation-based learning activities, whether or not educators purposefully include them. Patient-centered care, teamwork, and safety are easily incorporated into simulation, while evidence-based practice, quality improvement, and informatics may require more deliberate efforts (Pauly-O'Neill and Prion, 2013). The prelicensure (Appendix A) or graduate-level competencies (Appendix B), as appropriate, can often be integrated into current courses, skills labs, and simulation scenarios without significant revisions (Cronenwett *et al.*, 2007; Cronenwett *et al.*, 2009). Through careful examination of what is currently being done and re-envisioning the focus on QSEN competencies, educators can make meaningful additions to patient quality and safety. Helpful tools on the QSEN web site (www.QSEN.org) include a checklist that educators can use to examine existing scenarios for QSEN competencies; it can also be used to develop new scenarios (Alfes, 2010). In addition, Jarzemsky (2009) provides a template for development of scenarios that incorporate the competencies.

The following section will examine the incorporation of QSEN competencies in various simulation-based learning activities. Although this section is organized according to the QSEN competencies, it is important to note that the pedagogy of simulation allows for the integration of multiple QSEN competencies simultaneously. Table 12.2 provides examples of integration of the QSEN competencies into prelicensure and graduate education.

Patient-centered Care

Definition: *Recognize the patient or designee as the source of control and full partner in providing compassionate and coordinated care based on respect for patient's preferences, values, and needs* (Cronenwett *et al.*, 2007).

Table 12.2 Examples of select knowledge, skills, and attitudes and simulation learning activities for prelicensure and graduate students.

QSEN Competency	Prelicensure Knowledge, Skills, Attitudes (Cronenwett et al., 2007)	Simulation Learning Activity	Graduate Knowledge, Skills, Attitudes (Cronenwett et al., 2009)	Simulation Learning Activity
Patient-centered care	K: Integrate understanding of multiple dimensions of patient-centered care: physical comfort and emotional support. S: Elicit patient values, preferences, and expressed needs as part of clinical interview, implementation of care plan, and evaluation of care. A: Value seeing health care situations through patients' eyes.	*Presimulation:* Ostomy exercise. Students apply and wear ostomy appliance and reflect on experience. *Simulation:* Care for post-op patient with newly created ostomy, focus on comfort, emotional needs, teaching. *Postsimulation:* Debriefing: Discuss how pre-sim activity impacted nursing care; describe how having an ostomy affects all aspects of a patient's life.	K: Analyze multiple dimensions of patient-centered care. S: Elicit patient values, preferences, and expressed needs as part of clinical interview, diagnosis, implementation of care plan, and evaluation of care. A: Value the patient's expertise with own health and symptoms.	*Presimulation:* Learners reflect on care they or their family have received and examine where there were gaps in best practices for patient-centered care. *Simulation:* Imbedded patient-centered care opportunities around values, preference, and expressed needs with patient and family. *Postsimulation:* Ask advanced practice nurse to identify the patient's values, expressed needs they solicited during the interview, diagnosis, implementation of care, and evaluation of care. Solicit feedback on how they felt they were listened to, how they were integrated as a member of the team, and whether their values and expressed needs were considered in the plan of care.
Teamwork and collaboration	K: Describe scopes of practice and roles of health care team members. S: Function competently within own scope of practice as a member of the health care team. A: Value the perspectives and expertise of all health care team members.	*Presimulation:* Students view a TeamSTEPPS video on teamwork and collaboration, answer targeted questions. *Simulation:* Roles of team are assigned; primary nurse leads team huddle before simulation. Communicator uses SBAR (situation, background, assessment, recommendation) when contacting health care provider (HCP) about change in patient's condition. *Postsimulation:* Debriefing: Discuss effectiveness of team, how each member felt during scenario, interaction between members, use of SBAR.	K: Describe examples of the impact of team functioning on safety and quality of care. S: Follow communication practices that minimize risks associated with handoffs between providers, and across transitions in care. A: Value the solutions obtained through systematic, interprofessional collaborative efforts.	*Presimulation:* Learners receive training using the TeamSTEPPS curriculum. Analyze opportunity and success vignettes to highlight communication techniques. *Simulation:* Imbed communication opportunities for learners to provide handoffs involving interprofessional team members across a transition in care point for the patient. *Postsimulation:* Debrief interprofessional team members together to allow enhanced understanding of roles and effective communication techniques.

	K/S/A		Presimulation / Simulation / Postsimulation
Evidence-based practice	K: Explain the role of evidence in determining best clinical practice. S: Participate in structuring the work environment to facilitate integration of new evidence into standards of practice. A: Value the need for continuous improvement in clinical practice based on new knowledge.	K: Analyze how the strength of available evidence influences the provision of care (assessment, diagnosis, treatment, and evaluation). S: Develop guidelines for clinical decision-making regarding departure from established protocol/standards of care. A: Acknowledge own limitations in knowledge and clinical expertise before determining when to deviate from evidence-based best practices.	*Presimulation:* Assign specific policy or protocol used in clinical agency; have students search current nursing/medical literature to locate evidence to support policy and to identify inaccuracies, for example, protocol for patient with excessive bleeding postbirth. *Simulation:* In a postpartum hemorrhage (PPH) scenario, follow agency protocol, implement standing orders. *Postsimulation:* Debriefing: Discuss effectiveness of actions in protocol in stopping hemorrhage; discuss latest medications being used for PPH; revise protocol based on research evidence. *Presimulation:* Inform learner of the content areas for the simulation and ask them to come prepared with standards and protocols for the treatment of the patient. *Simulation:* Create controversy within the simulated case that causes the practitioner to consider departure from established protocols and standards of care. *Postsimulation:* Extend debriefing time to allow the practitioner to explain their decision-making based on the evidence they brought with them and what they, along with the patient, decided was the most appropriate plan of care. Allow time to reflect on how they felt, what concerns they have, and when this type of divergence would not be appropriate.
Quality improvement	K: Recognize that nursing and other health professions students are parts of systems of care and care processes that affect outcomes for patients and families. S: Participate in a root cause analysis of a sentinel event. A: Appreciate that continuous quality improvement is an essential part of the daily work of all health professionals.	K: Analyze the impact of context (such as access, cost, or team functioning) on improvement efforts. S: Assert leadership in shaping the dialogue about and providing leadership for the introduction of best practices. A: Appreciate that continuous quality improvement is an essential part of the daily work of all health professionals.	*Presimulation:* Read current journal article on root cause analysis. *Simulation:* In a capstone medical/surgical and leadership scenario, care for patient receiving blood transfusion after severe gastrointestinal (GI) bleeding; patient experiences transfusion reaction; students discover wrong blood is hanging. *Postsimulation:* Perform root cause analysis of the error, trace through EMR to point of care where error occurred; propose action/change in policy or procedure to prevent recurrence. *Presimulation:* Identify cases from the same type of systems the learner will be practicing in. *Simulation:* Create a leadership simulation based on the real cases and ask the learners to examine them in light of access, cost, or team functioning. Have student prepare a strategy for providing leadership around best practices. *Postsimulation:* Have teams of learners present their plan for change to you and other team faculty as though you are the people in the system that can bring about the change.

(Continued)

Table 12.2 (Continued)

QSEN Competency	Prelicensure Knowledge, Skills, Attitudes (Cronenwett et al., 2007)	Simulation Learning Activity	Graduate Knowledge, Skills, Attitudes (Cronenwett et al., 2009)	Simulation Learning Activity
Safety	K: Describe the benefits and limitations of selected safety-enhancing technologies (such as barcodes, computer provider order entry, medication pumps, and automatic alerts/alarms). S: Demonstrate effective use of strategies to reduce risk of harm to self or others. A: Value the contributions of standardization/reliability to safety.	*Presimulation:* Students complete self-study module on pediatric medication administration and medication calculations (including IV therapy). *Simulation:* In pediatric scenario, students care for 1-year-old with bacterial meningitis. Errors are embedded: ID band is missing; wrong IV fluid is hanging; alarm on IV pump is on silent; parent sitting in chair at bedside, side rail halfway up. IV antibiotic to be given; student must check calculation of dosage for weight of child; dosage is too high; must call HCP, communicate using SBAR, get order changed *Postsimulation:* Discuss risks to patient safety identified in scenario and actions that were taken or not taken; how to prevent similar errors in future.	K: Describe human factors and other basic safety design principles as well as commonly used unsafe practices (such as workaround and dangerous abbreviations). S: Participate as a team member to design, promote, and model effective use of technology and standardized practice that support safety and quality. A: Appreciate the cognitive and physical limits of human performance.	*Presimulation:* Readings on human factors and the cognitive and physical limits of human performance. *Simulation:* Embed confederates in the simulations who consistently use workarounds, inappropriate abbreviations, relying on memory, and other safety issues in the simulation. *Postsimulation:* Debrief the approaches and leadership exemplified by the advanced practice nurse in the scenario. Allow time for the embedded participant to talk about how the learner's approach felt and their likely response to a long-term change of habits.
Informatics	K: Identify essential information that must be available in a common database to support patient care. S: Navigate the electronic health record. Document and plan patient care in an electronic health record. A: Value technologies that support clinical decision-making, error prevention, and care coordination.	*Presimulation:* Practice locating information about a patient in the electronic health record (EHR). *Simulation:* Use EHR during handoff report to students; review last vital signs, assessment findings; current HCP orders; plan of care. Recorder documents using EHR during scenario. *Postsimulation:* Discuss importance of timely and thorough documentation, including ethical and legal implications.	K: Contrast benefits and limitation of common information technology strategies used in the delivery of care. S: Participate in the selection, design, implementation, and evaluation of information systems. A: Value the use of information and communication technologies in patient care.	*Presimulation:* Observe practitioners using common information technology; gather data on positive and negative effects of the technology, such as Alert Fatigue. *Simulation:* Design simulation as a panel of the system's personnel making a decision on a point of care technology to bring evidence-based information to the practitioner. Have the team come to consensus about what system to purchase, including its pros and cons. *Postsimulation:* Discuss roll out of new product, identify concerns about the implementation and its impact on patient safety.

Nurses are quick to affirm that the care they provide is patient centered, but the KSAs in the QSEN competencies broaden expectations (Walton and Barnsteiner, 2017). Patient-centered care goes beyond considering the patient's preferences for items such scheduling of care and management of pain to truly integrating the patient as part of the care team (see Chapter 3). Care management moves from those delivering the care to the patient receiving the care (Disch, Barnsteiner, and Walton, 2014). One of the 26 recommendations proposed by Benner and colleagues to transform nursing education is "Develop pedagogies that keep students focused on the patient's experience" (Benner *et al.*, 2010). The educator should teach pathology and psychosocial components of the illness in the context of the patient's experience.

The Joint Commission implemented Patient-Centered Communication standards in 2010 (Arocha and Moore, 2011). Patient-centered care goes beyond patient satisfaction; it contributes to safety and improved outcomes (Laird-Fick *et al.*, 2010). It is important to include the patient and/or family in their care decisions. In an effort to do this, nursing educators need to create opportunities for learners to apply patient-centered care approaches.

Disch, Barnsteiner, and Walton (2014) challenge us to consider "how health professionals are educated and the extent to which they develop competencies in delivering personalized care should be of paramount importance to individuals and their significant others. The traditional models of healthcare education have not served us well, and many advocate that health professionals' education must change...." The patient-centered care competency can easily be incorporated into simulation learning activities that create experiences that prompt students to consider health care issues from the point of view of the patient. In a medical/surgical nursing course for prelicensure students, a simulation can be created to help students gain a better understanding of many factors that affect a patient's daily life when they have an ostomy. Building on ostomy care content from didactic sessions and skills labs, a presimulation exercise helps students consider physical and emotional challenges associated with having an ostomy. Instructions for the students are presented in Textbox 12.1.

This exercise assists students to view an ostomy from a patient's perspective. Learning is enhanced by their reflection about the experience with a focus on patient-centered care. Students report insights about the impact of the ostomy on activities of daily living and gain an awareness of how placement of the stoma and ostomy appliance affects the fitting of clothing. They note discomforts associated with wearing the ostomy bag; the bag is hot, noisy, and bothersome, and there is constant concern about bag leakage. As a result of this exercise, students recognize that the ostomy affects all aspects of the patient's life and affects their family members. They appreciate the importance of optimizing skin care and adhesion of the ostomy bag. Students value patient input for stoma placement and recognize the importance of involving the patient in the care of the ostomy. They acknowledge and appreciate fears associated with having an ostomy and the need to provide quality patient teaching.

Textbox 12.1 Ostomy presimulation exercise

- Students work in pairs.
- Select site for ostomy and draw a stoma.
- Cut ostomy wafer to fit "stoma" and apply ostomy bag.
- Fill ostomy bag with wet brown paper towels with a drop of citrus extract to provide some weight, color, and odor.
- Students wear bag for as long as possible (usual length of time between bag changes for patient is 72 hours).

Following the presimulation exercise, students participate in a simulation activity to care for a postoperative patient with severe ulcerative colitis following abdominal surgery that resulted in the need for an ostomy. During this acute care, they are prompted to consider how to include the patient and spouse in care and discharge planning. A postsimulation exercise includes developing a discharge plan based on learning needs of the patient and family. In the debriefing, learners reflect on their performance and learning that occurred during the simulation. Providing experiences to assist the learners to look beyond the diagnosis and skills to the needs and desires of the patient can assist them in the delivery of patient-centered care.

Patient-centered care includes sensitivity to diversity of cultural, ethnic, and social backgrounds. Educators can intentionally vary the culture and ethnicity of patients and family members in high-fidelity scenarios. For example, in a medical/surgical scenario focused on care of acutely ill elders, the patient is Mr. Gonzalez, a recently widowed 79-year-old male from Mexico with poorly controlled type I diabetes who speaks only Spanish and lives with his daughter. Diversity in family structure can be addressed in simulation scenarios. In a maternity simulation, the mother and her partner may be a same sex couple.

Individual and family centered care communication skills can be rehearsed using simulation with individual professionals or in teams of care providers. Additionally, simulation can be used to develop healthcare negotiation skills with patients and their families.

Teamwork and Collaboration

Definition: *Function effectively within nursing and interprofessional teams, fostering open communication, mutual respect, and shared decision making to achieve quality patient care* (Cronenwett *et al.*, 2007).

Simulation provides a venue to allow various health care personnel to collaborate in a patient care scenario to deliver care within a team environment. This experience provides opportunities for learners to communicate and work with other members of the health care team, while also helping them see how their professional role interfaces with other members of the patient care team, described more fully by Disch in Chapter 5, Teamwork and Collaboration (2017).

Simulation-based learning activities most often occur with small groups or teams of learners. In each scenario, learners need to understand their roles prior to the start of the simulation. Assigning roles allows the learners to understand what is expected of them within the team and the roles of other members of the team. This allows the students to delegate appropriately, understand with whom to communicate, and how best to collaborate. Textbox 12.2 contains an example of team roles and responsibilities in a simulation-based learning activity for prelicensure students.

Teamwork and collaboration can easily be incorporated into simulation learning activities using an established, nationally recognized program known as TeamSTEPPS. This evidence-based program is designed to improve communication and teamwork skills among health care professionals. There is a national initiative to implement this program to improve the quality and safety of patient care with improved patient outcomes. TeamSTEPPS was developed by the U.S. Department of Defense and the AHRQ and can be obtained free of charge at the following web site: http://teamstepps.ahrq.gov/. The authors have used TeamSTEPPS in many different ways and find that it is essential to helping the learner understand the QSEN competency of teamwork and collaboration.

TeamSTEPPS defines teams broadly as either core teams (those you work with daily) or contingent teams (those who come together for a specific purpose or function such as emergency code team). Nurses usually recognize that they function within teams, whether nursing or interprofessional;

Textbox 12.2 Assigned roles for team members in simulation scenario

---

NOTE: Each team member wears a tag identifying his/her role in the scenario.

- Primary Nurse: directs the team, delegates tasks, stays at the bedside
- Secondary Nurse: collaborates with primary nurse in problem solving and care delivery, follows direction of primary nurse, may be assigned specific tasks such as managing IV therapy, administering medications, or starting oxygen
- Communicator: contacts health care provider, lab, blood bank, pharmacy, or other personnel as needed during scenarios; follows direction of primary nurse; communicates patient care data to primary nurse and team; communicates with patient's family/friends
- Recorder: documents time and results of assessments, medication administration, and other procedures, calls health care provider
- Observer (used in teams >5): completes scenario-specific form while quietly observing the performance of participants; contributes his or her observations during debriefing; provides thoughtful positive and constructive feedback in a professional manner

---

however, they may need to be reminded of the significant contributions of ancillary personnel (e.g., nursing assistants), patients, and families as sources of data and input about the plan of care.

Using the TeamSTEPPS model in simulation activities, learners huddle early in the simulation to plan strategies for patient care. During the simulation they apply TeamSTEPPS concepts and terminology. For example, the SBAR communication model can be used for information transfer during the scenario, such as during the hand-off report and when calling the health care provider (Lancaster, Westphal, and Jambunathan, 2015; Vecchia and Sparacino, 2015). In the debriefing, teamwork, communication, and collaboration are discussed.

TeamSTEPPS provides communication strategies that equip students with techniques needed to more effectively address power gradients within patient care settings. For example, when a learner calls the health care provider to report a worrisome change in the patient's condition, the learner is expected to use the following C-U-S words to communicate the seriousness of the patient's condition: "I am **C**oncerned that...", "I am **U**ncomfortable with...", "This is a patient **S**afety issue" (King *et al.*, 2006). These words empower nurses to express their concerns in a manner that are more likely heard. If the provider dismisses the information, the learner is instructed to use the "two-challenge rule" where they restate the concern (King *et al.*, 2006). If the provider does not respond to the patient care situation, then the nurse is instructed to go to the next level of command. These communication techniques may seem simple but have a powerful impact on the nurse's ability to be a voice for patient safety.

Faculty from schools of nursing, medicine, and pharmacy at a large public university collaborated to create interprofessional simulation learning experiences for their students. A group of nursing students from the maternal/newborn course, a group of medical students in a pediatric course, a group of medical students in an obstetrics course, and a group of pharmacy students were assigned to interprofessional teams to participate in two scenarios involving the birth of a compromised neonate. Nursing and obstetric medical students provided care for the laboring mother (using Noelle, the birthing simulator by Gaumard) and assisted her with birth. Pediatric medical students led the neonatal care team in resuscitation efforts for the compromised newborn infant. Pharmacy students in the simulations consulted with the health care providers in determining appropriate medications. Faculty from all disciplines facilitated the simulations and conducted debriefing sessions where students dialogued about teamwork and collaboration as well as clinical skills and care provided to the neonate.

At the same university, an interdisciplinary course focused on teamwork, communication, and patient safety is offered to nursing, medicine, and pharmacy students. Multiple simulation experiences (simulators and standardized patients) provide opportunities for students from the three professions to work together in patient care scenarios around issues such as medical errors, root cause analysis, error disclosure, teamwork, communication, and challenges associated with power gradients across disciplines.

Evidence-based Practice

Definition: *Integrate best current evidence with clinical expertise and patient/family preferences and values for delivery of optimal health care.* (Cronenwett *et al.*, 2007).

Simulation-based learning activities provide rich opportunities for learners to integrate evidence-based practice into their clinical practice, presented by Tracey and Barnsteiner in Chapter 7, Evidence-based Practice (2017). Research articles can be assigned, applied in the patient care scenario, and then discussed in debriefing.

Examination of research evidence that supports practice is ideally accomplished in presimulation or postsimulation activities. As part of presimulation activities, learners can be asked to find research evidence that supports a specific nursing care policy or protocol. For example, in a maternity scenario, learners may be asked to explore the literature for evidence to support the labor induction or augmentation protocol used in the clinical agency.

During the simulation, the learners can be asked to adopt a spirit of inquiry and make mental notes of things they want to know about or questions generated by the patient care scenario. In debriefing, they may be asked to consider whether or not procedures in the scenario were in accordance with policies, protocols, or research evidence surrounding a particular patient condition or problem. As a postsimulation assignment, learners may be asked to revise a policy, protocol, or procedure based on the latest evidence in the literature.

Quality Improvement

Definition: *Use data to monitor the outcomes of care processes and use improvement methods to design and test changes to continuously improve the quality and safety of health care systems* (Cronenwett *et al.*, 2007).

Quality improvement is a challenging competency to incorporate into simulation scenarios that include the KSAs as described by Johnson (2017). Educators need to be deliberate in integrating quality improvement into scenarios. A simulation can be created with embedded errors providing the learner the opportunity to identify and examine the root cause of the error, thus, bringing in the quality improvement science and assisting the learner to understand individual and systems contributions to healthcare errors. The set-up of the environment and the simulated patient allow for incorporating a variety of errors. For example, errors can be as simple as a missing identification or allergy band, an incorrect setting on the IV pump, wrong IV fluid infusing, or wrong medication or dose. More critical errors can be imbedded in the scenario, such as a transfusion reaction resulting from an incompatible blood transfusion. The learner assumes responsibility for patient care within the scenario unlike in traditional clinical where learners are often limited in their level of engagement in patient care (Moughrabi and Wallace, 2015).

During the debriefing session, error identification and recovery are discussed in detail. It is important to assist learners to recognize the interconnectedness of quality improvement and safety. Consequences of errors and the impact on patient safety are identified. Learners can compare their actions to standards of practice and agency policies/protocols. Recommendations can be made to prevent the errors from occurring in the actual patient care setting. Building on the root cause analysis of an adverse event, Just Culture principles can be applied to a discussion of the implications for health care professionals who commit medical errors. David Marx has developed the concept of Just Culture where the emphasis moves from blame to examining errors to improve patient care (Marx, 2001). Examining the behavior of errors, Marx differentiates them into three types: *Human Error*, which is inadvertent and the individual should be consoled; *At-Risk* behavior where risk is not recognized or may be mistakenly believed to be justified and the individual is coached; and *Reckless* behavior where there is conscious disregard of risk and the individual should be punished (Marx, 2001). He succinctly defines these concepts in a video found at the following web site: https://www.youtube.com/watch?v=ElNHdA_49Cs. North Carolina Board of Nursing has developed a Student Practice Event Evaluation Tool (SPEET), a rubric by which faculty can examine learner actions and determine if it warrants consoling, coaching, counseling, remediation, or disciplinary action (https://www.ncbon.com/myfiles/downloads/just-culture-speet.pdf). The use of the SPEET allows faculty to evaluate practice events with consistency and fairness and allows learners to learn from mistakes while enhancing patient safety (https://www.ncbon.com/myfiles/downloads/just-culture.pdf). A SPEET cue card assists faculty in the implementation of Just Culture in Education Programs (https://www.ncbon.com/myfiles/downloads/just-culture-speet-cue-card.pdf). Faculty can use this card to evaluate behavior in simulation and in debriefing assist students in the understanding of human error, at risk behavior, and reckless behavior.

As part of an interprofessional course focusing on teamwork, communication, and patient safety, students participate in a series of scenarios in which they discover an overdose of anticoagulant. The medicine, nursing, and pharmacy students collaborate to stabilize the patient. The error is documented using the hospital's policies and protocols, and students work with risk management officers to disclose the error to a standardized patient who assumes the role of the patient's family member. Students are equipped to disclose the error through course materials and Harvard School of Medicine's (2006) document *When Things Go Wrong: Responding to Adverse Events* (http://www.macoalition.org/documents/respondingToAdverseEvents.pdf). Each student receives written feedback from the standardized patient about his/her communication and skills during the error disclosure. Next, the students participate in a root cause analysis of the event to examine the error through the lens of each profession, discussing the individual and system factors that contributed to the error. Learners participate in the sequence of events across several weeks of class, allowing them to experience the discovery of the error, participate in a root cause analysis, and apply the quality improvement QSEN competency.

Safety

Definition: *Minimizes risk of harm to patients and providers through both system effectiveness and individual performance* (Cronenwett *et al.*, 2007).

Patient safety is a clear priority for nurses (Barnsteiner, 2017). Safety principles are inherent to all high-fidelity simulation learning activities. Learners are expected to adhere to practices that support safe patient care. Simulation provides an environment where learners can rehearse what they have learned and refine their KSAs based on reflection and feedback. Simulation can assist with the learners' transition from the "carefully controlled educational experiences to a fast paced clinical world of increasing patient complexity [which] requires a strong sense of self confidence, critical thinking, clinical reasoning, and teamwork" (Moughrabi and Wallace, 2015).

Medication errors are a major source of morbidity and mortality as reported by the IOM in *To Err Is Human* (Kohn *et al.*, 2000; James, 2013). The importance of reducing medication errors was further delineated in the IOM report *Preventing Medication Errors* (Aspden *et al.*, 2007). Simulation is an excellent medium for providing novice and experienced practitioners with learning opportunities focused on improving safety in medication administration. Factors associated with common errors include medications that have similar names or are packaged similarly, medications that are rarely used or prescribed, medications that are used often but have a high incidence of patient allergy, and medications that require monitoring therapeutic blood levels. In addition, high-alert medications and those with black box warnings have increased propensity for adverse patient outcomes and can raise awareness of safety concerns. Simulation scenarios focusing on any area of patient care or nursing specialty can easily incorporate principles of safe medication administration (Hayes *et al.*, 2015; Sears *et al.*, 2010). A person assigned as the "resource nurse" in scenarios can utilize a drug reference text or online resource to access information related to medications used in scenarios. Using simulation, students can learn about unpredictable interruptions that can occur during medication administration and that can contribute to medication errors (Hayes *et al.*, 2015).

Other safety concerns can be included in simulation scenarios. This can be as simple as the expectation that students will perform hand hygiene as they enter and depart the scenario. Students may be asked to identify safety concerns in the simulated patient room, for example, risk for falls.

Informatics

Definition: *Use information and technology to communicate, manage knowledge, mitigate error, and support decision-making* (Cronenwett *et al.*, 2007).

Shulman (2010) adeptly describes the significance of informatics in nursing: "One need only spend a few hours with nurses on a hospital floor or in a cancer treatment room, in an individual office or even during a home visit, before being struck by the varieties of technology with which the nurse must competently cope…. And computers are ubiquitous for record keeping, communication, and the monitoring of drugs. All these now fall within the nurse's responsibilities, and he or she is expected to understand what and how to perform in those circumstances." The expectations for all health care providers to competently use and adapt to various technologies continues to expand (Warren, 2012). Each simulation should incorporate informatics as appropriate and feasible. Learners should be able to access and document patient data in an electronic format. In presimulation activities, participants might be assigned a list of data to collect from the electronic health record so that they are aware of the patient's medical history. When possible, point of care information and alerts should be provided to assist learners in the care of the patient in the scenario.

In simulation scenarios, learners can practice using technology for dispensing and administering medications. Medications may be accessed through an electronic drug dispensing machine. Bar code scanners may be used to read patient identification bands and medications.

Conclusion

Simulation-based learning is an effective immersive, learner-centered, experiential instructional strategy that provides learners with opportunities to increase their KSAs related to the quality and safety of patient care. Because the foundations of nursing practice are the same concepts embodied in the QSEN competencies, it is not surprising that many of the KSAs are already imbedded in existing preprogrammed and original nursing scenarios. Educators can map those scenarios using the QSEN competencies and their KSAs. Moving forward, educators can deliberately design quality simulation cases to integrate QSEN competencies. The 2010 Carnegie report states that to do anything less has "grave implications for the extent to which students will develop skills of clinical inquiry and the ability to use knowledge in specific clinical situations" (Benner et al., 2010).

References

Alfes, C.M. (2010) Developing a QSEN competency checklist for simulation experiences. Retrieved from http://qsen.org/developing-a-qsen-competency-checklist-for-simulation-experiences/.

Arocha, O., and Moore, D.Y. (2011) The new Joint Commission standards for patient-centered communication. Retrieved from http://www.languageline.com/main/files/wp_joint_commission_012411.pdf.

Aspden, P., Wolcott, J.A., Bootman, J.L., and Cronenwett, L.R. (Eds.). (2007) *Preventing medication errors.* Institute of Medicine. Washington, DC: National Academies Press.

Barnsteiner, J. (2017) Safety. In G. Sherwood and J. Barnsteiner (Eds.), *Quality and safety in nursing: A competency approach to improving outcomes.* Hoboken, NJ: Wiley-Blackwell.

Benner, P. (1984) *From novice to expert: Excellence and power in clinical nursing practice.* Menlo Park, CA: Addison Wesley.

Benner, P., Sutphen, M., Leonard, V., and Day, L. (2010) *Educating nurses: A call for radical transformation.* San Francisco: Jossey-Bass.

Berndt, J. (2014) Patient safety and simulation in pre-licensure nursing education: An integrative review. *Teaching and Learning Nursing, 9,* 16–22.

Boese, T., Cato, M., Gonzalez, L., Jones, A., Kennedy, K., Reese, C., Decker, S., Franklin, A. E., Gloe, D., Lioce, L., Meakim, C., Sando, C. R., and Borum, J. C. (2013) Standards of Best Practice: Simulation Standard V: Facilitator. *Clinical Simulation in Nursing, 9*(6S), June, S22–S25. doi: http://dx.doi.org/10.1016/j.ecns.2013.04.010.

Bryant, K., (2013) Diabetes management-Nurse practitioner. In S.H. Campbell and K.M. Daley (Eds.), *Simulation scenarios for nursing educators: Making it real.* 2nd Ed. New York, NY: Springer.

Campbell, S.H. and LoGiudice, J. (2013) Abdominal pain in a woman of childbearing age. In S.H. Campbell and K.M. Daley (Eds.), *Simulation scenarios for nursing educators: Making it real.* 2nd Ed. New York: Springer.

Cronenwett, L., Sherwood, G., Barnsteiner, J., Disch, J., Johnson, J., Mitchell, P., *et al.* (2007) Quality and safety education for nurses. *Nursing Outlook, 55*(3), 122–131.

Cronenwett, L., Sherwood, G., Pohl, J., Barnsteiner, J., Moore S., Sullivan, D. T., *et al.* (2009) Quality and safety education for advanced nursing practice. *Nursing Outlook, 57*(6), 338–348.

Decker S. I., Anderson M., Boese T., Epps C., McCarthy J., Motola I., Palaganas J., Perry C., Puga F., Scolaro K., and Lioce L. (2015) Standards of best practice: Simulation standard VIII: Simulation-enhanced interprofessional education (sim-IPE). *Clinical Simulation in Nursing,* June, *11*(6), 293–297. doi: http://dx.doi.org/10.1016/j.ecns.2015.03.010.

Decker, S., Fey, M., Sideras, S., Caballero, S., Rockstraw, L. (R.), Boese, T., Franklin, A.E., Gloe, D., Lioce, L., Sando, C. R., Meakim, C., and Borum, J. C. (2013) Standards of Best Practice: Simulation Standard VI: The debriefing process. *Clinical Simulation in Nursing,* June, *9*(6S), S27–S29. doi: http://dx.doi.org/10.1016/j.ecns.2013.04.008.

Dearmon, V., Graves, R., Hayden, S., Mulekar, M., Lawrence, S., Jones, L., Smith, K., and Farmer, J. (2013) Effectiveness of simulation-based orientation of baccalaureate nursing students preparing for their first clinical experience. *Journal of Nursing Education, 52*(1), 29–38. doi: 10.3928/01484834-20121212-02.

Disch, J. (2017) Teamwork and collaboration. In G. Sherwood and J. Barnsteiner (Eds.), *Quality and safety in nursing: A competency approach to improving outcomes.* Hoboken, NJ: Wiley-Blackwell.

Disch, J., Barnsteiner, J.H., and Walton, M.K. (2014) The landscape for nurturing person- and family-centered care. In Barnsteiner, J., Disch, J., and Walton, M.K. *Person and Family Centered Care* (pp. 1–17). Indianapolis, IN: Sigma Theta Tau International.

Durham, C.F., and Alden, K.R. (2012) Integrating the QSEN competencies into simulations. In P.R. Jeffries (Ed.), Simulation in nursing education: From conceptualization to evaluation. 2nd Ed. New York: National League of Nursing.

Elliott, L., DeCristofaro, C., and Carpenter, A. (2012) Blending technology in teaching advanced health assessment in a family nurse practitioner program: Using personal digital assistants in a simulation laboratory. *Journal of the American Academy of Nurse Practitioners, 24,* 536–543.

Engum, S. A., and Jeffries, P.R. (2012) Interdisciplinary collisions: Bringing healthcare professionals together. *Collegian, 19*(3), 145–151. Retrieved from doi: http://dx.doi.org/10.1016/j.colegn.2012.05.005.

Franklin, A.E., Boese, T., Gloe, D., Lioce, L., Decker, S., Sando, C.R., Meakim, C., and Borum, J.C. (2013) Standards of Best Practice: Simulation Standard IV: Facilitation. *Clinical Simulation in Nursing,* June, *9*(6S), S19–S21. doi: http://dx.doi.org/10.1016/j.ecns.2013.04.011.

Franklin, A.E., and Lee, C.S. (2014) Effectiveness of simulation for improvement in self-efficacy among novice nurses: A meta-analysis. *Journal of Nursing Education, 53*(11), 607–614.

Gantt, L.T., and Webb-Corbett, R. (2010) Using simulation to teach patient safety behaviors in undergraduate nursing education. *Journal of Nursing Education, 49*(1), 48–51.

Garnett, S., Weise, J.A., and Winland-Brown, J.E. (2015) Simulation design: Engaging large groups of nurse practitioner students. *Journal of Nursing Education, 54*(9), 525–531.

Gloe, D., Sando, C.R., Franklin, A.E., Boese, T., Decker, S., Lioce, L., Meakim, C., and Borum, J.C. (2013). Standards of Best Practice: Simulation Standard II: Professional Integrity of Participant(s). *Clinical Simulation in Nursing,* June, *9*(6S), S12–S14. doi: http://dx.doi.org/10.1016/j.ecns.2013.04.004.

Hallenbeck, V.J., (2012) Use of high-fidelity simulation for staff education/development: A systematic review of the literature. *Journal for Nurses in Staff Development, 28*(6), 260–269.

Harvard School of Medicine. (2006) *When things go wrong: Responding to adverse events.* Retrieved from http://www.macoalition.org/documents/respondingToAdverseEvents.pdf.

Haut, C., Fey, M.K., Akintade, B., and Klepper, M. (2014) Using high-fidelity simulation to teach acute care pediatric nurse practitioner students. *The Journal for Nurse Practitioners, 10*(10), e87–e91.

Hayden, J. (2010) Use of simulation in nursing education: National survey results. *Journal of Nursing Regulation, 1*(3), 52–57.

Hayden, J.K., Smiley, R.A., Alexander, M., Kardong-Edgren, S., and Jeffries, P.R. (2014) The NCSBN National Simulation Study: A longitudinal, randomized, controlled study replacing clinical hours with simulation in prelicensure nursing education. *Journal of Nursing Regulation, 5*(2Suppl), S1–S64.

Hayes, C., Power, T., Davidson, P.M., Daly, J., and Jackson, D. (2015) Nurse interrupted: Development of a realistic medication administration simulation for undergraduate nurses. *Nurse Education Today, 35*(9), 981–986.

Henneman, E.A., Roche, J.P., Fisher, D.L., Cunningham, H., Reilly, C.A., Nathanson, B.H., and Henneman, P.L. (2010) Error identification and recovery by student nurses using human patient simulation: Opportunity to improve patient safety. *Applied Nursing Research, 23*(1), 11–21.

Hunt, C.W., Curtis, A.M., and Gore, T. (2015) Using simulation to promote professional development of clinical instructors. *Journal of Nursing Education, 54*(8), 468–471.

International Nursing Association of Clinical Simulation and Learning. (2011) Standards of Best Practice: Simulation. *Clinical Simulation in Nursing, 7*(4S), S1–S19.

Ironside, P.M., Jeffries, P.R., and Martin, A. (2009) Fostering patient safety competencies using multiple-patient simulation experiences. *Nursing Outlook, 57*(6), 332–337.

James, J.T. (2013) A new, evidence-based estimate of patient harms associated with hospital care. *Journal of Patient Safety, 9*(3), 122–128. Retrieved from http://journals.lww.com/journalpatientsafety/Fulltext/2013/09000/A_New,_Evidence_based_Estimate_of_Patient_Harms.2.aspx.

Jarzemsky, P. (2009) A template for simulation scenario development that incorporates QSEN competencies. Retrieved from http://qsen.org/a-template-for-simulation-scenario-development-that-incorporates-qsen-competencies/.

Jarzemsky, P., McCarthy, J., and Ellis, N. (2010) Incorporating quality and safety education for nurses competencies in simulation scenario design. *Nurse Educator, 35*(2), 90–92.

Johnson, J. (2017) Quality improvement. In G. Sherwood and J. Barnsteiner (Eds.), *Quality and safety in nursing: A competency approach to improving outcomes.* Hoboken, NJ: Wiley-Blackwell.

Kaddoura, M.A. (2010) New graduate nurses' perceptions of the effects of clinical simulation on their critical thinking, learning, and confidence. *The Journal of Continuing Education in Nursing, 41*(11), 506–516.

King, H.B., Toomey, L. Salisbury, M., Webster, J., and Almeida, S. (2006) TeamSTEPPS® [Team Strategies and Tools to Enhance Performance and Patient Safety], developed by the Department of Defense (DoD) in collaboration with the Agency for Healthcare Research and Quality (AHRQ).

Kohn, L.T., Corrigan, J.M., and Donaldson, M.S. (Eds.). (2000) *To err is human: Building a safer health system.* A report of the Committee on Quality of Health care in America, Institute of Medicine. Washington, DC: National Academies Press.

Laird-Fick, H.S., Solomon, D., Jodoin, C., Dwamena, F.C., Alexander, K., Rawsthorne, L., *et al.* (2010) Training residents and nurses to work as a patient-centered care team on a medical ward. *Patient Education and Counseling,* June 14.

Lancaster, R.J., Westphal, J., and Jambunathan, J. (2015). Using SBAR to promote clinical judgment in undergraduate nursing students. *Journal of Nursing Education, 54*(3 Suppl.), S31–S34.

Leigh, G. (2011) The simulation revolution: What are the implications for nurses in staff development? *Journal for Nurses in Staff Development, 27,* 54–57.

Lioce L., Meakim C.H., Fey M.K., Chmil J.V., Mariani B., and Alinier G. (2015). Standards of best practice: Simulation Standard IX: Simulation Design. *Clinical Simulation in Nursing,* June, *11*(6), 309–315. doi: http://dx.doi.org/10.1016/j.ecns.2015.03.005

Lioce, L., Reed, C.C., Lemon, D., King, M.A., Martinez, P.A., Franklin, A.E., Boese, T., Decker, S., Sando, C.R., Gloe, D., Meakim, C., and Borum, J.C. (2013) Standards of Best Practice: Simulation Standard III: Participant Objectives. *Clinical Simulation in Nursing,* June, *9*(6S), S15–S18. doi: http://dx.doi.org/10.1016/j.ecns.2013.04.005.

Lucas, A.N. (2014) Promoting continuing competence and confidence in nurses through high-fidelity simulation-based learning. *Journal of Continuing Education in Nursing, 45*(8), 360–365.

Marx, D. (2001) Patient safety and the "just culture": A primer for health care executives. Retrieved from http://www.safer.healthcare.ucla.edu/safer/archive/ahrq/FinalPrimerDoc.pdf.

Meakim, C., Boese, T., Decker, S., Franklin, A.E., Gloe, D., Lioce, L., Sando, C.R., and Borum, J.C. (2013) Standards of Best Practice: Simulation Standard I: Terminology. *Clinical Simulation in Nursing,* June, *9*(6S), S3–S11. doi: http://dx.doi.org/10.1016/j.ecns.2013.04.001.

Mompoint-Williams, D., Brooks, A., Lee, L., Watts, P., and Moss, J. (2014) Using high-fidelity simulation to prepare advanced practice nursing students. *Clinical Simulation in Nursing, 10,* e5–e10.

Moughrabi, S., and Wallace, D.R. (2015) The effectiveness of simulation in advancing quality and safety education for nurses-based competency in accelerated nursing students. *Journal of Nursing Education and Practice, 5*(8), pp 17–25. doi: http://dx.doi.org/10.5430/jnep.v5n8p17.

Pauly-O'Neill, S., and Prion, S. (2013) Using integrated simulation in a nursing program to improve medication administration skills in the pediatric population. *Nursing Education Perspectives, 34*(3), 148–153.

Piscotty, R., Grobbel, C., and Tzeng, H. (2011) Integrating quality and safety competencies into undergraduate nursing using student-designed simulation. *Journal of Nursing Education, 50*(8), 429–436.

Pittman, O.A. (2012) The use of simulation with advanced practice nursing students. *Journal of the American Association of Nurse Practitioners, 24*(9), 516–520.

Rutherford-Hemming, T., Lioce, L., and Durham, C.F. (2015) Implementing the Standards of Practice for Simulation. *Nurse Educator, 40*(3), 96–100.

Rutherford-Hemming, T., and Jennrich, J.A. (2013) Using standardized patients to strengthen nurse practitioner competency in the clinical setting. *Nursing Education Perspectives, 34*(2), 118–121.

Sando, C.R., Coggins, R.M., Meakim, C., Franklin, A.E., Gloe, D., Boese, T., Decker, S., Lioce, L., and Borum, J.C. (2013) Standards of Best Practice: Simulation Standard VII: Participant Assessment and Evaluation. *Clinical Simulation in Nursing*, June, 9(6S), S30–S32. doi: http://dx.doi.org/10.1016/j.ecns.2013.04.007.

Scolaro, K.L., Woodyard, D.J., Joyner, B.L, and Durham, C.F. (2015) Building interprofessional teams. In Sherwood, G.D. and Horton-Deutsch, S. *Reflective organizations: On the front lines of QSEN and reflective practice implementation*. Indianapolis, IN: Sigma Theta Tau International, 189–214.

Sears, K., Goldsworthy, S., and Goodman, W.M. (2010) The relationship between simulation in nursing education and medication safety. *Journal of Nursing Education*, 49(1), 52–55.

Shearer, J.E. (2013) High-fidelity simulation and safety: An integrative review. *Journal of Nursing Education*, 52(1), 39–45.

Shellenbarger, T., and Edwards, T. (2012) Nurse educator simulation: Preparing faculty for clinical nurse educator roles. *Clinical Simulation in Nursing*, 8(6), e249–e255.

Shulman, L.S. (2010) Foreword. In P. Benner, M. Sutphen, V. Leonard, and L. Day (Eds.), *Educating nurses: A call for radical transformation*. San Francisco: Jossey-Bass.

Smith, J.R., and Cole, F.S. (2009) Patient safety: Effective interdisciplinary teamwork through simulation and debriefing in the neonatal ICU. *Critical Care Clinics of North America*, 21, 163–179.

Stroup, C. (2014) Simulation usage in nursing fundamentals: integrative literature review. *Clinical Simulation in Nursing, March*, 10(3), e155–e164. doi: http://dx.doi.org/10.1016/j.ecns.2013.10.004

Strouse, A.C. (2010). Multidisciplinary simulation centers: Promoting safe practice. *Clinical Simulation in Nursing*, 6(4), e139–e142. doi: 10.1016/j. ecns.2009.08.007.

Tracey, M.F., and Barnsteiner, J. (2017) Evidence-based practice. In G. Sherwood and J. Barnsteiner (Eds.), *Quality and safety in nursing: A competency approach to improving outcomes*. Hoboken, NJ: Wiley-Blackwell.

Vecchia, E.D., and Sparacino, L. (2015) High fidelity simulator experience for enhancing communication effectiveness: Applications to quality and safety education for nurses. *Journal of Nursing Education and Practice*, 5(9), 78–82.

Walton, M.K., and Barnsteiner, J. (2017) Patient-centered care. In G. Sherwood and J. Barnsteiner (Eds.), *Quality and safety in nursing: A competency approach to improving outcomes*. Hoboken, NJ: Wiley-Blackwell.

Walton-Moss, B., O'Neill, S., Holland, W., Hull, R., and Marineau, L. (2012) Advanced practice nursing students: Pilot test of a simulation scenario. *Collegian*, 19, 171–176.

Warren, J. (2017) Informatics. In G. Sherwood and J. Barnsteiner (Eds.), *Quality and safety in nursing: A competency approach to improving outcomes*. Hoboken, NJ: Wiley-Blackwell.

Wilhaus, J. (2010) Interdepartmental simulation collaboration in academia: Exploring partnerships with other disciplines. *Clinical Simulation in Nursing*, 6(6), e231–e232. doi: 10.1016/j.ecns. 2010.02.011.

Resources

Agency for Healthcare Research and Quality (AHRQ)
This web site has a wealth of information and resources, including information on evidence-based
practice, relevant research, patient teaching information, and consumer information around quality
and safety. http://www.ahrq.gov/

Framework for Action on Interprofessional Education and Collaborative Practice Health
Professions Networks Nursing and Midwifery Human Resources for Health, World Health
Organization. http://whqlibdoc.who.int/hq/2010/WHO_HRH_HPN_10.3_eng.pdf

Institute for Healthcare Improvement (IHI)
The IHI is a not-for-profit organization leading the improvement of health care throughout the world.
The IHI web site has information about programs and links to patient safety information. http://www.
ihi.org/IHI/

Institute of Medicine (IOM)
The IOM is a nonprofit organization that provides science-based information about health and science
policy. http://www.iom.edu/

Institute for Safe Medication Practices (ISMP)
The ISMP is a nonprofit organization that educates health care providers and the public about safe
medication practices. It has a plethora of resources for safe medication practices. http://www.
ismp.org/

International Nursing Association for Clinical Simulation and Learning (INACSL)
The INACSL promotes research and disseminates evidence-based practice standards for clinical
simulation methodologies and learning environments. http://www.inacsl.org

Interprofessional Education Collaborative Expert Panel *Core competencies for interprofessional
collaborative practice: Report of an expert panel.* (2011) Washington, D.C.: Interprofessional
Education Collaborative. http://www.aacn.nche.edu/education-resources/IPECReport.pdf

National Center for Interprofessional Practice and Education
The National Center is discovering and sharing ways to improve health, engage people and communities,
enhance patient care and control costs by integrating health professions education and practice into a
transformative Nexus. https://nexusipe.org/

North Carolina Board of Nursing Just Culture
The purpose of the "Just Culture" program is to provide a mechanism for Nursing Education Program
faculty and the regulatory board to come together to develop a culture that promotes learning from
student practice errors while properly assigning accountability for behaviors and consistently
evaluating events. http://www.ncbon.com/dcp/i/nursing-education-resources-for-program-
directors-just-culture-information

National Patient Safety Foundation (NPSF)
The NPSF is a not-for-profit organization whose mission is to improve the safety of patients. http://
www.npsf.org/

Quality and Safety Education for Nurses (QSEN)
The quality and safety competencies are patient-centered care, teamwork and collaboration, evidence-based
practice, quality improvement, safety, and informatics. Knowledge, skills, and attitudes for
prelicensure education are outlined to clarify each competency. This site is a valuable resource
because it also offers free downloadable teaching strategies and annotated bibliographies for each of
the QSEN competencies. http://qsen.org/

Robert Wood Johnson Foundation Initiative on the Future of Nursing, at the Institute of Medicine.
The Future of Nursing: Leading Change, Advancing Health. (2010) http://www.iom.edu/Reports/2010/
The-Future-of-Nursing-Leading-Change-Advancing-Health.aspx

Simulation Innovation Resource Center (SIRC) National League for Nursing

The SIRC is an online e-learning site for nursing educators to learn about simulation and ways to integrate it into their curriculum. It provides various ways for educators to engage with experts and peers. http://sirc.nln.org/

TeamSTEPPS® (Team Strategies and Tools to Enhance Performance and Patient Safety)

Teamwork and communication curriculum developed by the Department of Defense in collaboration with AHRQ. http://teamstepps.ahrq.gov/

The Joint Commission

Accrediting body for many health care organizations, concerned with improving the safety and quality of patient care. http://www.jointcommission.org/

13

Quality and Safety Education in Clinical Learning Environments

Lisa Day, PhD, RN, CNE and Gwen Sherwood, PhD, RN, FAAN, ANEF

Jacob was in his first rotation on an acute hospital unit as a nursing student. One of the nurses on the unit asked if he would like to observe while she inserted a Foley catheter. Jacob, who had just learned this skill in the lab, agreed. Together they walked to the patient's room. They both washed their hands and approached the patient, who was comatose; the nurse greeted the patient and explained the procedure and why it was needed. The nurse then inserted the catheter following steps Jacob did not recognize as what he had learned in the skills lab. This disturbed Jacob. "She's not following the steps outlined in the skills textbook," he said to himself. "I had to follow those to the letter in order to pass. She's cutting corners just to save time like our teacher said nurses do all the time. "Recognizing that he was a guest on the unit for a learning experience, Jacob reflected to himself how best to handle the situation.

One important purpose of academic nursing education has always been to prepare student nurses to be safe and effective health care providers who are able to advocate effectively for patients, families, communities, and best nursing practice in clinical care settings. With the publication of the QSEN competencies for undergraduate and graduate nursing education, many nursing school curricula make clear reference to the importance of quality and safety in clinical nursing practice, and faculty strive to create learning environments where students can achieve these practice competencies (Cronenwett *et al.*, 2007). Most nurses involved in nursing education and practice agree that the best environment for this kind of practice-based learning is a clinical practice setting where students can work with real nurses who are providing care to real people in need of their services. For this reason, clinical learning has always been an integral part of academic nursing education. Even with the introduction of problem-based learning, classroom-based unfolding case study discussions and lab-based simulation exercises with realistic mannequins and live, standardized-patient actors, nurse educators agree that clinical learning experiences in the "real world" are vital to prepare student nurses for transition to practice (Ironside, McNelis, and Ebright, 2014).

Although all can agree that clinical practice settings offer the richest and most varied opportunities for students to learn about quality and safety practices, it has become more and more evident that learning in the real world is filled with risk and tension. One of the most important sources of tension is the absolute priority of providing the safest, highest quality care to patients while allowing learners, who are each at a different stage of development and each with a different level of knowledge and skill, to engage

Quality and Safety in Nursing: A Competency Approach to Improving Outcomes, Second Edition.
Edited by Gwen Sherwood and Jane Barnsteiner.
© 2017 John Wiley & Sons, Inc. Published 2017 by John Wiley & Sons, Inc.

in legitimate nursing practice while they are learning. The student, Jacob, in the scenario that opened this chapter was exposed to this tension as he observed the nurse complete a procedure – insertion of an indwelling urinary catheter – that he had demonstrated competency with in a skills lab.

Another source of tension arises from the cultural differences between academic schooling that takes place in classrooms and labs and involves clear roles for student learners and teachers with specific learning outcomes drawn from textbooks, and workplace learning that takes place on the job and involves students and employees learning together in primarily informal and more incidental ways. Jacob also experienced this tension as he watched the nurse in the workplace deviate from the steps he had learned in the lab for safe catheter placement.

In this chapter, we use the social learning theory of Lave and Wenger (1991) and theories of workplace learning (Manuti *et al.*, 2015) to discuss the current separation of academic and clinical learning in schools of nursing and suggest clinical assignments for undergraduate nursing students that optimize student learning about quality and safety in the clinical workplace. These clinical assignments are based on the QSEN prelicensure competencies and take best advantage of the real world setting while maintaining high expectations for student learning and expanding the possibilities for learning assessment (Cronenwett *et al.*, 2007). The assignments can be adapted to address the higher order learning to meet the graduate level competencies (Cronenwett *et al.*, 2009). By using the QSEN competencies as the framework for collaboration, faculty in schools of nursing and administrators and staff in health care facilities can narrow the academic-practice gap through closer association of academic and workplace learning (Sherwood and Drenkard, 2007). Bridging academic and workplace learning will advance learners' perceptions about clinical work and better prepare them for practice, advance graduate student practice capacity, and also help establish lifelong learning of staff nurses (Day and Sherwood, 2017a).

Workplace Learning and Social Learning Theory

The social learning theory proposed and developed by Lave and Wenger (1991) provides a suitable framework for thinking about nursing education that takes place in schools of nursing and on nursing care units (Lave and Wenger, 1991). These authors point out the inherently social nature of learning and the inherent learning that is always present in social environments. They define learning as the movement of the newcomer toward more full participation in a sociocultural community of practice. Social learning begins when learners engage in what Lave and Wenger (1991) term "legitimate peripheral participation." When a novice nurse takes responsibility for a part of nursing practice that is recognized by the community of nurses as authentic nursing work, she or he is engaged in legitimate peripheral participation. Nursing students and new nurses move toward full participation in the social community of nurses by starting with relatively simple work, for example, taking and reporting a patient's vital signs. Complexity and new responsibilities are added as the student develops new skills, for example, completing a full physical exam and health history and documenting it in the medical record. Clinical reasoning allows the student to recognize and act on abnormal patient data.

Using this definition of legitimate peripheral participation, the clinical setting is the perfect social environment for nurses to learn nursing practice. Academic nursing faculty demonstrate their support for this idea by building into their curricula learning experiences in actual clinical practice environments where student nurses participate in authentic nursing care within a community of working nurses. While engaged in this type of clinical learning, as Jacob was in the opening scenario, student nurses are closer to workplace learning models than models of academic schooling (Manuti *et al.*, 2015).

Formal and Informal Learning: Workplace Learning and Academic Schooling

Workplace learning and academic schooling each exist in formal and informal practices; formal and informal workplace learning have parallels in academic schooling. In-service and continuing education classes are examples of nurses' formal workplace learning; formal academic schooling consists of the courses that make up the official curriculum of a given program. Informal learning takes place in the work environment while nurses are engaged in practice and is often serendipitous or incidental to the goals of the work. Practicing nurses' informal workplace learning is in some ways similar to student nurses' learning from the "hidden curriculum" in schools of nursing (Day and Benner, 2014). The hidden curriculum contains values that are evident in faculty behaviors and expectations but not made explicit in the official curriculum and not found in course descriptions, objectives, or program outcomes. In the nurse's workplace, formal learning opportunities occur much less frequently than the informal opportunities nurses have for learning from and in practice.

Although there are important parallels with informal workplace learning, student nurses' clinical assignments are usually a combination of formal and informal schooling, and informal workplace learning. Instead of taking full advantage of the opportunities for students to learn in incidental ways from and in practice while engaging in legitimate peripheral participation, academic nurse educators structure student learning and the assessment of learning around formal school assignments. For example, student nurses are asked to initiate comprehensive formal nursing care plans while working nurses may adapt standardized, sometimes interprofessional, plans of care. Student nurses complete detailed written reports of the physical exam and history findings, however, working nurses document exam data by exception or by choosing from drop-down lists in EHRs. So, although the clinical environment provides many social and workplace learning opportunities for students, the assignments faculty often require students to complete take them away from the legitimate peripheral participation Lave and Wenger describe (1991). Students find themselves situated in a sociocultural community of practicing nurses where the work they are required to do for school seems to hold no importance and sometimes seems inconsistent with the dynamics of the practice setting. Learning to reflect on these contradictions is an important part of how student learners begin to make sense of practice.

Learning the Work of Nursing

The disconnection of academic schooling from what they see as the actual work of nurses creates a dissonance for students who have difficulty recognizing the value of academic assignments and often believe they learn more about real nursing practice through their exposure to the work environment and the informal role modeling of staff nurses (Benner *et al.*, 2010). Or, as in Jacob's experience, the student who works with a nurse whose practice deviates from what he or she learned in school may begin to mistrust the work environment and the nurses. But learning nursing practice is no longer a matter of simple on-the-job training through traditional forms of apprenticeship. Nursing practice has become complex and specialized, and professional nurses have a legitimate claim to a unique body of knowledge related to the human response to health, disease, and injury. It is this body of knowledge as well as the technical skills and appropriate professional behaviors and ethical comportment that academic nurse educators are charged with imparting to student nurses (Benner *et al.*, 2010; Sullivan, 2005; Sullivan and Rosin, 2008). To accomplish these goals, academic teachers expect students to develop clinical imagination and curiosity and to organize their thinking into active clinical reasoning and judgment skills as they learn to think like nurses. The task burden of working nurses, however, leaves little time for the development of curiosity or imagination. Staff nurses' clinical judgment often goes untapped and uncultivated from the pressure of the rule-based, procedure-driven practice managers and external regulators often demand. The practice student nurses sometimes witness in the workplace may not fully meet the expectations of academic nursing education. Like Jacob, students may be confused by the contradictions they sometimes witness in practice when experienced nurses take shortcuts and workarounds–practices that are difficult for students to understand and unsafe when adopted by beginners (Day and Sherwood, 2017b).

Building Clinically Relevant Assignments

Given the expectations of academic nursing education and the nature of nursing practice in the clinical environment, academic nurse educators find it difficult to build clinical assignments that create safe, legitimate peripheral participation for student nurses and also accomplish the goals of academic nursing education. Academic assignments that seem disconnected from real-world practice like writing nursing care plans and physical exam reports can be valuable methods to train students' minds in important ways. These assignments also can be important sources of information for the teacher in deciding the student's success in meeting the clinical course objectives. But it is also exciting to think about ways academic nurse educators and nurses in clinical practice can bring their worlds closer together and solve the academic-practice gap of which students are so acutely aware (Benner *et al.*, 2010). This gap is sustained by academic nurse educators' privileging of theoretical knowledge over the practical know-how and clinical wisdom demonstrated by nurses in practice (Benner, Kyriakidis, and Stannard, 2011). It is also sustained by nursing students' limited opportunities to engage in legitimate peripheral participation that contributes to their meeting clinical course requirements and compounded by the students' lack of access to and understanding of the expert nurse's flexible, thinking-in-action (Benner *et al.*, 2011). To change this entrenched paradigm means educators need to rethink ways to create clinical learning experiences that engage students in legitimate peripheral participation.

Clinical Assignments to Promote Quality and Safety

The most rewarding nursing education for students and practicing nurses involves the cultivation of academic-practice partnerships that contribute to growing the curiosity, imagination, and clinical reasoning and judgment skills of student and staff nurses while improving the safety and quality of care for patients, families, and staff. Clinical assignments for nursing students that are drawn from the competencies developed by the faculty of the QSEN project provide an excellent framework for creating academic-practice partnerships and for bringing academic and clinical practice worlds closer together (Cronenwett *et al.*, 2007; Day and Smith, 2007; Cronenwett *et al.*, 2009). They also can provide a mechanism for nursing students to engage in legitimate peripheral participation as part of the nursing community of practice while contributing to improving the quality and safety of the patient care unit. The QSEN-based clinical assignments described in this section are offered to suggest ways faculty, facility administrators, and staff can work together to bring student nurses into the community of nursing practice. Through this kind of legitimate peripheral participation student and new graduate nurses can engage in exciting work that prepares them for clinical practice environments and their role in promoting safety and quality.

Assignment #1: Awareness of Quality and Safety Standards. In the current health care environment, all staff RNs on a patient care unit, whether in ambulatory care, home care, nursing home, hospital, or behavioral health should be aware of current quality and safety standards and challenges for their patient population. Similarly, no student nurse should complete a clinical assignment in any patient care unit without knowing what is on the quality dashboard and where that unit stands in relation to its quality and safety benchmarks. Quality and safety standards and benchmarks are set by government and private accrediting agencies and regulators such as the AHRQ, the Joint Commission, and the Centers for Medicare and Medicaid Services and are available on each organizations' web site (AHRQ, 2015; Centers for Medicare and Medicaid Services, 2015; TheJoint Commission, 2015). Before the beginning of a clinical rotation, student nurses can be assigned to identify a population of patients served in the care setting and find quality and safety standards of one or more government or private agencies that apply to this population. Each student or group can work on a different population and/or a different standard, and the assignment can be altered depending on the level of the student. For example, if the students are early in their program like Jacob and his classmates, the teacher might assign them to work from the Joint Commission's NPSG for hospitalized patients with each pair of students focusing on a different goal. For example, Jacob and other students on the neurologic unit might investigate the NPSG, implement evidence-based practices to prevent health care-associated infections due to multidrug-resistant organisms in acute care hospitals in relation to a specific population like adults with severe alterations in consciousness. Or, for more advanced students, part of the assignment might be to identify a population and search government and agency web sites to find related standards. Once they have a list of quality and safety standards, the students can then talk with the unit manager and/or facility or unit quality improvement officer to hear what initiatives are in place or in development to monitor, maintain, and improve the quality and safety of care delivery and how the related outcomes of care are being measured. For the remainder of the rotation, as they engage in daily nursing work in the care setting, each student discusses patient care with staff and keeps notes about how they and the nurses and other staff are contributing to meeting quality and safety standards in their practices and how they are gathering and documenting data to determine the impact of quality and safety initiatives on patient outcomes.

Students can develop increased awareness of quality and safety standards and how these impact and guide practice in a real care setting. By focusing on how nurses support the quality and safety mission of the facility, it also draws the students' and staff members' attention to the important work nurses do every day to reduce risk and improve the quality of care. As a next step in the assignment, students can work with staff RNs to identify new areas of focus for quality and safety improvement initiatives as they encounter impediments to best practice and risks to patient and staff safety in the work environment. Students can then write a paper or present a unit in-service on the different practices they engaged in or witnessed that reduced risk and improved the quality of care. Students with artistic talents could even use these experiences to produce a comic book, a graphic novel, a YouTube video, or other type of story board with nurses and other staff as a superhero team in the quest for safety and quality!

This assignment addresses specific QSEN competencies:

- Quality Improvement and Safety: Students connect the data they collect on their patients to the unit's desired quality and safety outcomes.
- Informatics and Evidence-based Practice: Students seek information on quality and safety standards as they learn to navigate government and agency web sites and evaluate the quality of Internet sources. In addition, students' attention to collecting and recording data related to quality and safety outcomes can give them a new perspective on documentation.

Assignment #2: Evidence, Adaptation, and Innovation in the Practice Environment. Other areas of quality and safety learning that can be addressed in a clinical environment are evidence-based practice and patient-centered care. In classroom lectures and assignments, students learn about the value of using empirical evidence to guide and standardize practice; develop skills in how to find and interpret pre-appraised evidence, original research reports, and evidence-based nursing procedures; and hear from academic nurses and researchers about how research-based evidence should be translated into practice. What is sometimes missing from this learning is a realistic sense of the complexity and pace of the care delivery systems and clinical environments with multiple stakeholders, including patients and families, who sometimes have conflicting concerns and interests. Academic nurse educators can re-create these complexities to some extent in the simulation lab or with problem-solving activities in the classroom. Clinical learning activities can be the most effective way to capture the mix of tension, excitement, and frustration that can accompany the implementation of a new practice initiative or updating a familiar nursing procedure in order to match current best practice. Standardizing nursing procedures across units and individual nurses while adhering to the principles of evidence-based practice is always challenging. This is familiar to any clinician who has been through the transition from a paper to an EHR, or from one brand of intravenous pump to another, or who has participated in the staff education and competency validation associated with any universal change in practice.

Although it may not be possible for each nursing student to go through the real-life experience of a practice change while they are in school, clinical assignments can help students learn about this process while they are engaged in a real practice environment by drawing their attention to how nurses balance the best empirical evidence with their own expert judgment and patient and family preferences. By embedding this learning in clinical practice, students will be exposed to the many impediments to standardizing practice across units and across individual nurses and see for themselves how nurses and other staff adapt to change.

The "Staff Work-Arounds Assignment" published on the QSEN web site is an example of an assignment focused in this area (QSEN, 2011). In this assignment, student nurses search for standardized nursing policies, procedures, standards of care, and other evidence-based nursing practice guidelines, and reflect on why the nurses' actual practice that they observe may deviate from the standards through the use of various "work arounds" (QSEN, 2011). This assignment would have been good for Jacob. Had he discussed urinary catheterization technique with the nurse, he would have found that the nurse knew the institution's written procedure for this but had made adaptations in order to better match the preferences of the patient's family members who care for her, which includes regular urinary catheterizations, at home. He also may have found that the institution's written procedure was based on more current evidence and did not match that found in his textbook.

As a variation of the Staff Work-Arounds assignment, student nurses assigned to different facilities or to different units within a facility can select a common nursing procedure (for example, administering medications or completing a urinary catheterization) and observe several nurses on the unit completing this task with different patients. Students then come together to compare and discuss the policies and procedures of different facilities and compare the practices of different nurses on the same unit, nurses from different units in the same facility, and nurses from different facilities. This can also be completed as a writing assignment for pairs or groups of students assigned to different units or facilities, or as an online discussion forum. The students collaborate to write a paper comparing the practices of nurses working in different units or facilities and exploring the interactions of evidence-based practice and nurses' work culture including the possibility of innovations staff nurses develop that result in practices that are equally safe but more efficient or, like the nurse Jacob was working with, more patient/family centered.

Assessing Student Learning: QSEN Competencies and Evaluation of Student Performance

There are many excellent resources on assessing and evaluating learning available to faculty (Billings and Halstead, 2012; Gaberson, Oermann, and Shellenbarger, 2015; Oermann and Gaberson, 2014). It is not our intent to replicate these efforts here but to consider how the focus on quality and safety competencies warrant re-thinking assessment methods consistent with new teaching and learning paradigms. Assessing student learning with the specific assignments described in this chapter will require faculty members to develop grading rubrics that include criteria for KSAs specific to the goals of the course. These assignments can provide valuable information on students' engagement with, and KSAs in, quality and safety. In addition to these specific assignments, the clinical learning environment presents many excellent opportunities for students to develop KSAs related to quality and safety as they participate in everyday patient care activities. While nursing students obviously have opportunities to learn in informal ways while participating in the social environment on the patient care unit, assessing this type of learning often is difficult for clinical nurse educators, and there are few, if any, valid and reliable tools to help with this important work. The QSEN competencies serve as excellent learning outcomes but do not offer specific criteria or methods for determining student success in achieving these outcomes. The best methods for assessing informal clinical learning will use multiple sources of data and take into account all the diverse ways students who have had different experiences might demonstrate their competence in quality and safety. Staff, patients/clients, and family members are other important sources of information for clinical faculty as they evaluate students' clinical learning.

Including staff, patient/client, and family members' feedback can be challenging for clinical faculty. Even though they can provide valuable input on students' performance, nurses and other staff members often are reluctant to participate in evaluating a student's learning. They may feel they do not have the time or skills to collect and interpret data on student nurses' performance or they do not want to feel responsible if a student fails. Also, attending to student performance criteria may feel overly burdensome to staff. Similarly, patients and family members may not be able to provide any details on a student's behavior and may hesitate to give a student nurse a "bad" report. Clinical faculty may be able to overcome this resistance by reassuring staff members, patients, and family members that the purpose of assessment is to foster professional growth and development; any input they provide will contribute to student development and is not intended as the deciding factor on whether a student passes or fails a clinical assignment but provides a more comprehensive perspective.

It is also important to make it as easy as possible for staff members, patients/clients, and family members to provide feedback on student performance. Rather than expecting them to complete a written evaluation based on specific course objectives and criteria, clinical faculty members can develop a short list of questions with which to interview staff, patients/clients, and family members. Some teachers or the students themselves can then write down or audio record the answers at the end of each clinical shift as a requirement of the clinical evaluation process. It is then up to clinical faculty and students to interpret these data based on course objectives and performance criteria. For example, a QSEN competency related to teamwork and collaboration skills is to "Initiate requests for help when appropriate to situation." A question for staff members that can assist clinical faculty and students in evaluating this competency might be, "When and how did the student ask for your help today? When did the student exceed expectations?" Another QSEN skill competency related to patient-centered care is "Remove barriers to presence of families and other designated surrogates based on patient preferences." Questions for patients/clients and family members to evaluate student competency include, "How did the student attend to your/your family's comfort today?" and, "What would you have liked the student to do that he/she didn't do?" The responses to these simple questions elicited by faculty members or by the students themselves can provide valuable data students can use to improve their practice and that clinical faculty can consider in forming the final evaluation of student performance.

Bringing Academic and Workplace Learning Together

The importance of life-long learning to the professional nurse's success in delivering safe and effective care is evident in the AACN's *Essentials of Baccalaureate Education for Professional Nursing Practice* (AACN, 2008). The learning environments of school and the workplace are quite different and the type of learning that takes place in each, while both are essential to the success of new nurses, can appear to be unrelated. For this reason, it is now commonly accepted that new graduate nurses need the support of a new graduate nurse residency as they make the transition from school to practice. This is at least partly because academic nursing education and practice, that is, academic learning and workplace learning, have been separated during nursing students' academic schooling. Academic and clinical nurse educators as well as clinical nurses often think of academic learning environments like classrooms and labs as the sites where students acquire new learning and think of clinical environments as the sites where students then should be able to apply their new knowledge in providing care to patients/clients. Nurse educators and clinical nurses who are able to help students see practice as a source for new knowledge and skills and the social context of the workplace as a valuable environment for students to learn new KSAs will prod them toward life-long learning as they get ready to transition to the work role (Spector, Ulrich and Barnsteiner, 2017).

Reflective Practice: Debriefing to Learn

A commitment to quality and safety requires nurses to engage in ongoing education and professional development beyond what is included in academic schooling. Combining academic and workplace learning in both the school and work environments will ready new nurses to take up their responsibilities as life-long learners and will help practicing nurses renew their commitment to current best practices. This will require robust partnerships of academic nurse educators, students, and clinical and administrative nurses and collaborations across schools and clinical facilities. It will require academic educators to stay in touch with clinical practice and stay apprised of what nurses confront in their current work environments. And it will require clinical and administrative nurses to stay informed of the current trends in evidence-based practice and collaborate with academia to adapt practices so that they meet the current standards of the wider community of nursing.

One good model for academic-practice partnerships in nursing is the dedicated education unit (DEU) about which much has been published (Claeys *et al.*, 2015; Devereaux Melillo *et al.*, 2014; Hill, Foster, and Oermann, 2015; McVey *et al.*, 2014; Mulready-Shick and Flanagan, 2014; Nishioka *et al.*, 2014a, 2014b; Sharpnack, Koppelman, and Fellows, 2014; Smyer, Tejada, and Tan, 2015). The success of the DEU depends on a mutual commitment from academic and clinical nurse educators, clinicians, and administrators to create work-place learning environments that are supportive of student nurses and attentive to their learning needs while also maintaining the best quality and safest care for patients/clients and their families. The DEU creates a role for the student nurse that integrates her/him into the community of practice of a patient/client care unit and encourages legitimate peripheral participation and provides an excellent opportunity to implement the QSEN competencies and bring academic and work-place learning settings closer together.

Summary

Clinical learning has always been an integral part of academic nursing education, yet orientations for new graduates continue to lengthen. This chapter considers approaches to clinical learning that situate the learner and faculty to have a real world experience by integrating into the work of the unit. Integrating the QSEN competencies offers new opportunities in forming clinical academic partnerships. Nurse educators and clinical nurses can work together to help students see practice as a source for new knowledge and skills and experience the social context of the workplace as a valuable learning environment that will foster learners to develop habits of life-long learning and have smooth transition to the work role.

References

AACN. (2008) *Essentials of baccalaureate education for professional nursing practice*. Washington D.C.: AACN.

AHRQ. (2015) *2014 National Healthcare Quality and Disparities Report chartbook on patient safety*. Rockville, MD: Agency for Healthcare Research and Quality.

Benner, P., Kyriakidis, P., and Stannard, D. (2011) *Clinical wisdom and interventions in acute and critical care: A thinking-in-action approach*. 2nd Ed. New York: Springer Publishing Company.

Benner, P., Sutphen, M., Leonard, V., and Day, L. (2010) *Educating nurses: A call for radical transformation*. San Francisco: Jossey-Bass.

Billings, D.M., and Halstead, J.A. (2012) *Teaching in nursing: A guide for faculty*. 4th Ed. St. Louis, MO: Elsevier Saunders.

Centers for Medicare and Medicaid Services. (2015) Regulations and Guidance. Retrieved August 5, 2015, from https://www.cms.gov/Regulations-and-Guidance/Regulations-and-Guidance.html.

Claeys, M., Deplaecie, M., Vanderplancke, T., Delbaere, I., Myny, D., Beeckman, D., and Verhaeghe, S. (2015) The difference in learning culture and learning performance between a traditional clinical placement, a dedicated education unit and work-based learning. *Nurse Educ Today, 35*(9), e70–77. doi: 10.1016/j.nedt.2015.06.016.

Cronenwett, L., Sherwood, G. Barnsteiner, J., Disch, J., Johnson, J., Mitchell, P., Taylor Sullivan, D., and Warren, J. (2007) Quality and safety education for nurses. *Nursing Outlook, 55*(3), 122–131.

Cronenwett, L., Sherwood, G., Pohl, J., Barnsteiner, J., Moore, S., Taylor Sullivan, D., Ward, D., and Warren, J. (2009) Quality and safety education for advanced practice nursing practice. *Nursing Outlook, 57*(6), 338–348.

Day, L., and Benner, P. (2014) The hidden curriculum in nursing education. In F.W. Hafferty and J.F. O'Donnell (Eds.), *The Hidden Curriculum in Health Professional Education*. Lebanon, NH: University Press of New England.

Day, L., and Sherwood, G. L. (2017a) Transforming Education to Transform Practice: Using Unfolding Case Studies to Integrate Quality and Safety in Subject Centered Classrooms. In G. Sherwood and J. Barnsteiner (Eds.), *Quality and safety in nursing: A competency approach to improving outcomes*, 2nd Ed. Hoboken, NJ: Wiley-Blackwell.

Day, L., and Sherwood, G. (2017b) Quality and Safety in Clinical Learning Environments. In G. Sherwood and J. Barnsteiner (Eds.), *Quality and safety in nursing: A competency approach to improving outcomes*, 2nd Ed. Hoboken, NJ: Wiley-Blackwell.

Devereaux Melillo, K., Abdallah, L., Dodge, L., Dowling, J. S., Prendergast, N., Rathbone, A., Thornton, C. *et al*., (2014) Developing a dedicated education unit in long-term care: a pilot project. *Geriatr Nurs*, *35*(4), 264–271. doi: 10.1016/j.gerinurse.2014.02.022.

Gaberson, K.B., Oermann, M.H., and Shellenbarger, T. (2015) *Clinical teaching strategies in nursing*. New York: Springer Publishing Company.

Hill, R.Y., Foster, B., and Oermann, M. (2015) Dedicated education unit model for a transition into practice course. *J Contin Educ Nurs*, *46*(9), 403–408. doi: 10.3928/00220124-20150821-02.

Ironside, P.M., Ebright, P., and McNelis, A.M. (2014) Clinical education in nursing: Rethinking learning in clinical settings. *Nursing Outlook*, *62*(3):185–191.

Lave, J., and Wenger, E. (1991) *Situated learning: Legitimate peripheral participation*. Cambridge: Cambridge University Press.

Manuti, A., Pastore, S., Scardigno, A.F., Giancaspro, M.L., and Morciano, D. (2015) Formal and informal learning in the workplace: A research review. *International Journal of Training and Development*, *19*(1), 1–17.

McVey, C., Vessey, J.A., Kenner, C.A., and Pressler, J.L. (2014) Interprofessional dedicated education unit: an academic practice partnership. *Nurse Educ*, *39*(4), 153–154. doi: 10.1097/nne.0000000000000051.

Mulready-Shick, J., and Flanagan, K. (2014) Building the evidence for dedicated education unit sustainability and partnership success. *Nurs Educ Perspect*, *35*(5), 287–293.

Nishioka, V.M., Coe, M.T., Hanita, M., and Moscato, S.R. (2014a) Dedicated education unit: nurse perspectives on their clinical teaching role. *Nurs Educ Perspect*, *35*(5), 294–300.

Nishioka, V.M., Coe, M.T., Hanita, M., and Moscato, S.R. (2014b) Dedicated education unit: student perspectives. *Nurs Educ Perspect*, *35*(5), 301–307.

Oermann, M.H., and Gaberson, K.B. (2014) *Evaluation and testing in nursing education*. 4th Ed. New York: Springer Publishing Company.

QSEN. (2011) Quality and Safety Education for Nursing. Retrieved 1/7/11, from http://www.qsen.org/

Sharpnack, P.A., Koppelman, C., and Fellows, B. (2014) Using a dedicated education unit clinical education model with second-degree accelerated nursing program students. *J Nurs Educ*, *53*(12), 685–691. doi: 10.3928/01484834-20141120-01.

Smith, E., and Day, L. (2007) Integrating quality and safety content into clinical teaching in the acute care setting. *Nursing Outlook.*, *55*(3):138–143.

Smyer, T., Tejada, M.B., and Tan, R.A. (2015) Systematic and deliberate orientation and instruction for dedicated education unit staff. *J Nurs Educ*, *54*(3), 165–168. doi: 10.3928/01484834-20150218-17.

Spector, N., Ulrich, B., and Barnsteiner, J. (2017) Improving Quality and Safety with Transition to Practice. In G. Sherwood and J. Barnsteiner (Eds.), *Quality and safety in nursing: A competency approach to improving outcomes*, 2nd Ed. Hoboken, NJ: Wiley-Blackwell.

Sullivan, W. (2005) *Work and integrity: The crisis and promise of professionalism in america* (2 ed.). San Francisco: Jossey-Bass.

Sullivan, W., and Rosin, M.S. (2008) *A new agenda for higher education: Shaping a life of the mind for practice* San Francisco: Jossey-Bass/Carnegie Foundation for the Advancement of Teaching.

The Joint Commission. (2015) Core Measure Sets. Retrieved July 25, 2015, from http://www.jointcommission.org/core_measure_sets.aspx

Resources

Agency for Healthcare Research and Quality (AHRQ)
This web site has a wealth of information and resources, including information on evidence-based practice, relevant research, patient teaching information, and consumer information around quality and safety including the TeamSTEPPS curriculum. http://www.ahrq.gov/

American Association of Colleges of Nursing (AACN)
This national association of deans was a strategic partner in developing QSEN, and the QSEN competencies are embedded in the essentials for baccalaureate, Master's, and Doctor of Nursing Practice programs. Their web page offers educational resources including several web sources of information about QSEN. AACN led regional faculty development conferences for faculty and continues to offer leadership to improving quality and safety. **http://www.aacn.nche.edu/**

Institute for Healthcare Improvement (IHI)
The IHI is a not-for-profit organization leading the improvement of health care throughout the world. IHI web site has information about programs and links to patient safety information. http://www.ihi.org/IHI/

Institute of Medicine (IOM)
The IOM is a nonprofit organization that provides science-based information about health and science policy. http://www.iom.edu/

Institute for Safe Medication Practices (ISMP)
The ISMP is a nonprofit organization that educates health care providers and the public about safe medication practices. It has a plethora of resources for safe medication practices. http://www.ismp.org/

International Nursing Association for Clinical Simulation and Learning (INACSL)
This group promotes research and disseminate evidence-based practice standards for clinical simulation methodologies and learning environments. http://www.inacsl.org

National League for Nursing (NLN)
This national organization was a partner in helping launch QSEN, and offers a wealth of resources for nurse educators, offers accreditation to member schools, and sponsors numerous educational conferences. The QSEN competencies are embedded in all nursing education programs from practical nursing through PhD. (**http://www.nln.org/**)

North Carolina Board of Nursing: Just Culture
The purpose of the "Just Culture" program is to provide a mechanism for Nursing Education Program faculty and the regulatory board to come together to develop a culture that promotes learning from student practice errors while properly assigning accountability for behaviors and consistently evaluating events. http://www.ncbon.com/dcp/i/nursing-education-resources-for-program-directors-just-culture-information

National Patient Safety Foundation (NPSF)
The NPSF is a not-for-profit organization whose mission is to improve the safety of patients. http://www.npsf.org/

Quality and Safety Education for Nurses (QSEN)
The quality and safety competencies are patient-centered care, teamwork and collaboration, evidenced-based practice, quality improvement, safety, and informatics. Knowledge, skills, and attitudes for prelicensure education are outlined to clarify each competency. This site is a valuable resource because it also offers free downloadable teaching strategies and annotated bibliographies for each of the QSEN competencies. http://qsen.org/

Robert Wood Johnson Foundation Initiative on the Future of Nursing, at the Institute of Medicine. *The Future of Nursing: Leading Change, Advancing Health* (2010). http://www.iom.edu/Reports/2010/The-Future-of-Nursing-Leading-Change-Advancing-Health.aspx

Simulation Innovation Resource Center (SIRC) National League for Nursing

The SIRC is an online e-learning site for nursing educators to learn about simulation and ways to integrate it into their curriculum. It provides various ways for educators to engage with experts and peers. http://sirc.nln.org/

14

Interprofessional Approaches to Quality and Safety Education

Mary A. Dolansky, PhD, RN, FAAN, Ellen Luebbers, MD, Mamta K. Singh, MD, MS and Shirley M. Moore, PhD, RN, FAAN

"Taking care of patients is so complicated and I am thankful that I have learned what people from other professions can do. Together we are able to do so much more for the patient and do it faster and safer. I do not know if I could last if I did not have a team to help me. Our patient may have died if we were not all communicating and working together." Quote from a student

Quality and safety education equips and enables health professionals to not only provide care but to improve it in the process. It has been well documented that to improve patient safety and the quality of care health professionals must work collaboratively with members of other professions. Learning to work collaboratively is a unique skill and facilitated by the use of interprofessional education (IPE) approaches. In this chapter we define interprofessional education as: "Occasions when two or more professions learn with, from and about each other to improve collaboration and the quality of care" (CAIPE, 1997). Interprofessional collaboration is an essential component in all the *QSEN competencies.* The QSEN competencies are described elsewhere in great detail in this book. These competencies are displayed in Appendices A and B and can be accessed at the QSEN web site: www.qsen.org. This chapter addresses the most recent evidence regarding IPE in quality and safety. It includes exemplar programs that are achieving IPE, and provides information on examples of effective pedagogies for planning, implementing, and evaluating learning experiences across professions. Specifically, we address three questions:

1) What is the added value of IPE to the quality and safety learning process?
2) What does it mean to learn with, from, and about another profession?
3) What are the best-practice considerations to take into account when designing IPE strategies for quality and safety?

The Added Value of Interprofessional Education to the Quality and Safety Learning Process

If students are to learn and practice the knowledge and skills associated with quality and safety, they must also learn how to work together collaboratively. In reviews of the literature and national reports, IPE was shown to promote interprofessional collaboration (IOM, 2015; Zwarenstein, Goldman, and

Reeves, 2009; Zwarenstein *et al.*, 2001). To consider the added value of IPE to quality and safety education, faculty should start by identifying those outcomes that may *only* be achieved through IPE. Thistlethwaite and colleagues (2010), on behalf on the World Health Organization (WHO) Study Group on Interprofessional Education and Collaborative Practice, conducted a review of the literature on learning outcomes associated with IPE and identified six broad themes:

- teamwork
- roles and responsibilities
- communication
- learning and reflection
- the patient/client (patient-centered care, quality and safety, coordination of care)
- ethics and attitudes

These outcomes are also consistent with those needed to prepare students for collaborative, patient-centered practice and the improvement of care in a complex health care environment.

Other learning outcomes include understanding the scopes of practice of other professionals, role negotiation, priority setting, conflict management, and understanding, cooperating, and valuing the contributions of other professionals. In addition to interprofessional collaboration, beginning evidence demonstrates the positive effects of IPE on other professional practice and health care outcomes.Examples include the impact of IPE on ED culture and patient satisfaction; clinical team behavior and reduction of clinical error rates for emergency department teams; management of care delivered to domestic violence victims; and mental health practitioner competencies related to the delivery of patient care. Although examples exist, more rigorous IPE studies to provide better evidence of the impact of IPE on professional practice and health care outcomes are needed (IOM, 2015). A call to action from the National Center for Interprofessional Education is for IPE to address the Triple Aim, a framework developed by the IHI that consists of improving population health, costs, and quality of care (Brandt *et al.*, 2014).

Learning With, From, and About Each Other

What does it mean to learn with, from, and about each other? A major goal of IPE is to increase positive attitudes among individuals of different professions. Conditions to support this follow: clear roles and responsibilities, positive expectations, a cooperative environment, successful joint work, and a perception that members of the other group are typical (Oandasan and Reeves, 2005a). Specific strategies can be built into education programs to enhance *learning with, from, and about each other*. An important strategy is the creation of a non-threatening learning environment in which learners feel psychologically safe to express themselves freely. This includes the provision of safe places for discussing and dealing with issues of power in education and practice settings. Another approach to promote *learning with, from, and about* is planning space and time for reflection. Students need to be able to reflect on their role in a team, and a team needs to be able to reflect together upon itself. Both self and group reflections are most useful if students have been exposed to issues that they must grapple with, such as issues related to hierarchy, respect, communication, role delineation, and decision-making in groups. These reflections are best when based on subject matter that relates to learners' immediate interests and concerns. See Textbox 14.1.

Giving students the opportunity to have input into the teaching design can facilitate this relevance for them. Lastly, *learning with, from, and about* each other is facilitated by faculty modeling distributive leadership instead of top-down hierarchical models of leadership. Faculty can facilitate interprofessional collaboration by including the following approaches in learning activities: (a) Ensure clarity

---

Textbox 14.1 Learning Roles and Responsibilities

An undergraduate nursing student and a first year medical student participate in an obesity and hypertension screening program in the Cleveland Public schools. It was critical in the development of this program to create an authentic team structure for the learning to occur. Without that structure, chaos of the activity prevented learning. Nursing students function as leaders for the day, and the medical students are team members. Each is oriented and trained for these roles. Briefing, huddles, and debriefing are built into the day, and students are asked to reflect on what they have learned.

---

of roles and responsibilities that includes scope of practice; (b) Respect, trust, and communicate; and (c) Provide attention to heirchical organizational structures (McInnes *et al.*, 2015) and understand the mental models or views of all professions (Senge, 1990). A simple strategy to achieve understanding the mental models or views of others is to facilitate interprofessional awareness by having students practice (a) hearing the views (mental models) of others, (b) sharing their views (mental models) and (c) being willing to change their mind in order to achieve a shared vision (Senge, 1990). The strategy can be introduced to interprofessional students after listening to a story. An appropriate story about nurse/physician communication related to the concerns a nurse has about a patient but chooses not to assert her concerns can be found on the QSEN web site from StoryCare (http://qsen.org/faculty-resources/interprofessional).

> "This experience helped me learn that I can gain a lot from working with team members from a different profession, as they have different skills and knowledge that can be used to complement my own skills and knowledge."
>
> *Quote from a student*

Best-Practice Considerations to take into Account when Designing IPE Strategies for Quality and Safety

Organizing Frameworks for IPE in Quality and Safety Education

In IPE, faculty have two purposes: achieving the goals of a particular content area of education, such as quality and safety, as well as achieving the goals associated with learning to collaborate across different professions. Either of these two content areas can be the "foreground" or the "background" in a particular learning initiative. When teaching quality and safety in an interprofessional education format, faculty can consciously shift quality and safety content and interprofessional collaboration content from the "background" or implicit learning to the "foreground" or a more explicit curriculum. The models and competencies described below address IPE and IPE for quality and safety. The goal is to promote competency in the skills of quality and safety improvement and/or working together in health care teams.

Models of IPE

Several Models of IPE have been applied to quality and safety education. Common elements of these models are role clarification, communication, team training (including group process and conflict management skills), and leadership training. A predominant model is the WHO Framework for Action on Interprofessional Education and Collaborative Practice (FAIECP) (World Health Organization, 2010). This model calls for the collaboration of local health systems and educational systems to promote processes for shared decision-making and governance that support collaboration for the improvement of health. Another model is the Canadian

Interprofessional Health Collaborative Competency Framework that focuses on role clarification, team functioning, interprofessional conflict resolution, and collaborative leadership to promote interprofessional collaboration. The model also describes the influence of quality improvement and contextual environmental factors on IPE. The web site of the Canadian Interprofessional Health Collaborative contains a particularly rich set of teaching and evaluation strategies and tools for IPE that can be accessed at www.cihc.ca.

A third IPE model that focuses on health care team training for safety and quality improvement is Team STEPPS, an evidence-based framework to improve communication and teamwork skills among health care professionals (King *et al.*, 2008). At the core of the framework are four teachable-learnable skills:

- *leadership* (ability to coordinate the activities of team members by ensuring team actions are understood, changes in information are shared, and that team members have the necessary resources)
- *situation monitoring* (process of actively scanning and assessing situational elements to gain information, understanding, or maintain awareness to support functioning of the team)
- *mutual support* (ability to anticipate and support other team members' needs through accurate knowledge about their responsibilities and workload)
- *communication*

Developed by the Department of Defense Patient Safety program in collaboration with AHRQ, TeamSTEPPS provides a source for ready-to-use materials and training curriculum to successfully integrate teamwork principles into all areas of the health care system. Materials are free and can be obtained at http://teamstepps.ahrq.gov. The TeamSTEPPS program consists of a pretraining assessment for site readiness, training tools and modules, an implementation and sustainability plan, and psychometrically validated instruments to measure outcomes. Research testing the effect of the TeamSTEPPS program has demonstrated a relationship to improvement in teamwork skills and outcomes in both operating room (Weaver *et al.*, 2010) and trauma teams (Capella *et al.*, 2010).

Interprofessional Core Competencies

Core competencies also provide organizing frameworks for IPE. Core competencies for interprofessional practice have been developed in several countries and were developed by the Interprofessional Education Collaborative (IPEC) in 2011 in the United States. The work was sponsored jointly by the American Association of Colleges of Nursing, the American Association of Colleges of Osteopathic Medicine, the American Association of Pharmacy, the American Dental Association, the Association of American Medical Colleges, and the Association of Schools of Public Health (Interprofessional Education Collaborative Expert Panel, 2011). These competencies were designed to support the achievement of interprofessional collaborative practice of health professionals toward a vision of safe high quality accessible patient-centered care. The competencies build on each profession's expected disciplinary competencies by adding the ability to work effectively as members of interprofessional clinical teams. The competencies are structured in four interprofessional practice domains:

1) Values/Ethics for Interprofessional Practice
2) Roles/Responsibilities
3) Interprofessional Communications
4) Teams and Teamwork

These competencies represent a comprehensive set of interprofessional collaboration competences and have been distributed to be used and assessed for their usefulness to guide IPE initiatives.

Design of IPE Strategies

Numerous reviews have synthesized Key elements of IPE and pedagogical approaches to successful IPE (Oandasan *et al.*, 2005a; Oandasan and Reeves, 2005b). Textbox 14.2 describes key elements in planning interprofessional learning experiences. In a review of team training, Weaver and colleagues (2010) found that team training is being implemented across a wide spectrum of providers and is primarily targeting intra- and interprofessional communication, situational awareness, leadership, and role clarity. Evidence exists that structured IPE activities need to have clinical relevance to be valued by the students (Gilligan, Outram, and Levett-Jones, 2014; Hean *et al.*, 2012) and be theoretically based (Abu-Rish, 2012; Barr, 2013; Hean *et al.*, 2012; Suter *et al.*, 2013). Textbox 14.3 displays an example of a program at the VA that integrates these features. A set of core features has been identified that contributes to successful interprofessional learning: cooperative learning, reflective learning, experiential learning, and the promotion of transfer of learning. Each of these core features is expanded upon below.

Textbox 14.2 Key Factors in Planning Interprofessional Learning Experiences

What is driving the development of this program?
What are the opportunities and barriers in the current learning environment?
What professions will (should) be involved?
What is the level of the learner?
What size group?
Where will learning take place?
Are there explicit learning objectives (content and process)?
What content will be included (emphasized)?
What instructional methods will be used (information-based, practice-based, simulation-based)?
How will cooperative learning be built into the program?
How will learner and faculty reflections be built into the program?
How will experiences to promote transfer of the skills learned be included?
Who is delivering the educational programming?
How will performance feedback be accomplished?
How will evaluation of training experiences be done?
How will learning be assessed?
What is the level of the learner?

Textbox 14.3 Example of an Interprofessional Education Program that Integrates Clinical Relevance and that Is Theory-based

VA Centers of Excellence in Primary Care Education (http://www.va.gov/OAA/coepce/index.asp)

The Office of Academic Affiliation of the Veterans Administration (VA) in 2010 funded five sites for $5 million each over five years to develop innovative interprofessional curriculum to train future health care professionals to work in patient-centered medical home models within the VA. The five original sites in Boise, Cleveland, San Francisco, Seattle, and New Haven VA hospitals have worked closely with their health professional affiliates to develop and study a novel curriculum to deliver patient-centered care. The core competencies or educational domains that are expected of all learners of the program follow:

- **Shared Decision-Making**: Care is aligned with the values, preferences, and cultural perspectives of the patient. Curricula focus is on communication skills necessary to promote patient's self-efficacy.

- **Sustained Relationships**: Care is designated to promote continuity of care, and curricula focus on longitudinal learning relationships.
- **Interprofessional Collaboration**: Care is team based, efficient, and coordinated. Curricula focus is on developing trustful, collaborative relationships.
- **Performance Improvement**: Care is designed to optimize the health of populations. Curricula focus is on using the methodology of continuous improvement in redesigning care to achieve quality outcomes.

The curriculum has resulted in interprofessional learners engaging in meaningful quality improvement efforts along with clinical nurse managers and schedulers in the clinic thus linking learning with clinical improvement work. Examples of quality improvement work include reducing emergency department visits for low acuity musculoskeletal pain, improving human immunodeficiency virus (HIV) screening in veterans, reducing unnecessary lab testing, and reducing no show rates. These QI projects and many others have also been presented at national meetings thus illustrating how ground-level QI work can also serve as scholarly work thus aligning key goals of academics and clinical quality experiences.

Cooperative Learning

D'Eon (2005) describes five elements of best-practice cooperative learning: 1) positive interdependence, 2) face-to-face interactions, 3) individual accountability, 4) interpersonal and small group skills, and 5) group processing. Textbox 14.4 provides a description of each of these factors. One effective way of promoting cooperative learning in the classroom is to use a series of case studies of increasing complexity. A structured approach to raise awareness of the interdependence among health professionals is key to collaborative work. Recently this concept has been taken a step further to move from simple cooperative learning to team learning, which is a dynamic process of sharing, co-construction, and constructive conflict (Decuyper *et al.*, 2010).

Small group learning formats have been especially successful to promote cooperative learning and for developing an understanding of roles and responsibilities and changing attitudes. In designing group learning, the faculty needs to consider group balance (an evenly distributed mix of health professionals and levels of learners as possible), group size (eight to ten members is desirable), and group stability (extent to which there are established members leaving and new ones joining). Small groups are a convenient place for students to practice reflections as a group and as individuals.

Additionally, using problem-based learning (PBL) and team-based learning (TBL) are effective approaches that make the learning process more meaningful and engaging, while returning the responsibility for learning back to the learners. In PBL, learning occurs in response to learning deficits identified through small group problem-solving. In TBL, groups of six to seven students initially learn by preparing for and taking readiness assessment tests and then by building on that foundation through in-class, group application activities (Michaelson, Knight, and Fink, 2002).

Reflection

There is wide agreement on the importance of building and promoting mechanisms for reflective learning into IPE (Hall and Zierler, 2015). Such skills can be applied to reflective practice (and are inherent in quality and safety processes). Reflective activities are those activities that assist the learner to "stand back from an experience and make meaning of it." The transformative learning that can result from IPE occurs from the metacognitive insights gained from reflective processes. Specific methods to promote reflection include self-assessments, structured journaling, and written papers based on the journals (Clark, 2009). It is important to create an opportunity for a group or a team to reflect upon itself together in addition to individual reflection.

Textbox 14.4 Features of Cooperative Learning

Positive interdependence means being interconnected. It consists of having roles that complement each other and working together toward shared goals.

  Promotive interactions consist of close, purposeful activity, such as discussion, debate, case studies, or patient care that involves joint decision-making and where members help each other to succeed.

  Individual accountability means each person is held accountable for learning the content and contributing their fair share to the group success.

  Interpersonal and small group skills refer to team skills, usually involving communication, leadership, group decision-making, situation awareness, and management of conflict.

  Group processing skills refers to reflecting on the actions of individuals and groups that contribute to the effectiveness of the group process and deciding what to do about it.

  Adapted from D'Eon (2005). Reproduced with permission of Taylor & Francis.

Self-assessments provide self-knowledge and insights for participants about what they bring to an IPE experience. These self-assessments, in addition to determining strengths and needs regarding a particular content area such as quality and safety, also may assess an individual's skills related to group process, such as learning style preferences, personality type, conflict management style or leadership abilities. Reflective activities provide opportunities in IPE for a learner to engage in reflection of self as well as reflection of how others are the same or different from themselves. Reflective activities, however, must be planned; both space and time for reflection are needed. Specific strategies and tools to promote both individual and group reflection are described on the QSEN web site. Lastly, educators need to "reflect more on reflection" if they are to be effective teachers in ensuring the learning outcomes essential for teamwork and interprofessional practice, including incorporating both theory and practice into the development of interprofessional educational interventions.

Experiential Learning
Experiential learning is especially important in IPE. Experiential learning is based on the tenet of learning through action in the real world. John Dewey introduced the "learn by doing" philosophy (Dewey, 1938). Dewey believed that problem-solving calls for new responses; especially in situations involving conflict or challenge. Habitual actions and thoughts do not solve these problems, but active experimentation and trying out new processes might. David Kolb introduced the Kolb Experiential Learning Cycle (Kolb, 1984), which is the foundation for current methods of experiential learning. The process of making sense out of experience, that is, learning on a deeper, more integrated level, is articulated in the Experiential Learning Model (1984). Schon described a learning-in-action approach as a way for professionals to reflect on how their practice experiences contribute to professional knowledge acquisition and application (Schon, 1987). Through this structured reflection process, practitioners gain insights that challenge and guide professional practice. Schon later added the reflection-in-action and the reflection-on-action components as also being important to experiential learning.

  In IPE, experiential learning focused on quality and safety is done by having students from two or more health professions schools work on a real health care problem. The implementation of quality improvement projects in which students plan, carry out the plan (with varying levels of supervision), gather observations of the outcomes, and reflect in such a way as to create generalizations about how they would handle similar situations in the future is ideal for learning (Hands *et al.*, 2014). A positive byproduct of the use of practice-based projects in quality and safety education is the increased attention paid to, and recognition of, the practitioners in the field. Textbox 14.5 describes a recent IPE project that includes experiential learning that has impacted practice.

Textbox 14.5 Example of an Interprofessional Education Project that Includes Experiential Learning and Impacts Clinical Care

At the University of Colorado, work is being done on the Anschutz Medical Campus to coordinate quality and safety education for students and clinicians. This initiative is known as The Institute for Healthcare Quality, Safety and Efficiency (IHQSE). IHQSE is a partnership among the University of Colorado School of Medicine, University of Colorado College of Nursing, University Physicians, Inc., Children's Hospital Colorado, and the University of Colorado Hospital. The overarching goal of IHQSE is to fundamentally improve the outcomes of the care provided to patients.

The first offering of the IHQSE is a 12-month Certificate Training Program (CTP) for interprofessional teams of clinicians, which launched in January of 2013. The mission of the CTP is to create a capable work force to improve and create innovative models of care to transform our entire clinical enterprise. The CTP is run by eight faculty members with support from six process improvement and data analyst staff and an administrative assistant. The CTP faculty, who teaches the classroom sessions and coaches the teams, is composed of six physicians, one nurse, and one process improvement expert. Interprofessional clinical teams must be composed of three different professions (most teams have a physician and a nurse) to apply to the program, and demonstrate administrative support for release time to accommodate the rigorous time commitment. Participating teams meet weekly for the year, which includes twice monthly for four-hour-long didactic sessions, and twice monthly with CTP faculty, process improvement specialists or data analysts for coaching. The CTP curriculum focuses on enhancing team performance, leadership development, and process improvement. The combination of exposure to updated quality improvement, patient safety, and leadership content, with concurrent application of this knowledge to improvement work in their microsystem produces empowered, effective leaders. Often these clinical experts have had insights into system gaps for years but have not had the knowledge of how to lead effective, enduring improvement efforts. At the conclusion of the CTP, teams present their improvement work to key administrative stakeholders. Upon graduation from the CTP, teams maintain their coaching, process improvement specialist and data analyst support for two years in order to pursue continuous quality improvement.

Two cohorts consisting of 82 participants representing 25 teams completed the CTP in 2013 and 2014. Comparing before and after program surveys reveal significant improvements in self-perceptions of leadership, team-building, quality improvement, patient safety, and efficiency skills. Examples of improvement project outcomes are provided in Table 14.1.

Table 14.1 Examples of IHQSE certificate training program teams and outcomes.

Certificate Training Program Team	Improvement Project Outcomes
Cancer Clinics	13% reduction in time from referral to patient being seen
Emergency Department	10% reduction in CT turnaround time 87% reduction in door-to-EKG time for chest pain patients
Infusion Center	20% decrease in patient chair time
Neonatal Intensive Care Unit	Reduction in readmissions from 3.3% to 0%
Operating Room	43% improvement in urologic first case on-time starts
Orthopedics	33% reduction in length of stay (LOS) for geriatric hip fracture patients
Palliative Care	15% reduction in LOS for patients receiving palliative care consultation

Transfer of Learning

Learning must prepare students for the real world in which they will work. Students must be able to transfer what they have learned in one or more situations to other situations that are not exactly the same. One approach to foster transfer of learning is to expose students to relevant cases that actively challenge them to search for meanings at increasing levels of abstraction with feedback (D'Eon, 2005). Faculty needs to structure the progression of increasingly complex cases representing learning tasks associated with giving and improving care. Factors that can increase the complexity of learning cases include different co-morbidities, more departments involved, more professionals involved, simulated to real environments, more complex systems, conflicting values, greater number of confounding factors, urgency to make decisions, and data that are more complex. Learning experiences that assist students to identify recurring patterns and salient features of situations requires a conscious effort on the part of the faculty. For the transfer of learning to be successful, skilled faculty must be available to facilitate the transfer. An example of transferred learning is noted in Textbox 14.6.

Assessment

Continual assessment of formative and summative learning is an essential component of IPE. Kirkpatrick's Four-Level Training Evaluation Model is a useful framework to guide the evaluation of an IPE experience (Kirkpatrick, 2015). Resources, products, and a certification program can be found at the following web site: http:www.kirkpatrickpartners.com. The four levels of evaluation follow: 1) reaction (satisfaction), 2) knowledge (skills acquired), 3) behavior (transfer of learning to the workplace),

---

Textbox 14.6: Example of Transfer of Learning

The Case Western Reserve University (CWRU) Student-Run Free Clinic (SRFC) is an interprofessional student organization and is run by a board of students that consists of second year medical students, second year graduate nursing students, and graduate social work students. Every committee has students from every school, and the leadership team is responsible for all aspects of running the clinic and the public health outreach program. Continual quality improvement is an overarching goal of the board. The following is an example of interprofessional quality improvement within their own clinic.

The interprofessional clinical teams consist of volunteers who are not there every week and do not understand the system. The students were learning from each other and serving a struggling population of patients, but there was increasing stress on the clinic days due to teams leaving before all the work was completed. Volunteers were very well intentioned but did not understand the process well enough to know that two or three people were staying long after clinic hours were over to complete the unfinished work of chart completion and follow up of labs. The increasing stress was causing problems within the board, and there were disagreements on clinic day as people were leaving. The clinical coordinator team from all three schools gathered data to find out what work was not being completed and decided to aim for 100% work completion from each team at the end of every clinic day. They created a checklist of the jobs that were not being done and now require every team to check out with a clinical coordinator before they leave. The checklist must be completed before anyone leaves. This process requires the team to support each other and work together to accomplish the work. The stress in the clinic has decreased, and 100% of the teams complete their work every clinic day. The faculty reflected with the students on their process in preparation for a presentation. This learning led the students to understand the value of QI and working together to find additional ways to improve their clinic, transferring their learning from the first project.

and 4) results (impact on society). The complexity of behavioral change increases as evaluation of intervention ascends. To date, the majority of IPE assessments have been limited to self-reporting of attitudes and beliefs. The National Center for Interprofessional Practice has assembled a web-based collection of existing IPE measurement instruments (https://nexusipe.org/measurement-instruments). An IPE evaluation guide was developed by Reeves and colleagues (2015) that provides the following suggestions: think about evaluation first and be clear with the purpose of the evaluation, consider the outcomes, and use models and theoretical perspectives. They also suggest carefully selecting an evaluation design using qualitative and quantitative methods and provide ideas about disseminating evaluation results to the broader IPE community.

Examples of National Interprofessional Training Programs in Quality and Safety Education

Two national interprofessional training programs stand out as exemplary models of large-scale, comprehensive IPE in health care quality and safety education. Interestingly, both of these programs rely heavily on virtual learning approaches that connect learners across geographical distances.

The first of these "virtual" training programs is the IHI Open School. The IHI Open School for health professions is a virtual school to teach quality improvement skills and patient safety to the next generation in pharmacy, nursing, dentistry, medicine, health management, health policy, and allied health. The IHI Open School is the "other school" that students attend at their convenience while enrolled in their current educational programs. There are no applications, no admissions requirements, and no fees for students or faculty. Online offerings including courses, case studies, videos, podcasts, and discussions designed to help students develop competencies in quality improvement and patient safety at beginner, intermediate, and advanced levels. There is also a mentored practicum experience. Certification for completion of the online modules is available.

To supplement the IHI Open School's online delivery system (www.ihi.org/OpenSchool), a network of local chapters offers students the chance to learn and compare notes with students from different health care professions and to undertake projects with other students to apply quality improvement knowledge. The IHI Open School promotes organizations (health care and academic institutions) to start local chapters as a way for interprofessional students to discuss the common goal of increasing quality and safety in health care. Local chapters host a variety of activities from safety conferences to participating in quality improvement activities. Monthly telephone calls are coordinated by IHI, and chapters share their activities and work.

Another exemplary model of national interprofessional training programs in quality and safety education is the VAQS. Unlike the IHI Open School that focuses on health professionals in training, the mission of the VAQS program is to develop leaders who can apply knowledge and methods of health care improvement to the care of veterans and non-veterans, innovate and continually improve health care, teach health professionals about health care improvement, and perform research and develop new knowledge for the ongoing improvement of the quality and value of health care services.

Traditionally started as a physician-only fellowship program, the two-year VAQS curriculum was revised in 2010 to include pre- and postdoctoral nurses. There are nine sites across the United States, and eight sites are located at a VA medical center and partnered with an academic medical center and nursing school. One site is in Canada. Local "senior" quality scholars (experienced faculty in quality improvement) facilitate the learning activities (Splaine *et al.*, 2009). Additionally, local improvement projects at the respective participating VA centers that are led by the interprofessional team of scholars are an important dimension of this training program. Further information about the VA Quality Scholar program can be found at www.vaqs.org.

Educator Development for IPE

In this chapter we have described approaches to IPE with varying levels of evidence regarding their use. The approaches represent best practices that educators should use in designing IPE for quality and safety. Educators have several roles in IPE for which they must be adequately prepared. First, faculty must model collaborative teamwork. This is done in interdisciplinary faculty teams during planning, implementing, and evaluating IPE learning experiences. They must demonstrate flexibility and compromise with faculty from other professions. This includes reducing professional territoriality and modeling conflict management in constructive ways. To promote effective communication across the "cultural" differences among professions, faculty needs to demonstrate the use of techniques to share their views (mental models) and uncover the views (mental models) of others.

Faculty needs to understand how power dynamics issues in society related to gender, social class, and race need to be taken into account in IPE, particularly how they affect professional identity formation and power distribution. For example, an understanding of how the historical power and hierarchy differences among physicians and nurses (physicians historically being upper-middle class men, and nurses historically being middle working class women) can affect their respect and regard for the opinions of each other (Ho *et al.*, 2008). This means paying attention to the language that is embedded in the power within communications among learners of different professions. Faculty who facilitate IPE must be prepared to examine and address these inherent social issues, and students need to see the desired behaviors modeled by faculty. The most effective faculty will be those who are able to reflect on these issues with the learners as they arise.

A key to successful IPE is to have IPE champions serve as coaches or mentors in their organizations. There is wide agreement in the literature that champions are an essential factor of successful IPE programs. Faculty champions promote peer learning and a faculty development community so that adaptation of curricula fit the local context (Hall and Zierler, 2014). Champions make connections with other faculty, make connections with students, and generally promote the program's initiatives (Ho *et al.*, 2008). Formal leaders can use their power to influence structures, promote resources, stimulate interest, and provide reward systems. Faculty champions can also influence governance structures such as bylaws and faculty approval of curriculum to support IPE approaches. Champions play a role in creating a climate for change, cooperation, and flexibility.

Gaining organizational support for IPE is essential for long-term sustainability of this approach to learning. Barnsteiner and colleagues (Barnsteiner *et al.*, 2007) propose six criteria that reflect full engagement by an organization in IPE: 1) an explicit philosophy of IPE that permeates the organization; 2) faculty from the different professions co-creating the learning experiences; 3) students having integrated and experiential opportunities to learn collaboration and teamwork and how it relates to safe, quality care delivery; 4) IPE learning experiences embedded in the curricula and made part of the required caseload for students; 5) demonstrated competence by students with a single set of interprofessional competencies; and 6) an organizational infrastructure that fosters IPE, including support for faculty time to develop IPE options, incentive systems for faculty to engage in IPE, and integrated activities across schools and professions for students and faculty.

Summary

In this chapter we present the current evidence for the added value of teaching quality and safety using interprofessional learning approaches. Conceptual frameworks and sets of core competencies relevant to IPE in quality and safety that faculty can use to design, implement, and evaluate are described. In particular, the processes of cooperative learning, reflective learning, experiential learning, and transfer of learning are highlighted as key elements of IPE that we believe will promote successful quality and safety education. We also described the need for adequate preparation of faculty to facilitate successful interprofessional education experiences in quality and safety. Cooke and colleagues (Cooke, Ironside, and Ogrinc, 2011) and the IOM (2015) call for a transformation reorientation to quality and safety education that focuses on how the care team's patients fared and how the systems of care were improved. What is needed is a national agenda to conduct purposive IPE research linked to improvement in outcomes (Lutifyya *et al.*, 2015). We believe this transformation can best be accomplished using a collaborative approach between academia and practice. Never has the need to prepare students for collaborative, patient-centered practice and the improvement of care been greater.

References

Abu-Rish, E., Kim, S., Choe, L., Varpio, L., Malik, E., White A., *et al.*, Zierler, B. (2012) Current trends in interprofessional education of health sciences students: A literature review. *Journal of Interprofessional Care*, *26*(6), 444–451. doi:10.3109/13561820.2012.715604.

Barnsteiner, J.H., Disch, J.M., Hall, L., Mayer, D., and Moore, S.M. (2007) Promoting interprofessional education. *Nurs.Outlook*, *55*, 144–150.

Brandt, B., Lutfiyya, M.N., King, J.A., and Chioreso, C. (2014) A scoping review of interprofessional collaborative practice and education using the lens of the Triple Aim. *Journal of Interprofessional Care*, *28*(5), 393–399.

Barr, H. (2013) Toward a theoretical framework for interprofessional education. *Journal of Interprofessional Care*, *27*(1), 4–9.

Brashers, V., Owen, J., and Haizlip, J. (2015) Interprofessional education and practice guide No. 2: Developing and implementing a center for interprofessional education *J Interprof Care*; *29*(2): 95–99.

CAIPE. (1997) Interprofessional Education–A Definition. *CAIPE Bulletin No.13.*

Capella, J., Smith, S., Philp, A., Putnam, T., Gilbert, C., Fry, W. *et al.* (2010) Teamwork training improves the clinical care of trauma patients. *J Surg. Educ*, *67*, 439–443.

Clark, P.G. (2009) Reflecting on reflection in interprofessional education: implications for theory and practice. *J Interprof. Care*, *23*, 213–223.

Cooke, M., Ironside, P.M., and Ogrinc, G.S. (2011) Mainstreaming quality and safety: a reformulation of quality and safety education for health professions students. *BMJ Qual. Saf*, *20* Suppl 1, i79–i82.

Cronenwett, L., Sherwood, G., Barnsteiner, J., Disch, J., Johnson, J., Mitchell, P., *et al.* (2007) Quality and Safety Education for Nurses. *Nurs.Outlook*, *55*, 122–131.

D'Eon, M. (2005) A blueprint for interprofessional learning. *J Interprof.Care*, *19* Suppl 1, 49–59.

Dewey, J. (1938) *Experience and Education*. New York: Collier Books.

Gilligan, C., Outram, S., and Levett-Jones, T. (2014) Recommendations from recent graduates in medicine, nursing and pharmacy on improving interprofessional education in university programs: a qualitative study. *BMC Medical Education*, *14*(1), 52.

Gittell, J.H., Beswick, J., Goldmann, D., and Wallack, S. (2014) Teamwork Methods for Accountable Care: Relational Coordination and TeamSTEPPS. Health Management Review. doi: 10.1097/HMR.0000000000000021. See more at: https://nexusipe.org/resource-exchange/relational-coordination-scale-rcs#sthash.lLZ1uDIc.dpuf.

Hall, L.W. and Zierler, B.K. (2014) Interprofessional education and practice guide No.1; Developing faculty to effectively facilitate interprofessional education. *J Interprof Care*, Early Online: 1–5.

Hand, R., Dolansky, M.A., Hanahan, E., and Tinsley, N. (2014) Quality Comes Alive: An Interdisciplinary Student Team's Quality Improvement Experience in Learning by Doing–Health Care Education Case Study. *Quality Approaches in Higher Education*, 5(1), 26–32. Awarded the journal's 2014 Best Paper.

Hean, S., Craddock, D., Hammick, M., and Hammick, M. (2012) Theoretical insights into interprofessional education: AMEE Guide No. 62. *Medical Teacher*, 34(2), e78–e101.

Ho, K., Jarvis-Selinger, S., Borduas, F., Frank, B., Hall, P., and Handfield-Jones, R. *et al.* (2008) Making interprofessional education work: the strategic roles of the academy. *Acad.Med.*, 83, 934–940.

Interprofessional Education Collaborative Expert Panel. (2011) *Core competencies for interprofessional collaborative practice: Report of an expert panel* Washington, DC: Interprofessional Education Collaborative.

Institute of Medicine. (2013) Interprofessional Education for Collaboration: Learning How to Improve Health from Interprofessional Models Across the Continuum of Education to Practice: Workshop Summary. Editors: Global Forum on Innovation in Health Professional Education; Board on Global Health; Institute of Medicine. Washington (DC): National Academies Press (US); Oct.

Institute of Medicine. (2015) Measuring the impact of interprofessional education on collaborative practice and patient outcomes. The National Academies Press at http://www.nap.edu/catalog.php?record_id=21726

Lutfiyya, M.N., Brandt, B., Delaney, C., Pechacek, J., and Cerra, F. (2015) Setting a research agenda for interprofessional education and collaborative practice in the context of United States health system reform. *J Interprof Care*, (31)-8.

Logan, J., and Graham, I.D. (1998) Toward a comprehensive interdisciplinary model of healthcare Research Use. *Science Communication*, 20(2) 227–246.

King, H.B., Battles, J., Baker, D.P., Alonso, A., Salas, E., Webster, J., *et al.* (2008) TeamSTEPPS: Team Strategies and Tools to Enhance Performance and Patient Safety.

Kirkpatrick model of evaluation. (2015) Retrieved from http://www.isixsigma.com/dictionary/kirkpatrick-four-levels-evaluation-model/Kirkpatrick's four-level training evaluation model: Analyzing training effectiveness. Retrieved from http://www.midtools.com/pages/article/kirkpatrick.htm.

Kolb, D. (1984) *Experiential learning: Experience as the source of learning and development*. New Jersey: Prentice-Hall.

Mciness, S., Peters, K., Bonney, A. and Halcomb, E. (2015) An integrative review of facilitators and barriers influencing collaboration and teamwork between general practitioners and nurses working in general practice. *Journal of Advanced Nursing*, 71(9), 1973–1985. doi: 10.1111/jan.12647.

Michaelsen, L.K., Knight, A.B., and Fink, L.D. (2002) Team Based Learning: A Transformative use of Small Groups. Library of Congress.

Oandasan, I., and Reeves, S. (2005a) Key elements for interprofessional education. Part 1: the learner, the educator and the learning context. *J Interprof. Care*, 19 Suppl 1, 21–38.

Oandasan, I., and Reeves, S. (2005b) Key elements of interprofessional education. Part 2: factors, processes and outcomes. *J Interprof. Care*, 19 Suppl 1, 39–48.

Reeves, S., Zwarenstein, M., Goldman, J., Barr, H., Freeth, D., Hammick, M., *et al.* (2008) Interprofessional education: effects on professional practice and health care outcomes. *Cochrane. Database. Syst. Rev.*, CD002213.

Reeves, S., Tassone, M., Parker, K., Wagner, S.J., and Simmons, B. (2012) Interprofessional education: An overview of key developments in the past three decades. *Work: A Journal of Prevention, Assessment and Rehabilitation*, 41(3), 233–245.

Reeves, S., Boet, S., Zierler, B., and Kitto, S. (2015) Interprofessional education and practice guide No. 3: Evaluating Interprofessional Education. *Journal of Interprofessional Care*, 29(4), 305–312.

Schon, D. (1987) *Educating the reflective practitioner: How professionals think in action*. London: Jossey-Bass.

Senge, P. (1990) The Leader's New World: Building learning organizations. Sloan Management Review 32(1) http://www.simpsonexecutivecoaching.com/pdf/orglearning/leaders-new-work-building-learning-organizations-peter-senge.pdf.

Splaine, M.E., Ogrinc, G., Gilman, S.C., Aron, D.C., Estrada, C.A., Rosenthal, G.E., *et al.* (2009) The Department of Veterans Affairs National Quality Scholars Fellowship Program: experience from 10 years of training quality scholars. *Acad Med.*, 84, 1741–1748.

Storycare 108. (2016) Nurse/physician communication related to the concerns a nurse has about a patient but chooses not to assert her concerns. Retrieved September 19 from http://qsen.org/faculty-resources/interprofessional.

Suter, E., Goldman, J., Martimianakis, T., Chatalalsingh, C., DeMatteo, D.J., and Reeves, S. (2013) The use of systems and organizational theories in the interprofessional field: Findings from a scoping review. *Journal of Interprofessional Care*, 27(1), 57–64.

Thistlethwaite, J. and Moran, M. (2010) Learning outcomes for interprofessional education (IPE): Literature review and synthesis. *J Interprofessional Care*, 24, 503–513.

U.S. Department of Health and Human Services. (2015) HHS Education and Training Resources on Multiple Chronic Conditions for the Healthcare Workforce. Retrieved September 19 from http://www.hhs.gov/ash/initiatives/mcc/education-and-training/framework-curriculum/module-4.html.

Weaver, S.J., Lyons, R., DiazGranados, D., Rosen, M.A., Salas, E., Oglesby, J. *et al.* (2010) The anatomy of health care team training and the state of practice: a critical review. *Acad.Med.*, 85, 1746–1760.

Weaver, S.J., Rosen, M.A., Salas, E., Baum, K.D., and King, H.B. (2010) Integrating the science of team training: guidelines for continuing education. *J Contin.Educ.Health Prof.*, 30, 208–220.

World Health Organization. (2010) *A framework for action on interprofessional education and collaborative practice*. Geneva 27, Switzerland: WHO Department of Human Resources for Health, CH-1211.

Zwarenstein, M., Goldman, J., and Reeves, S. (2009) Interprofessional collaboration: effects of practice-based interventions on professional practice and healthcare outcomes. *Cochrane.Database.Syst.Rev.*, CD000072.

Zwarenstein, M., Reeves, S., Barr, H., Hammick, M., Koppel, I., and Atkins, J. (2001) Interprofessional education: effects on professional practice and health care outcomes. *Cochrane.Database.Syst.Rev.*, CD002213.

Resources

QSEN Website and Teaching Strategies

An interprofessional page is located on the QSEN web site that includes links to key resources (http://qsen.org/faculty-resources/academia/interprofessional-education/). The QSEN web site includes bibliographies, video presentations, and learning modules for curricular innovation for explicit clinical content for interprofessional activities. The QSEN web site is the largest repository of teaching strategies and resources related to quality and safety in nursing; faculty are invited to post successful strategies to share with others.

MedED Portal (American Association of Medical Colleges)

The interprofessional education portal reflects the Core Competencies for Interprofessional Collaborative Practice and is designed to create a national clearinghouse of competency-linked learning resources for interprofessional education and models of team-based or collaborative care. See more at https://www.mededportal.org/about/initiatives/ipe/#sthash.hJ7ZYhKG.dpuf

Multiple Chronic Conditions

In 2013, the Office of the Assistant Secretary for Health in collaboration with the Health Resources and Services Administration published an online interprofessional healthcare education and training initiative on Multiple Chronic Conditions (MCC). Module 4 includes an interprofessional curriculum and competencies for healthcare professionals and paraprofessionals http://www.hhs.gov/ash/initiatives/mcc/education-and-training/framework-curriculum/module-4.html). The training materials are appropriate for learners of health care professionals across the educational continuum (undergraduate, graduate, and post-graduate).

The National Center for Interprofessional Practice and Education (https://nexusipe.org/)

The NCIPE leads, coordinates the advancement of collaborative, team-based health professions education and patient care as an efficient model for improving quality, outcomes and cost (Triple Aim). It is the only organization in the United States, designated by the Health Resources and Services Administration (HRSA) of the US Department of Health and Human Services to provide coordination and national visibility to advance interprofessional education and practice as a viable and efficient health care delivery model. By aligning the needs and interests of education with health care practice, they created a new shared responsibility–"Nexus"–for better care, added value and healthier communities. The center, housed at the University of Minnesota, is a public-private partnership created in October 2012.

Institute of Medicine (2013)

The Global Forum hosted two conferences on "interprofessional education" in 2012. Both workshops focused on linkages between interprofessional education (IPE) and collaborative practice. Topics covered include curricular innovations, pedagogic innovations, cultural elements, and human resources for health and metrics. The summary of the workshops is available at http://www.ncbi.nlm.nih.gov/books/NBK207110/?report=reader.

Starting a Center at your University

If your institution is interested in starting an Interprofessional Center, a guide is available (Brasher, Owen, and Haizlip, 2015). The authors provide success tips that include building upon past success, engaging support at the highest levels, applying for grant funding, integrating required IPE into the core curricula, providing evidence that it is effective, creating a framework for developing new IPE activities, engaging in continuous engagement, making faculty development a high priority, aligning center goals with national and local health systems priorities, and making a business case.

Faculty Development Resources

University of Missouri–Columbia and University of Washington have a funded faculty development resource center that includes a faculty development interprofessional tool kit based on the IPE competencies by the Interprofessional Education Collaborative (IPEC). Using a variety of techniques, including didactic teaching, small group exercises, immersion participation in interprofessional education, local implementation of new IPE projects, and peer learning, the program positioned each site to successfully introduce an interprofessional innovation faculty training center. Find information at http://collaborate.uw.edu/educators-toolkit/faculty-development-training-toolkit/faculty-development-ipe-training-toolkit.html

15

Improving Quality and Safety with Transition-to-Practice Programs

Nancy Spector, PhD, RN, FAAN, Beth T. Ulrich, EdD, RN, FACHE, FAAN and Jane Barnsteiner, PhD, RN, FAAN

The evidence creates a compelling case for all newly licensed registered nurses (NLRNs) to have a transition to practice (TTP) program from the student to the professional role. Evidence has linked TTP programs to improved safety and quality patient outcomes as well as to the retention of new graduate RNs. As a result, NCSBN has developed a TTP model that incorporates the QSEN competencies. This chapter provides current evidence for implementing successful TTP programs in hospitals for NLRNs along with implications for nonhospital sites, and information for nurse educators who are preparing students for their nursing careers and practice organizations.

The following NLRN experiences illustrate the support that formal TTP programs provide, compared to the lack of support in facilities that don't have these programs. (These were qualitative data from the *Spector et al.* [2015a] multisite, TTP study of NLRNs. The comment from the control nurse was provided on the survey he/she completed, and the data from the three intervention NLRNs were obtained from focus groups that were held with the intervention NLRNs.)

These verbatim survey comments are from a nurse in the control group with no structured transition program:

> Some nurses view new nurses as incompetent and are unwilling to help and answer questions. Recently an older nurse pointed to a phone and explained to me how to use it and what it was because I asked a question. My question never got answered.

Yet, a different picture of support is painted by the intervention group nurses who were in an evidence-based TTP program (verbatim focus group comments):

> I think when people are nice and approachable, you can go to someone and you're not afraid and you have support ... even your coworkers. That makes a world of difference. That's how you learn.

Similarly, here are verbatim focus group comments from two new nurses in the TTP program who felt supported by their preceptors:

> #1 It makes it a lot easier to have a preceptor kind of looking over your shoulder, because it's pretty much like taking the training wheels off. I've learned all this theory, but it's really nice

Quality and Safety in Nursing: A Competency Approach to Improving Outcomes, Second Edition.
Edited by Gwen Sherwood and Jane Barnsteiner.

having somebody looking over my shoulder saying, wait, are you sure you want to do it that way? Are you sure there's not a better way? Should you have done that? Because you're learning this very specific skill set.

#2 "But you need somebody there to make it feel like it's fine. Like I had my preceptor's phone number and I would call her, and I was like, 'I can't believe that I'd do that.' And she was like, 'calm down and go to sleep.' You know, you need that, somebody that says, 'now go to sleep and we'll talk about it tomorrow, you'll be fine.' It can be really, really stressful.

Transition-to-Practice Programs: Definition and Extent

A TTP program is a formal program of active learning implemented across all settings for all newly licensed nurses (registered nurses and licensed practical/vocational nurses) designed to support their progression from education to practice (Spector *et al.*, 2015a). These are comprehensive, evidence-based programs that are integrated throughout the health system, thus being supported at all levels of the organization.

Questions have arisen about the difference between nurse residency programs and TTP programs. These terms are now being used synonymously. For example, recommendation number three from the IOM's Future of Nursing report, which advoca*tes for nurse residency programs, states:*

> State boards of nursing, accrediting bodies, the federal government, and health care organizations should take actions to support nurses' completion of a transition-to-practice program (nurse residency) after they have completed a prelicensure or advanced practice degree program or when they are transitioning into new clinical practice areas (Institute of Medicine, 2011).

Orientation, on the other hand, is a separate process that is focused on the hiring institution, and not on transitioning the new nurses to their futures in nursing practice. The American Nurses Association (2010) defines orientation as the process of introducing staff to the philosophy, goals, policies, procedures, role expectations, and other factors needed to function in a specific work setting. Orientation takes place both for new employees and when changes in nurses' roles, responsibilities, and practice settings occur.

What is the extent of these comprehensive residency or TTP programs? One study (Budden, 2011), using the NCSBN definition of TTP programs and the ANA definition of orientation found that currently only 9–31% of all nursing employers, across all settings, reported offering a TTP program, and 1–8% of employers did not even offer an orientation program to their new graduates. Fewer than 50% of hospitals report having TTP programs. A survey of chief nurse officers and chief nurse executives who are members of the AONE reported that 36.9% of this sample offered nurse residencies in 2011 (Pittman *et al.*, 2013). They found that residencies were more common in urban (85%), midsized, not-for-profit hospitals located in the South, whereas the Northeast had a greater share of hospitals without residencies. Similarly, Barnett, Minnick, and Norman (2014) found that in hospitals with more than 250 beds, 48% had nurse residency programs.

In nonhospital sites, the situation is more concerning. A white paper written by the American Academy of Ambulatory Care Nursing (AAACN, 2014) stated that nurse residency programs are rare in that setting, and this severely limits effective patient care and succession planning. Likewise,

Pittman and colleagues (2015) report that, of their sample of the Visiting Nurse Associations of America, only 14.7% of home health agencies or hospices have transition programs for new graduates. Even though more programs are developing in long-term care (University of Wisconsin School of Nursing, 2015), a national survey conducted in 2006 found only 5.6% of RNs and 8.8% of LPNs had TTP programs in long-term care facilities.

TTP programs are not limited to NLRNs. Successful TTP programs for experienced nurses transitioning to new specialties and new roles have been reported in specialty areas such as critical care (Gohery and Meany, 2013), emergency departments (Bongiovanni and Laidlow, 2010) and for new nurse practitioners (Sargent and Olmeda, 2013). While the needs are broad, this chapter focuses on the evidence and implications for TTP program for NLRNs.

Although TTP programs are not available to a majority of new nurses, many professions such as medicine, pharmacy, pastoral care, physical therapy, and teaching require formalized transition to practice programs for their graduates. Many of these programs receive either federal or state assistance; nursing does not.

Evidence Linking Transition-to-Practice Programs to Quality and Safety

There is a growing evidence base, from research reviews and three large multisite studies, on how TTP programs promote quality and safety by improving new nurses' competence, safety, and retention. Data are presented on both hospital and nonhospital settings.

Competence

Employers report new graduates are not ready to practice. In the early 2000s, NCSBN studies found that fewer than 50% of employers reported "yes definitely" when asked if new graduates are ready to provide safe and effective care (NCSBN, 2002; 2004); these studies prompted NCSBN's TTP initiative. Similarly, Berkow and colleagues (2008), from the Nursing Executive Center, conducted a survey of more than 5,700 frontline nurse leaders, asking about employer perceptions of new graduates on 36 competencies. Improvement was needed across levels of education (associates degree in nursing [ADN] and BSN). For example, 53% of employers were satisfied with the top-rated competency (utilization of information technologies), while only 10% were satisfied with the last-rated competencies, such as delegation of tasks. Berkow and colleagues (2008) noted that the bottom-rated competencies would be better taught in an experiential environment, such as a TTP program. Berman *et al.* (2014) assessed the competence of NLRNs entering a TTP program using the QSEN practice tool. Of the 36 criteria, the lowest competence was found in the understanding of quality improvement methodologies, followed by the ability to anticipate risks related to assessment data; evaluation and system improvements based on clinical practice data; location, review, and application of scientific evidence and medical literature; and prioritization of actions related to patient needs and delegation of actions if appropriate.

Reviews of the research on TTP programs (Anderson, Hair, and Todero, 2012; Edwards *et al.*, 2015; Rush *et al.*, 2013) have found improvement in competency when these programs are implemented (Goode, Ponte & Havens, 2016). Similarly, Chappell and Richards (2015), in a systematic review evaluating clinical leadership skills in new graduates, found there was a positive impact of TTP programs on their clinical leadership skills. A summary of the competency evidence that was found in these research reviews is shown in Table 15.1. However, there is a critical need for more rigorous research

Table 15.1 Evidence on competency from research reviews of TTP programs.

Research Review	Number of Studies	Competency findings
Anderson, Hair, and Todero (2012)	20	Positive impact on new RN graduates' performance include critical thinking, control over practice, nursing skills, confidence, autonomy, behavioral performance, improved safe patient care.
Chappell and Richards (2015)	17	TTP programs at least 24 weeks long significantly increase clinical leadership skill in the new nurse.
Edwards *et al.* (2015)	30	Separate analysis of internship/residency, graduate nurse orientation, mentorship/preceptorship, and simulation programs found increased self-reported competence (general and clinical); perceived confidence; knowledge; and readiness to practice with a TTP program.
Goode *et al.* (2016)	23	Systematic review, rating evidence from level 2-6, finding TTP programs improve NLRN competency.
Rush *et al.* (2012)	47	Increased competency, regardless of rater, duration of program or type of program. Qualitatively, one study found students didn't feel independent until a year in practice; the TTP program acted as a shelter for them.
Theisen and Sandau (2013)	26	Improved communication, including delegation and when handling workplace conflict.

on TTP programs, particularly in nonhospital settings. The authors of these research reviews reported several major limitations with the studies of TTP programs, including the following:

- Lack of detail on the content of the TTP programs
- Lack of control groups
- Lack of valid and reliable measurement tools and an inconsistent use of research tools across the studies
- Using only new nurse self-reports
- Small samples
- Lack of multisite studies with diverse settings
- Lack of scientific rigor when conducting the studies

Three multisite national studies of TTP programs provide further insight into the effect of these programs on competency, as well. One of the studies used the University HealthSystem Consortium (UHC)/AACN residency program to compare start, mid-program, and completion competency measures (Goode *et al.*, 2013). Another compared outcomes after implementing the Versant program to a comparison group in each hospital from two years prior to implementing the residency program and compared residency outcomes by cohort, facility, and organization to the outcomes from the Versant National Database (Ulrich *et al.*, 2010). The third was a multistate TTP program, which randomly assigned new nurses to a control group (the organization's traditional onboarding program) or the NCSBN TTP program (Figure 15.1) (Spector *et al.*, 2015a). In the latter study, the researchers further divided the control group into those with established programs and limited programs, based on criteria cited in the TTP literature. The established programs were supported by the institution, had been in place for a while, and were comprehensive, evidence-based programs, whereas the limited programs were sparse and did not have many of the evidence-based elements of a TTP program.

Analyzing 10 years of data (approximately 31,000 nurses) from the UHC/AACN residency program and using a standardized measurement tool (Casey-Fink Graduate Nurse Experience Survey), Goode

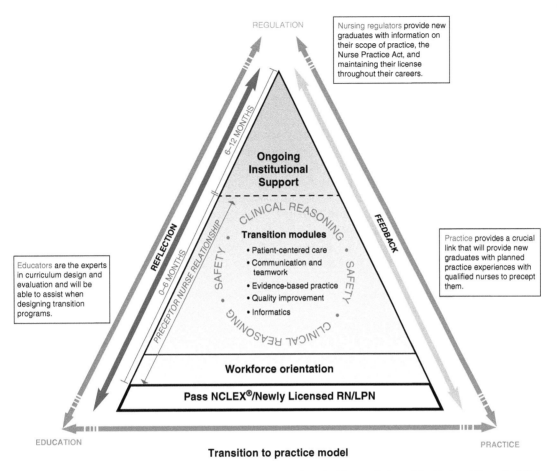

Figure 15.1 NCSBN's TTP model. Source: Spector 2015. Reproduced with permission of the National Council of State Boards of Nursing.

et al. (2013) found that new nurses' perceptions of their overall confidence and competence, ability to organize and prioritize their work, and ability to communicate and provide leadership significantly increased over the one-year residency program.

Ulrich *et al.* (2010) analyzed 10 years of resident data (more than 6000 residents) from the Versant program, using a number of previously validated instruments to measure outcomes such as competence, confidence, satisfaction, organizational commitment, leader empowering behavior, conditions for work effectiveness, etc. In a random sample of the residents and the comparison group, trained observers measured their competence, and these were compared. The residents rated themselves higher than the trained observers in week 2 and at the end of the residency. The trained observers found significant improvement in new nurse competency from the beginning to the end of the RN residency.

Spector *et al.* (2015a) studied 1088 new nurses over a one-year period. These researchers used two competency scales (Overall Competency and Specific Competency), which were modified from previously published scales, and piloted by the researchers before conducting the study. The ratings were completed by the new nurses and their preceptors (or managers in the control group, if they had no preceptors). There were no differences in the ratings between the new nurses and the preceptors, except the preceptors consistently rated the new nurses higher than the new nurses rated themselves, and this was statistically significant for the Overall Competency Scale. This was consistent with NCSBN's National Simulation Study, where the managers rated the NLRNs higher than they rated themselves in their first six months of practice (Hayden *et al.*, 2014). However, it was not consistent with Ulrich and colleague's (2013) findings cited above, where the NLRNs rated themselves higher than their preceptors did.

Although the nurses in the NCSBN TTP program and in the control group significantly improved in overall competence over the year-long period, there was no significant difference in overall competence among the groups. However, related to specific competencies, the NCSBN TTP group scored significantly higher over the year-long period, compared to the control group, for patient-centered care, use of technology, communication, and teamwork. When the researchers divided the control group into the Limited and Established programs, they found that the Established group scored significantly higher in overall competence, the NCSBN TTP group was in the middle, and the Limited group lagged behind. However, there were then little differences among the three groups in the specific competency measures, except that the NCSBN TTP group scored higher on the use of technology domain. It could be that the TTP group scored significantly higher in the specific competencies because the modules they had completed incorporated the QSEN competencies.

Simulation is a common strategy in TTP programs to improve competency (Beyea, Slattery, and von Reyn, 2010; Everett-Thomas *et al.*, 2015). Beyea *et al.* (2010) studied an experiential transition program using simulation and measuring confidence, competence, and readiness to practice, all of which significantly increased after their program. This program uses simulation vignettes that highlight high-risk and low-frequency events (such as cardiac arrests), as well as commonly occurring clinical situations. According to this study, a transition program incorporating active learning is a highly effective way of developing competency and confidence in new graduates. Everett-Thomas *et al.* (2015) similarly found that in a 10-week simulation program, the new nurses had significant improvement in both applied knowledge in clinical skills and in overall clinical performance.

Safety

Research links new nurses to patient safety issues, such as near misses, adverse events, and practice errors. Bjørk and Kirkevold (1999), in a classic study, found that patient safety can be compromised when there are no effective TTP programs in place. They conducted a prospective, longitudinal study in Norway, videotaping nursing practice and interviewing nurses and patients. Even though the nurses reported they had become more efficient and rated themselves as better nurses over time, the analysis of their practice revealed that they made the same practice errors (such as contaminating wounds and unsafely removing wound drains) at the end of the study as they made at the beginning. The authors reported that because there were limited opportunities for feedback and reflection, the new nurses did not learn from their mistakes. However, they did not compare these findings to institutions where TTP programs were in place.

Likewise, Ebright and colleagues (2004) have cited near misses as a problem for new graduates. They interviewed new nurses and found that of 12 recruited new nurse participants, seven reported at least one near-miss event, while one new nurse described two near-miss events. Themes identified related to near misses/adverse events, for example, included difficulty with first-time experiences, handing off patients, and novices assisting novices, among others. Similar to the Bjørk and Kirkevold (1999) study, without supportive TTP programs, new graduates did not learn from their near misses.

Inexperienced nurses who lack on the job support may also adversely affect patient safety because of missed nursing care. When nursing care is omitted, patient outcomes can be negatively affected, thus promoting falls, failure to rescue, pressure ulcers, or other adverse events. Using focus groups, Kalisch (2006) identified seven themes for why care is missed; some of these included the poor use of existing staff resources and ineffective delegation. Further, subthemes included inadequate orientations for new nurses and inconsistent assignments. Without consistent patient assignments and opportunities for follow-through, novice nurses don't have the opportunity to get to know their patients well enough to recognize changes. Similarly, Benner *et al.*, (2010) cited student nurses' lack of opportunities for patient follow-up as one reason for implementing TTP programs in nursing.

New nurses have significant job stress (Elfering, Semmer, and Grebner, 2006 ; Goode *et al.*, 2013; Spector *et al.*, 2015a), and this stress has been linked to patient errors (Elfering *et al.*, 2006; Nielson *et al.*, 2013; Park and Kim, 2013; Spector *et al.*, 2015a). In an observational study using multilevel modeling, Elfering *et al.* (2006) studied 23 "young" nurses for two weeks in 19 hospitals in Switzerland and found that patient safety events (such as wrong dose of medication, patient falls, etc.) were significantly related to job stressors in nurses, as measured by trained observers. Similarly, using a descriptive correlation design, Park and Kim (2013) studied 279 nurses who had worked for at least six months in five hospitals in Korea and found that job stress was a significant predictor of patient safety incidents. In another study of workplace stress, Nielson *et al.* (2013) conducted in the ED of a Danish regional hospital, researchers found a significant association between stress and adverse events.

Spector *et al.* (2015a) also reported a link between increased job stress in new nurses and adverse events. In all three groups (Limited, Established, and NCSBN's TTP program), the NLRN reports of work stress increased at six months of practice but decreased at 9 to 12 months. Similarly at six months, their reports of errors increased and their satisfaction decreased, but improved at 9 to 12 months. Goode *et al.* (2013) found a similar trend with satisfaction, though not with stress; they did not measure errors or safe practices.

NLRN reports of their job satisfaction are linked to other outcomes of interest in TTP programs. Studies have found that there is a moderately strong relationship between job satisfaction and intent to leave (Hairr *et al.*, 2014) and a moderate relationship between satisfaction and job performance (Judge *et al.*, 2001). For NLRNs in a TTP program, Ulrich *et al.* (2010) reported significant correlations between job satisfaction and turnover intent and, further, that turnover intent was a meaningful predictor ($p < 0.0001$) of actual turnover. In a population of 63,034 RNs in acute hospitals, Choi and Boyle (2014) found that lower job satisfaction was significantly related to increased patient falls. This was one of the first studies to link job satisfaction to patient safety outcomes. More studies exploring the relationship between job satisfaction and patient safety should be conducted.

Until recently, no study reported on errors and near misses when new nurses were in a comprehensive TTP program versus when they were not. In a systematic review (Edwards *et al.*, 2015) and in critical reviews (Anderson, Hair, and Todero, 2012; Rush *et al.*, 2013; Theisen and Sandau, 2013) of the research on TTP programs, the authors highlighted key findings of studies, but there were no data reported on patient safety. However, Spector *et al.* (2015a) did investigate patient safety outcomes in new nurses. The researchers found significantly lower reports of errors and near misses and the use of negative safety practices (such as not using universal precautions) when new nurses were in an Established TTP program with evidence-based components, compared to those in a Limited program. Additional research on patient safety and TTP programs is needed.

Retention/Turnover

For this chapter, retention is defined as the percentage of new graduates remaining at their organization after one year, and turnover is the percentage of new graduates leaving an organization after the same time period. Some articles report retention, while others report turnover.

NLRNs who do not participate in comprehensive TTP programs have a higher turnover rate than those who do (Spector, 2015a). In this year-long, multisite study of NLRNs hired in hospitals, the researchers prospectively tracked turnover rates. They found that when a hospital had a limited TTP program that did not include many of the evidence-based components, the voluntary, year-long turnover rate was 25.0%. However, when the new nurses participated in an established evidence-based program that was integrated into the institution, the turnover rate was 12.0%. When NCSBN's TTP program was introduced to the institution and implemented over a year, the turnover rate was slightly higher at 14.7%. Both the Established and NCSBN TTP programs had statistically higher turnover rates than the limited programs. A possible explanation for the higher turnover rate in NCSBN's program could be that the program had not been in place long enough to be incorporated into the hospital's system. Ulrich *et al.* (2010) found that as a TTP program becomes assimilated into the system, the turnover rate drops even further. Turnover from the Versant program was 7.1% in the first year of the program, but it dropped to 4.3% after five cohorts had been through the program. Pre-Versant turnover rates averaged 27.0% among all sites. Similarly, Goode *et al.* (2013), in their multisite study of the UHC/AACN residency program, reported turnover rates of 12% in the first annual evaluation, though, once integrated into the system, the turnover rate decreased to 5.4%.

Of related research reviews, Edwards *et al.* (2015) reported retention rates in internship/residency programs varied from 73 to 94% in four studies, and turnover rates ranged from 8.0 to 16.5% in five studies. The review did not report the retention or turnover rates before the programs were in place. Edwards *et al.* (2015) reported on one study of NLRNs (Newhouse *et al.*, 2007) where the retention was significantly improved after the first year of practice when compared to a comparison group. However, the significant improvement did not hold for 18 and 24 months in practice, possibly indicating that extending the program into the second year would be important. Similarly, Rush *et al.* (2013) reviewed publications on retention and turnover rates in TTP programs. Of those studies reporting on retention rates, the average was 90.1%, while those reporting on turnover had an average rate of 10.5%. When studies examined pre- and post-program rates, every program had improved retention or turnover rates, though Rush *et al.* (2013) did not indicate if these improvements were statistically significant. While Goss (2015) focused on the effect of implementing preceptorships on retention rates, she presented few details on the actual retention/turnover rates when implementing preceptorships as compared to either pre-preceptorship or comparison group data.

This first-year turnover may adversely affect patient quality and safety, though the research is not conclusive on this. Replacing new nurses who leave the agency with temporary staff may be associated with adverse events and decreased quality of care. Mazurenko, Liu, and Perna (2015) conducted a systematic review of studies investigating the effect of temporary nurses on the quality of care. Some of the 25 studies met their research criteria and reported adverse effects with temporary nurses, others did not. It is likely a complex association, where the quality of the work environment has an effect as well. That is, it could be that hospitals with poorer work environments are unable to recruit or retain nurses and therefore the adverse effects are from the poor work environment, rather than the turnover. Indeed, Aiken *et al.* (2013) looked at whether temporary nurses lead to higher mortality or failure to rescue. They used 2006 primary survey data from 40,356 registered nurses in 665 hospitals in four states, linked with American Hospital Association and inpatient mortality data from state agencies for approximately 1.3 million patients. Before controlling for hospital environment, they found that a higher proportion of agency nurses in hospitals was significantly associated with a higher mortality. However, once they controlled for hospital environment, this association was rendered insignificant. Future studies on the use of temporary nurses should address the hospital environment.

Mazurenko *et al.* (2015) suggest that the differences in study findings may also relate to how the researchers define quality of care outcomes. Aiken *et al.* (2013) used mortality and failure to rescue and found no significant differences. However, other studies found that the use of temporary nurses had an adverse effect on care when measuring nurse-sensitive patient outcomes or when quality of care was measured as the nursing process (Bae, Mark, and Fried, 2010; Hass, Coyer, and Theobald, 2006; Hurst and Smith, 2011; Wu and Lee, 2006).

Another issue with using temporary staff is continuity of care. Duffield *et al.* (2009) examined staff consistency on 40 wards. They used the word "churn" to describe the constant movement of staff, thus creating changes to skill mix and challenges in scheduling, performance management, and supervision. They illustrate how the impact on one ward, with a high degree of "churn," had a higher rate of adverse outcomes than the majority of wards in the study. Even though the literature is mixed on whether turnover adversely affects quality and safety, coordination of care is affected, as well as management and economic issues for the hospital.

Bae *et al.* (2010) have developed a formula that hospitals may consider. They studied the relationship between temporary nurses and patient safety outcomes (patient falls and medication errors) and found that when nurses worked on units with high levels of temporary nurses (15% or more), there were greater numbers of patient falls. Interestingly, when there were moderate levels of temporary nurses (5 to 15%) there were fewer medication errors. This, Bae *et al.* (2010) suggest, is likely because the temporary nurses relieve a shortage, though using high proportions of temporary nurses can harm patients.

Quality and Safety in Nonhospital Sites

Most of the evidence linking retention, quality, and safety has been done in hospitals. Since 18% of new nurses are employed in nonhospital sites (NCSBN, 2014), more research on new nurses should be conducted in these settings. In articles describing model programs for transitioning new nurses into home care delivery (Carignan *et al.*, 2007; Meadows, 2009), higher retention rates were reported when organizations used their models. Carignan *et al.* (2007) reported on preliminary findings from three self-report scales (satisfaction, control over practice, and new graduate experience), though statistical differences were not reported. Although there are no published data about competence and retention in ambulatory care, anecdotal data indicate that many new nurses leave in the first year, though when these employers develop TTP programs, they report improved retention rates (AAACN, 2014).

Similarly, in long-term care, there is a paucity of published data on whether transition programs improved safety and quality. Researchers in Wisconsin (Nolet *et al.*, 2015) report on their experiences with providing a nurse internship program for junior and senior nursing students, finding challenges in creating interest in new nurses for working in long-term care. Additionally, Wisconsin and New Jersey are developing nurse residency programs for new graduates who work in long-term care (Cadmus, Salmond, Hassler, Black & Bohnarczyk, 2016; University of Wisconsin School of Nursing, 2015). While these programs have been successful, at this point, they are only able to reach a small proportion of nurses in these environments often limiting them to settings with the most resources.

In the NCSBN study of transition programs in nonhospital sites, 17 nursing homes hired new nurses (Spector *et al.*, 2015b). Although the numbers of new nurses hired were too low (16 LPNs and 21 RNs) for statistical analysis, the data provided were illustrative. As with the hospital part of this study, the new nurses in nursing homes self-reported their errors or near misses and use of safety practices. The use of safety practices was similar to those reported by the new nurses in hospitals, however, the new nurses' reports of errors were much higher in nursing homes than those reported in hospitals. The 12-month retention data in the nursing home sites were tracked, though with dismal results. Overall, 35% of the new nurses were still employed in nursing homes after one year in practice. When comparing the groups, 29% of the control group nurses remained, and 40% of those participating in the NCSBN TTP program remained. Of the nurses who left, a much greater percentage left involuntarily than those in the hospital sites. The qualitative reports of the new nurses hired in nursing homes, along with their preceptors and the site coordinators, provided some insight into the challenges of implementing a transition program in nursing homes. There was little support from their employers and no time for the new nurses to complete the program. Likewise, the preceptors, while interested in participating in the program, were too busy to provide work with the new nurses and received little administrative support. A priority for the nursing community should be to strategize on how to better support new graduates in long-term care.

Standardized TTP Programs

Research reviews and large datasets, as described above, provide evidence that formal TTP programs improve outcomes in new nurses. This section outlines the evidence that supports the TTP program elements and describes the design of three standardized national programs. Additionally, the standards of two national residency accreditation programs will be outlined.

Systematic and other research reviews are valuable for identifying key components of transition programs (see Table 15.2). One review focused on preceptor support (Goss, 2015); another on outcomes of program types, such as residency, simulation, etc. (Edwards *et al.*, 2015); two identified specific elements of TTP programs (Anderson *et al.*, 2012; Theisen and Sandau, 2013); and two reported on the best practices of TTP programs (Goode *et al.*, 2016, Rush *et al.*, 2012). There were many recurring themes among all of these reviews, such as the importance of implementing preceptorships and preceptor training. Indeed, the focus of Goss's systematic review was solely on the preceptor role affecting retention. Although Goss concluded that implementing preceptorships has a positive effect on retention, few specifics were provided of actual differences in retention rates based on provision of preceptorships or not. Other common components cited in these reviews included content and experience in patient safety, evidence-based practice, communication and teamwork, critical thinking, leadership, time management/organization skills, and access to specialty content educational experiences. Administrative support for a TTP program was also seen as an important aspect across these reviews. Related to length of program time, implementing a one-year TTP program and a three- to six-month preceptorship was supported by the research. However, it is important to point out that many of the studies reviewed had significant limitations, as identified earlier. More rigorous research on TTP programs should be conducted.

Although many health care organizations have well-planned, homegrown TTP programs, as demonstrated in the multisite study by Spector *et al.* (2015a), three national programs will be described. Each has been studied extensively (Goode *et al.*, 2013; Spector *et al.*, 2015a; Ulrich *et al.*, 2010), and while specific results were described previously, the major results will be outlined.

NCSBN TTP Program

After reviewing national studies (NCSBN, 2002; 2004) where more than 50% of the employers reported that newly licensed nurses were not prepared to provide safe and effective care, NCSBN's membership saw the lack of TTP programs to be a safety issue. Therefore, NCSBN's board of

Table 15.2 Elements of TTP programs from research reviews of TTP studies.

Research Review	Number of Studies	Elements of TTP Programs
Anderson, Hair, and Todero (2012)	20	<ul><li>Communication</li><li>Teamwork and collaboration</li><li>Patient safety</li><li>Evidence-based practice</li><li>Time management</li><li>Critical thinking</li><li>Delegation</li><li>Patient outcomes</li><li>Leadership and professional development</li><li>One-year in length</li><li>Preceptorship</li></ul>
Edwards *et al.* (2015)	30	Four support strategies:<ul><li>Internship/residency</li><li>Graduate nurse orientation</li><li>Mentorship/preceptorship</li><li>Simulation</li></ul>
Goode *et al.* (2016)	23	<ul><li>Evidence-based and structured program, national accreditation, 6-12 months in length.</li></ul>
Goss (2015)	20	Focus on a preceptor support system:<ul><li>Support and recognize the preceptor</li><li>Foster communication</li><li>Provide educational opportunities</li><li>Provide preceptor training programs</li><li>Model caring behaviors</li><li>Apply 3 to 6 month preceptorship</li><li>Provide administrative support</li><li>Use preceptor programs to positively impact new nurse retention</li></ul>
Rush *et al.* (2012)	47	<ul><li>Defined resource person</li><li>Mentorship</li><li>Peer support opportunities</li><li>Strong prelicensure nursing programs</li><li>Formal education during the TTP program</li><li>Paired with a trained preceptor</li><li>Specialty content and skills</li><li>Workplace environment</li></ul>
Theisen and Sandau (2013)	26	<ul><li>Communication</li><li>Leadership skills</li><li>Conflict resolution</li><li>Prioritization, organization, and time management skills</li><li>Critical thinking and clinical reasoning</li><li>Stress management</li><li>One-year in length</li><li>Preceptorship</li></ul>

directors convened a committee to develop a TTP program. A committee of NCSBN's membership, with representatives from AONE, spent a year reviewing the evidence to develop a standardized TTP model. The model was designed to be flexible so that any program (independently developed or in partnership with other institutions) that meets the requirements of this model could be used. It was developed to be robust; that is, it could be used across all settings and with all levels of education, from practical nursing to master's entry nursing. Additionally, the NCSBN TTP program was planned as a "no-blame" model. The NCSBN TTP model assumes that education programs are adequately preparing our nurses for practice and that practice settings are not unfairly expecting new nurses to move immediately into skilled practice. Instead, there was a missing piece in nursing: no standardized TTP program.

NCSBN's TTP model was collaboratively planned, with input from a variety of nursing and health care organizations, and many changes were made based on their insight. For example, the original model was re-categorized to highlight the QSEN competencies so that it would be in line with national nursing initiatives (Cronenwett *et al.*, 2007; Sherwood and Barnsteiner, 2012).

The elements of NCSBN's TTP evidence-based program include the following features (see Figure 15.1):

- **An institutional-based orientation program**. Orientation is defined as the process of introducing staff to the philosophy, goals, policies, procedures, role expectations, and other factors needed to function in a specific work setting. Orientation takes place both for new employees and when changes in nurses' roles, responsibilities, and practice settings occur (ANA, 2010).
- **Trained preceptors**. A key to the TTP model is that a *trained* preceptor is assigned to the new nurse for the first six months, ideally to work with and train the new nurse. The preceptors complete training before working with the NLRN.
- **Learning modules**. In the first six months of the program, the new nurse completes five modules. However, because this program was designed to be flexible, this content could be presented using a number of teaching strategies. Indeed, a hybrid model (face-to-face and online strategies) would be an excellent methodology to consider. Because this program was studied (Spector *et al.*, 2015a), online modules were designed for the study to control for the teaching methodology.
  - *Communication and teamwork* with major subcategories such as transitioning from student to an accountable nurse (role socialization); communicating to ensure safe and quality care (TeamSTEPPS, 2014); delegating and decision-making; experiencing work environment and conflicts; growing as a professional nurse.
  - *Patient-centered care* with major subcategories such as content specialty (work with preceptor); multiple dimensions of patients; prioritizing and organizing; just culture; moral/ethical concerns; health care systems; professional boundaries.
  - *Evidence-based practice* with major subcategories such as defining evidence-based practice with scenarios; using databases; critically appraising the literature; using clinical practice guidelines; using evidence-based practice models; implementing evidence-based practice in practice settings.
  - *Quality improvement* with major subcategories such as an overview of quality improvement; identifying improvement gap opportunities; quality improvement tools; measuring and monitoring the data; using quality improvement in practice (case study); keys to successful improvement.
  - *Informatics* with major subcategories such as informatics as the foundation of nursing; computer and information literacy skills; information management skills with cases; informatics; and the nurse's role in delivering safe patient care.

- **Safety and clinical reasoning.** This is threaded throughout the modules.
- **Institutional support**. Support is provided during the second six months of the program when the new nurse participates in system activities, such as committees, unit projects, grand rounds, and other learning opportunities offered by the institution.
- **Feedback and reflection.** This is threaded throughout the entire year.

Major Study Findings

As compared to a limited transition program, when a formalized evidence-based TTP program is integrated into the hospital and has administrative support, it is associated significantly with the following results (Spector *et al.*, 2015a):

1) Decreased self-reported errors and use of negative safety practices
2) Increased overall competency (preceptor and new nurse ratings)
3) Decreased self-reported work stress
4) Increased self-reported job satisfaction
5) Increased retention

Additional findings follow:

1) There was a positive return on investment when NCSBN's TTP hospital program was compared to a Limited program (not comprehensive and without many evidence-based criteria) (Silvestre, Ulrich, Johnson, Spector & Blegen, in press)
2) There are significantly better outcomes when hospital preceptorships are supported by the institution so that preceptors have few preceptees and time for the dyad to work together, and they share shifts and assignments (Blegen *et al.*, 2015).
3) More work needs to be done with nonhospital settings, particularly long-term care, to find resources to implement and study transition programs.

UHC/AACN Residency Program

In 2002, six hospitals and their partner school piloted the UHC/AACN Nurse Residency Program. As of August 2012, 31,000 nurses and 86 organizations representing 100 hospitals have participated in the UHC/AACN residency program (Goode *et al.*, 2013). This year-long program considers orientation and specialty content (e.g., telemetry or emergency nursing) as the responsibility of the hospital and not the residency program, similar to the NCSBN TTP program.

The UHC/AACN TTP program content includes the following:

- Leadership, with a focus on patient-centered care and interprofessional collaboration
- Quality and safety and related nurse sensitive outcomes
- Professional role, which includes professional issues and managing changing patient conditions
- An evidence-based practice project, which positively impacts their units
- Face-to-face seminar sessions and facilitated peer discussions

Major study findings over the one-year period of the program follow (Goode *et al.*, 2013):

- The perception of overall competence, confidence, ability to organize and prioritize, and ability to communicate and provide leadership significantly improved.
- Satisfaction significantly decreased at six months and then stabilized.

- Scores on organizing, prioritizing, communication, and leadership were significant predictors of commitment to current position and to nursing.
- The top three skills residents were uncomfortable with included code/emergency response, and chest tube and ventilator care.
- The evidence-based projects were highly rated by the organizations and had an impact on improving nursing practice.

Versant

The Versant program was instituted in 1999, and their researchers have reported the first 10 years of program outcome data (N = 6000 new graduates) (Ulrich *et al.*, 2010).

The program began in children's hospitals with didactic courses and guided clinical experience with a one-on-one preceptor. In 2004, the residency was expanded to general acute care hospitals with successful results, using didactic courses and 18 weeks of clinical immersion. In 2013, the residency period was extended to one year, which included ongoing structured mentoring and debriefing beyond the immersion period, and recently the immersion period (with the one-on-one preceptor) was condensed to 420 hours with 100% of competencies validated (L. Africa, personal communication, November 12, 2015). The Versant program includes the following:

- A structured immersion program with a preceptor for each resident
- Knowledge assessment and validation, with education available as needed
- Case studies
- Self-care sessions
- Rotations to related departments
- Detailed competency validation
- A structured mentoring model, where the new graduates have structured meetings and mentoring sessions

This program acknowledges the importance of active participation of everyone throughout the organization, which is facilitated by an RN residency architecture that delineates roles and systems for implementation and management of the residency.

Major study findings include the following:

- Turnover of the NLRNs in the program was improved significantly when compared to pre-Versant turnover.
- Competency (self-assessed and of a random sample of residents observed by trained observers) improved significantly from the beginning to the end of the residency.
- Total satisfaction increased in a stepwise fashion from the end of the residency to months 12 and 24.
- Self-confidence grew across time.
- Higher satisfaction correlated significantly with lower intent to leave.

Commission on Collegiate Nursing Education (CCNE) Accreditation Standards

In 2008, the CCNE began approving post-baccalaureate nurse residency programs, and in 2015, the focus changed from just post-baccalaureate programs to entry-to-practice programs, regardless of education (CCNE, 2015). CCNE accredits two types of entry into practice residency programs:

1) Employee-based programs that hire newly licensed nurses
2) Federally funded traineeship residency programs that engage newly licensed nurses for the residency program, but make no commitment for ongoing employment

CCNE defines a residency program as a series of learning experiences that occur continuously over a minimum of 12 months through a partnership between a health care organization and an academic nursing program. As of this writing, 25 residency programs have been accredited by CCNE. Key curricular elements include the following:

- *Management and delivery of quality patient care* – quality and safety, patient and family centered care, management of patient care delivery, management of the changing patient condition, communication and conflict measurement and informatics and technology
- *Professional role and leadership* – Performance improvement and evidence-based practice, professional development, ethical decision-making, stress management, business of healthcare

The accreditation requirements stress appropriate education and experience for the program educators/faculty. Further, they require that preceptors are oriented to their roles and responsibilities. The requirements call for evidence of administration support, from the top down, and a systematic process for determining program effectiveness.

ANCC Accreditation Standards

In 2014, the American Nurses Credentialing Center (ANCC) instituted the Practice Transition Accreditation Program (PTAP), which accredits three types of transition programs (ANCC, 2015):

1) RN Residency, which is a planned, comprehensive program for newly licensed nurses with less than 12 months of experience. The program must be at least six months in length.
2) RN Fellowship, which is a planned, comprehensive program for currently licensed nurses with 12 or more months of experience. This program is generally for those nurses who change specialties.
3) APRN Fellowship, which is a planned comprehensive program for licensed APRNs.

As of this writing, ANCC has accredited four sites. Key curriculum elements include communication, critical thinking/clinical reasoning, ethics, evidence-based practice, informatics, interprofessional collaboration, patient-centered care, quality improvement, role transition, safety, stress management, and time management.

The programs must demonstrate administrative support, and program faculty must have appropriate preparation. Additionally, practice-based learning takes place under the guidance of preceptors (or other experienced health professionals), who also must be prepared to work with residents.

Summary

In summary, the evidence supports TTP programs of 9 to 12 months in length. Administrative support, from the top down, is essential for promoting the program and for providing adequate resources. Program content supported by the literature, and structured, includes the QSEN competencies and their related KSAs (http://qsen.org/competencies/pre-licensure-ksas/), clinical reasoning, stress management, and specialty content. Preceptors who are trained for the role provide expertise in experiential learning and are key to the program.

Implications for Educators and Practice Partners

Transition to practice should be a seamless journey, from education to competent practice, for NLRNs. This section provides ideas for both educators and their practice partners for accomplishing this.

Educators

Partnerships between clinical practice organizations and schools of nursing are critical links to successful new graduate transition (Spector, 2015). Educators are an integral part of transitioning new nurses to practice, both in preparing their students for practice, but also in collaborating with clinical practice organizations as they plan and implement transition programs.

What specifically can educators do to facilitate transition to practice? The evidence from TTP studies suggests that integrating the QSEN competencies into prelicensure nursing curricula, along with their accompanying KSAs, will assist with TTP. Additionally, robust clinical immersion courses during the last semester of the academic program, using trained preceptors, are strongly recommended because of the experiential learning they provide. Participating in dedicated education units is a strategy that some nursing programs have used to collaborate with clinical practice partners. In this model, nurse executives, faculty, and staff nurses partner to transform patient care units into supportive environments for nursing students and staff nurses, while continuing to provide quality care to patients. This partnership between education and clinical sites is mutually beneficial and enhances the collaboration between academe and practice (Murray and James, 2012).

Educators are strongly encouraged to work with clinical practice organizations to design clinical and simulation experiences that will foster a more seamless transition to practice. Educators can use their expertise in teaching-learning strategies to design effective, evidence-based TTP programs and preceptorships. Since many educators also are experienced researchers, they can assist the clinical practice organizations to study the outcomes of their TTP programs, thus providing more evidence on effective programs.

Practice

As can be seen from the collective research findings on TTP programs (see Table 15.1, Goode *et al.*, 2013; Spector *et al.*, 2015a; Ulrich *et al.*, 2010), comprehensive, evidence-based TTP programs provide significantly higher retention rates, improved new nurse competencies, higher satisfaction, less stress, and increased confidence. One study (Spector *et al.*, 2015a) found significantly fewer reports of patient errors and increased use of safety practices when new nurses participated in an established, evidence-based TTP program, versus those who were in a limited program. Therefore, it is incumbent upon practice settings to provide TTP programs to their new graduates.

It is essential that the TTP program be enculturated into the system and supported from the top down. There must be adequate and timely channels of communication among the preceptor, resident, charge nurses, and the resident's frontline nurse manager so that meaningful assignments can be made for the NLRN. These communication channels are important to ensure that experiences are maximized and that competency validations and development needs are known. The content of the TTP program should provide the elements supported in the research, and partnering with nursing programs can facilitate planning evidence-based programs.

The evidence supports pairing trained preceptors with new nurses to provide experiential learning. Haggerty, Holloway, and Wilson (2013) conducted a longitudinal evaluation of preceptor support for NLRNs and reported a quality preceptorship benefits the development of competence and confidence of NLRNs. The key components of successful preceptor support were access to preceptors, how preceptors met NLRN learning needs, the importance of the preceptor-preceptee relationship, preceptor preparation for the role, and an overall culture of support. Preceptors play many roles: teacher/coach, leader/influencer, facilitator, evaluator, socialization agent, protector, and role model (Ulrich, 2012), and therefore, a structured preceptor training and support program is a necessary component of a TTP program (Blegen *et al.*, 2015; Bradley *et al.*, 2012; Bratt, 2009; Goode *et al.*, 2013;

Spector, 2015a; Ulrich *et al.*, 2010). One analysis found that new nurse outcomes were significantly improved when preceptors had few preceptees, worked one-on-one with the preceptees, and shared shifts and assignments (Blegen *et al.*, 2015). Additional studies on preceptorship needs are important to understand how to promote the best outcomes.

Oftentimes, practice settings cite cost as a reason for not implementing TTP programs, yet there is evidence to support the return on investment of TTP programs. Ulrich *et al.* (2010) reported that Versant Residency hospitals experienced significant savings for their systems as turnover decreased. For example, in one hospital the 12-month turnover rate of new nurses improved from 35.00% to 5.36%, which translated to an estimated savings of $2,706,000 to $2,904,000 for the hospital. In a study of 15 hospitals, Trepanier and colleagues (2012) found major cost savings in decreased turnover and decreased contract labor usage as the result of implementing a TTP program. Silvestre and colleagues (in press) analyzed return on investment (ROI) of the multistate NCSBN multisite TTP study and found a positive ROI, largely due to decreased turnover-even when smaller organizations only hire low numbers of nurses. Decreased nurse-related litigation costs have also been reported as an outcome of a TTP program in an ED (Bongiovanni and Laidlow, 2010).

Conclusion

There have been national calls for nursing to implement TTP programs in nursing (Benner *et al.*, 2010; The Joint Commission on Accreditation of Healthcare Organizations, 2005; IOM, 2003, 2011). This chapter has presented the evidence supporting TTP programs for all NLRNs to improve quality and safety of patient care. Evidence-based TTP program elements are presented, encouraging practice/education partnerships to design the programs and study the outcomes.

References

American Nurses Association. (2010) Nursing Professional Development: Scope and Standards of Practice. MD: Author.

American Nurses Credentialing Center. (2015) Practice transition accreditation program. Retrieved from http://www.nursecredentialing.org/Accreditation/PracticeTransition.

Advance Healthcare Network for Nurses. (2014) Impacting long-term in New Jersey. Retrieved from http://nursing.advanceweb.com/Features/Articles/Impacting-Long-Term-Care-in-New-Jersey.aspx.

Aiken, L.H., Shang, J., Xue, Y., and Sloane, D.M. (2013) Hospital use of agency-employed supplemental nurses and patient mortality and failure to rescue. *Health Services Research*, *48*(3), 931–948.

American Academy of Ambulatory Care Nursing (AAACN). (2014) Ambulatory registered nurse residency white paper – The need for an ambulatory nurse residency program. Pitman, NJ: Author.

Anderson, B., Hair, C., and Todero, C. (2012) Nurse residency programs: An evidence-based review of theory, process, and outcomes. *Journal of Professional Nursing*, *28*(4), 203–212.

Bae, S.H., Mark, B., and Fried, B. (2010) Use of temporary nurses and nurse and patient safety outcomes in acute care hospital units. *Health Care Management Review*, *35*(3), 333–344.

Barnett, J.S., Minnick, A.F., and Norman, L.D. (2014) A description of U.S. post-graduation nurse residency programs. *Nursing Outlook*, *62*(3), 174–184.

Benner, P., Sutphen, M., Leonard, V., and Day, L. (2010) *Educating nurses: A call for radical transformation.* San Francisco, CA: Jossey-Bass.

Berkow, S., Virkstis, K., Stewart, J., and Conway, L. (2008) Assessing new graduate nurse performance. *Journal of Nursing Administration, 38*(11), 468474.

Berman, A., Beazley, B., Karshmer, J., Prion, S., Van, P., Wallace, J., and West, N. (2014) Competence gaps among unemployed new nursing graduates entering a community-based transition-to-practice program. *Nurse Educator, 39*(2), 56–61.

Beyea, S.C., Slattery, M.J., and von Reyn, L.J. (2010). Outcomes of a simulation-based residency program. *Clinical Simulation in Nursing, 6*(5), 169–175.

Bjørk, I.T., and Kirkevold, M. (1999) Issues in nurses' practical skill development in the clinical setting. *Journal of Nursing Care Quality, 14*(1), 72–84.

Blegen, M.A., Spector, N., Ulrich, B.T., Lynn, M.R., and Barnsteiner, J. (2015) Preceptor Support in Hospital Transition to Practice Programs. *Journal of Nursing Administration,* December.

Bongiovanni, D., and Laidlow, T. (2010). *Bridging the gap: A practice-academic partnership orientation model with critical thinking clinical simulation.* 43rd Annual Meeting and Exposition, American Organization of Nurse Executives, April 12, Indianapolis, IN.

Bradley, C.A., Doepken, A.K., Fall, D.D., Feldt, M.L., Thornburgh, J.L., and Zook, C.J. (2012) For managers: Selecting Supporting, and sustaining preceptors. In B.T. Ulrich (Ed.), *Mastering precepting: A nurse's handbook for success* (pp. 213–231). Indianapolis, IN: Sigma Theta Tau International.

Bratt, M.M. (2009) Retaining the next generation of nurses: the Wisconsin nurse residency program provides a continuum of support. *The Journal of Continuing Education in Nursing, 40*(9), 416–425.

Budden, J.S. (2011) A survey of nurse employers on professional and practice issues affecting nursing. *Journal of Nursing Regulation, 1*(4), 17–25.

Cadmus, E., Salmond, S.W., Hassler, L.J., Black, K., and Bohnarczyk. (2016) Creating a long-term care new nurse residency model. *The Journal of Continuing Education in Nursing. 47*(5), 234–240.

Carignan, S., Baker, L., Demers, K., and Samar, A. (2007) Home healthcare internship and preceptor programs: One organization's journey. *Home Healthcare Nurse, 29*(7), 439–447.

Chappel, K.B. and Richards, K.C. (2015) New graduate nurses, new graduate nurse transition programs, and leadership skill. *Journal for Nurses in Professional Development, 31*(3), 128–137.

Choi, J., and Boyle, D.K. (2013) RN workgroup job satisfaction and patient falls in acute hospital units. *Journal of Nursing Administration, 43*(11), 586–591.

Commission on Collegiate Nursing Education. (2015) Standards for accreditation of entry-to-practice residency programs. Retrieved from (http://www.aacn.nche.edu/ccne-accreditation/CCNE-Entry-to-Practice-Residency-Standards-2015.pdf).

Cronenwett, L., Sherwood, G., Barnsteiner, J., Disch, J., Johnson, J., Mitchell, P., Sullivan, D.T. and Warren, J. (2007) Quality and safety education for nurses. *Nursing Outlook, 55,* 122–131.

Duffield, C., Roche, M., O'Brien-Pallas, L., and Catling-Paull, C. (2009) The implication of staff 'churn' for nurse managers, staff, and patients. *Nursing Economic$, 27*(2), 103–110.

Ebright, P.R., Urden, L., Patterson, E., and Chalko, B. (2004) Themes surrounding novice nurse near-miss and adverse-event situations. *JONA, 34*(11), 531–538.

Edwards, D., Hawker, C., Carrier, J., and Rees, C. (2015) A systematic review of the effectiveness of strategies and interventions to improve the transition from student to newly qualified nurse. *International Journal of Nursing Studies, 52,* 1254–1268.

Elfering, A., Semmer, K., and Grebner, S. (2006) Work stress and patient safety: Observer-rated work stressors as predictors of characteristics of safety-related events reported by young nurses. *Ergonomics, 49*(5–6), 457–469.

Everett-Thomas, R., Valdez, B., Valdez, G.R., Shekhter, I., Fitzpatrick, M., Rosen, L.S., Arheart, K.L., and Birnbach, D.J. (2015) Using simulation technology to identify gaps between education and practice among new graduate nurses. *Journal of Continuing Education, 46*(1), 34–40.

Gohery, P., and Meaney, T. (2013) Nurses' role transition from the clinical ward environment to the critical care environment. *Intensive and Critical Care Nursing, 29*, 321–328.

Goode, C.J., Lynn, M.R., McElroy, D., Bednash, G.D., and Murray, B. (2013) Lessons learned from 10 years of research on a post-baccalaureate nurse residency program. *Journal of Nursing Administration, 43*(2), 73–79.

Goode, C.J., Ponte, P.R., and Havens, D.S. (2016) Residency for transition to practice: An essential requirement for new graduates from basic RN programs. *Journal of Nursing Administration, 46*(2), 71–79.

Goss, C.R. (2015) Systematic review building a preceptor support system. *Journal for Nurses in Professional Development, 31*(1), E7–E14.

Haggerty, C., Holloway, K., and Wilson, D. (2013) How to grow our own: An evaluation of preceptorship in New Zealand graduate nurse programs. *Contemporary Nurse, 43*(2), 162–171.

Hairr, D.C., Salisbury, H., Johannsson, M., and Redfern-Vance, N. (2014) Nurse staffing and the relationship to job satisfaction and retention. *Nursing Economic$, 32*(3), 142–147.

Hass, H., Coyer, F.M., and Theobald, K.A. (2006) The experience of agency nurses working in a London teaching hospital. *Intensive Critical Care Nursing, 22*(3),144–153.

Hayden, J.K., Smiley, R.A., Alexander, M., Kardong-Edgren, S., and Jeffries, P.R. (2014) The NCSBN national simulation study: A longitudinal, randomized, controlled study replacing clinical hours with simulation in prelicensure nursing education. *Journal of Nursing Regulation, 5*(2), S3–S64.

Hurst, K., and Smith, A. (2011) Temporary nursing staff – cost and quality issues. *Journal of Advanced Nursing, 67*(2), 287–296.

Institute of Medicine. (2003) *Health professions education: A bridge to quality*. Washington, DC: The National Academies Press. Retrieved from http://www.iom.edu/Reports/2003/Health-Professions-Education-A-Bridge-to-Quality.aspx.

Institute of Medicine. (2011) The future of nursing: Leading change, advocating health. Washington, DC: National Academies Press. Retrieved from http://www.thefutureofnursing.org/IOM-Report.

The Joint Commission on Accreditation of Healthcare Organizations (JCAHO). (2005) *Health care at the crossroads: Strategies for addressing the evolving nursing crisis*. Chicago, IL: Author. Retrieved from http://www.jointcommission.org/Strategies_for_Addressing_the_Evolving_Nursing_Crisis_/.

Judge, T.A., Thorsen, C.J., Bono, J.E., and Patton, G.K. (2001) The job satisfaction-job performance relationship: A qualitative and quantitative review. *Psychological Bulletin, 127*(3), 376–407.

Kalisch, B.J. (2006) Missed nursing care: A qualitative study. *Journal of Nursing Care Quality, 21*(4), 306–313.

Mazurenko, O., Liu, D., and Perna, C. (2015) Patient care outcomes and temporary nurses. *Nursing Management, 46*(8), 32–38.

Meadows, CA. (2009) Integrating new graduate nurses in home health care. *Home Healthcare Nurse, 27*(9), 561–568.

Murray, T.A. and James, D.C. (2012) Evaluation of an academic service partnership using a strategic alliance partnership. *Nursing Outlook, 60*(4), e17–e22.

National Council of State Boards of Nursing. (2002) *Report of findings from the 2001 employers survey*. Chicago, IL: Author.

National Council of State Boards of Nursing. (2004) *Report of findings from the 2003 employers survey*. Chicago, IL: Author.

National Council of State Boards of Nursing. (2014) 2014 RN practice analysis: Linking the NCLEX-RN examination to practice. Chicago, IL: Author. Retrieved from https://www.ncsbn.org/15_RN_Practice_Analysis_Vol62_web.pdf.

Newhouse, R.P., Hoffman, J.J., Suflita, J., and Hairston, D.P. (2007) Evaluating an innovative program to improve new nurse graduate socialization into the acute healthcare setting. *Nursing Administration Quarterly*, *31* (1), 50–60.

Nielson, K.J., Pedersen, A.H., Rasmussen, K., Pape, L. and Mikkelsen, K.L. (2013) Work-related stressors and occurrence of adverse events in an ED. *American Journal of Emergency Medicine*, *31*, 504–508.

Nolet, K., Roberts, T., Gilmore-Bykovskyi, A., Roiland, R., Gullickson, C., Ryther, B., and Bowers, B.J. (2015) Preparing tomorrow's nursing home nurses: The Wisconsin long term care clinical scholars program. *Gerontology & Geriatrics Education*, *36*(4), 396–415.

Park, Y.M., and Kim, S.K. (2013) Impacts of job stress and cognitive failure on patient safety incidents among hospital nurses. *Safety and Health at Work*, *4*, 2010–2015.

Pittman, P., Bass, E., Hargraves, J., Herrara, C., and Thompson, P. (2015) The future of nursing: Monitoring the progress of recommended change in hospitals, nurse-led clinics, and home health and hospice agencies. *Journal of Nursing Administration*, *45*(2), 93–99.

Pittman, P., Herrera, C., Bass, E., and Thompson, P. (2013) Residency programs for new nurse graduates. 43(11), 597–602.

Rush, K.L., Adamack, M., Gordon, J., Lilly, M., and Janke, R. (2013) Best practices of formal new graduate nurse transition programs: An integrated review. *International Journal of Nursing Studies*, *50*(3), 345–356.

Sargent, L., and Olmedo, M. (2013) Meeting the needs of new-graduate nurse practitioners. *Journal of Nursing Administration*, *43*(11), 603–610. doi: 10.1097/01.NNA.0000434506.77052.d2.

Sherwood, G., and Barnsteiner, J. (2012) *Quality and safety in nursing: A competency approach to improving outcomes*. West Sussex, UK: Wiley-Blackwell Publishing.

Silvestre, J., Ulrich, B. Johnson, T., Spector, N., and Blegen, M. (in press) A multisite study on a new graduate registered nurse transition to practice program: Return on investment, *Nursing Economic$*.

Spector, N., Blegen, M.A., Silvestre, J., Barnsteiner, J., Lynn, M.R., Ulrich, B., Fogg, L., and Alexander, M. (2015a) Transition to practice in hospital settings. *Journal of Nursing Regulation*, *5*(4), 24–38.

Spector, N., Blegen, M.A., Silvestre, J., Barnsteiner, J., Lynn, M.R., and Ulrich, B. (2015b) Transition to practice in nonhospital settings. *Journal of Nursing Regulation*, *6*(1), 4–13.

Spector, N. (2015) The National Council of State Boards of Nursing's transition to practice study: Implications for educators. *Journal of Nursing Education*, *54*(3), 119–120.

TeamSTEPPS. (2014) TeamSTEPPS National Implementation. Retrieved from http://teamstepps. ahrq.gov/.

Theisen, J.L., and Sandau, K.E. (2013) Competency of new graduate nurses: A review of their weaknesses and strategies for success. *Journal of Continuing Education in Nursing*, *44*(9), 406–414.

Trepanier, S., Early, S., Ulrich, B., and Cherry, B. (2012) New graduate nurse residency program: A cost-benefit analysis based on turnover and contract labor usage. *Nursing Economic$*, *30*(4), 207–214.

Ulrich, B. (2012) The preceptor role. In B. Ulrich (Ed.), *Mastering precepting: A nurse's handbook for success* (pp. 1–15). Indianapolis, IN: Sigma Theta Tau International.

Ulrich, B., Krozek, C., Early, S., Ashlock, C.H., Africa, L.M., and Carman, M.L. (2010) Improving retention, confidence, and competence of new graduate nurses: Results from a 10-year longitudinal database. *Nursing Economic$*, *28*(6), 363–376.

University of Wisconsin School of Nursing. (2015) Nurse residencies: Now coming to long-term care. Retrieved from http://www.son.wisc.edu/1110.htm.

Wu, S.H., and Lee, J.L. (2006) A comparison study of nursing care quality in different working status nursing staffs: an example of one local hospital. *Journal of Nursing Research*, *14*(3), 181–189.

16

Leadership to Create Change

Joanne Disch, PhD, RN, FAAN

"There's got to be a better way."

Amir was a senior nursing student in his last semester of nursing school. He had been working on a med-surg nursing unit during his final clinical rotation and was working with the charge nurse today. He sensed her frustration and found out that this was the third time this week that a patient was being suddenly discharged without prior warning and with the expectation that the patients' families would be able to come within an hour to take the patient home. Amir quickly appreciated the frustration to the patient, family and nursing staff as well as possible adverse events to the patient due to the poor, or nonexistent, discharge teaching as the patient was going out the door. Using a Fishbone Diagram framework, he interviewed several attending physicians, house staff, nurses, social workers, and three patients and plotted out the factors that each person identified. He then went back to each group and shared what he had found. It quickly became apparent that the physicians were being pressured to discharge patients as early as possible, and they usually forgot to alert the nurses on rounds. To try and improve the situation, Amir had read in the American Journal of Nursing that adding a question to the Rounding Script had helped another hospital. So he proposed to the senior attending on service that week and to the charge nurse that, for two weeks, they would ask at the end of rounds, "What's the likelihood Mr X will be discharged tomorrow?" If the answer was "a good possibility," the nurses were to begin planning as though discharge were occurring tomorrow. After two weeks, only one discharge order had been written for that day without prior notice.

"Leadership is a critical function in promoting high quality, safe health care" (Joint Commission, 2009). In Chapter 6, Johnson (2017) examines the role of nurses in quality improvement. This chapter will review research findings on the relationship between leadership and quality/safety; offer a new way to think about leadership, particularly as it relates to quality and safety; and provide a framework for creating change. A basic premise of this chapter is that all nurses are leaders in some way if leadership means *working with and through others to improve something*. This underscores the fundamental responsibility that *all* nurses have when, for example, working with patients to better manage their pain, communicating clearly with other members of the health care team to revise the plan of care, or developing a better staffing plan. We work with and through others to improve patient health, health care delivery, the education of our students, and the nursing profession. Although much of the research that exists focuses on the role of nurses as leaders in formal roles, the principles and concepts apply to all nurses.

Quality and Safety in Nursing: A Competency Approach to Improving Outcomes, Second Edition.
Edited by Gwen Sherwood and Jane Barnsteiner.
© 2017 John Wiley & Sons, Inc. Published 2017 by John Wiley & Sons, Inc.

The Evolution of Leadership

Northouse (2016) describes leadership as a "process whereby an individual influences a group of individuals to achieve a common goal." He notes that there are four components central to the concept: 1) leadership is a process; 2) leadership involves influence; 3) leadership occurs in a group context; and 4) leadership involves goal attainment. Historically, the emphasis of leadership was originally on the individual and his/her characteristics and attributes. The belief was that an individual was innately a leader that could translate into most situations. Eventually, the focus shifted to leadership as arising from the nature of the relationship between the leader and the follower, and the recognition that, without followers, there is no leader.

More recently, the emphasis has shifted toward leadership being more context-dependent, or for a particular purpose, and that an individual is not necessarily equipped to be a leader in any and all situations. The definition that we will use in this chapter is that leadership is *working with and through others to improve something*. At first glance, this seems to be an extremely simple concept, yet it is also very comprehensive. It contains two powerful elements:

1) The leader has a goal of improving something which infers that the leader is knowledgeable about current trends and preferred courses of action; understands the alternatives and the evidence supporting each; has a big picture and systems orientation; and possesses expertise in change management and quality improvement principles and methods.
2) The leader has an ability to work with and through others, which requires excellent interpersonal skills; an ability to listen and elicit ideas from others; and to create a sense of team and a healthy work environment within which people can do their very best work and feel comfortable speaking up and respectfully disagreeing.

Given the need for transformative change in health care today, the framework of generative leadership fits particularly well here. Generative leaders are "individuals who create new options or new approaches to old problems, and work with and through others to effect needed change" (Disch, 2009). The goal is change for the purpose of improvement and working with and through others to improve quality and patient safety. Disch (2009) describes generative leaders as:

> … intellectually curious and never satisfied with the status quo; they are resilient and optimistic, seeing opportunities where others see insolvable problems … [they] recognize there are multiple ways of knowing, and surround themselves with other thought leaders, including those with whom they disagree. They use a holistic, systems perspective in their thinking and move beyond perceived limitations of time, space, traditional thought, and their own views of the world.

The Relationship Between Leadership and Safety

The role of leadership in promoting safety has been a focus in occupational settings for years (Cooper, 2000; Geller, 2000; Zohar, 2002a, 2002b). In a comprehensive review of the topic, Hofmann and Morgeson (2004) differentiated safety-specific leader behaviors from general leader behaviors. They found that when supervisors engaged in more safety-related behavior, such as undergoing training, developing positive-negative contingencies, and demonstrating safe practices, followers engaged in more safety-related behavior. When leaders had cooperative relationships with their employees, safety compliance was also enhanced.

Several researchers have posited that leadership and safety are actually independent of each other and found support for safety being positively related to leadership when the supervisor clearly valued safety as a priority (Hofmann, Morgeson, and Gerras, 2003; Zohar, 2002a). Alternatively, when there was a poor safety climate (little value for safety) and positive leader/follower exchange, employees engaged in safety behaviors less frequently. This suggests that leadership alone is not enough, but that a culture of safety must also be created and expectations conveyed. Furthermore, Mullen and Kelloway (2009) found that leaders' safety attitudes (and employees' ratings of leader safety-specific behaviors) were highest when the leaders received safety-specific leadership training, as compared to when they received general leadership training.

In health care, it is becomingly increasingly clear that leaders throughout the organization have to be accountable for safety and quality. The scope of accountability varies, depending on their particular roles. This responsibility is increasingly complex due to the dynamic nature of health care, competing demands for resources, the escalating pressure for achieving quality and safety goals, and the proliferation of criteria that must be monitored and reported.

This emphasis on leadership is critically important. The Joint Commission (2009) established clear expectations for leaders in healthcare organizations:

> It is the leaders who can together establish and promulgate the organization's mission, vision, and goals. It is the leaders who can strategically plan for the provision of services, acquire and allocate resources, and set priorities for improved performance. And it is the leaders who establish the organization's culture through their words, expectations for action, and behavior–a culture that values high-quality, safe patient care, responsible use of resources, community service, and ethical behavior; or a culture in which these goals are not valued.

Yet problems continue. Through its review of root cause analyses of sentinel events from years 2011 to 2015, the Joint Commission has identified leadership as one of the three most frequently cited contributory factors in sentinel events (2015). This past year, the NPSF (2015) identified leadership as the number one factor in a set of eight factors identified as being critical to improving health care safety. And in a national Rand report (Schneider *et al.*, 2014), on patient safety in the Commonwealth of Massachusetts, authors noted that we have "a vacuum in leadership–and vacuum is not too strong a word–a very major obstacle in making progress in safety." They attributed this to safety not being an institutional priority, and that insufficient attention was paid to creating a safety culture, generating patient engagement, or dealing with health information technology issues.

Creating a Culture of Safety

Of paramount importance for the leader is creating and sustaining a culture of safety, whether it be across the organization or within sub-units. The concept of a safety culture originally emerged from industries such as aviation and nuclear power in studies of HROs, which "consistently minimize adverse events despite carrying out intrinsically complex and hazardous work. HROs maintain a commitment to safety at all levels, from frontline providers to managers and executives" (AHRQ, 2014). See Chapter 8 in this book for a description of the principles and processes associated with HROs.

Translating this to health care, a strong safety culture is one that is fair and just, in which health care professionals and leaders are held accountable for unprofessional conduct yet not punished for human mistakes; errors are identified and addressed before they harm patients or if harm occurs, it is acknowledged and used for improving processes and systems; where strong feedback loops enable frontline staff to learn from previous errors and alter care processes to prevent recurrences. Indeed, "improving the culture of safety within health care is an essential component of preventing or reducing errors and improving overall health care quality" (AHRQ, 2014).

Cultures of safety possess three essential elements: 1) environmental structures and processes, 2) safety-promoting attitudes and perceptions, and 3) safety-related behaviors of individuals, both leaders and followers (Cooper, 2000). Specific to health care, Sammer and colleagues (2010) conducted a comprehensive review of the literature on safety culture in US hospitals and found seven dimensions that formed the basis of an actionable model for a culture of safety: leadership, teamwork, an evidence base, communication, learning, a philosophy of being just, and a patient-centered approach. Rather than just focusing on the behavior of individuals, leaders know that safety is based in the culture and the system. In organizations that are highly reliable in being safe (HROs), there is a continual drive toward the goal of maximum attainable safety, and there is recognition that the goal is not to eliminate errors but to prevent harm to the patient (Bagian, 2005). In these organizations, everyone is aware of the interconnected and dynamic nature of daily operations, and that a change in one area or process can ripple out to other areas within the organization.

Reason and Hobbs (2003) caution that a safety culture should be "a wary one" with a "collective mindfulness" of the things that can go wrong. Safe clinical environments rely on leaders and staff to connect frequently, through such mechanisms as daily check-ins and huddles, to learn from and update each other on how things are going and what might be safety threats. Leaders who are committed to safety talk directly with frontline caregivers, through opportunities such as executive rounds and open forums, and keep the focus on what the employees and medical staff need to provide safe care to patients and families. Leaders who are committed to safety demonstrate this on a daily basis through their questions, decisions, and priorities. In an organization where concerns for patient safety are paramount, even members of the board of directors know the key quality indicators as well as the financial metrics, and the board agenda often starts with the quality/safety content rather than being covered at the end of the meeting when time allows. An emphasis on openness, mutual respect, listening and learning permeates the entire organization.

The Role of Nurses in Quality and Safety

"Nurses are the key caregivers in hospitals [and] significantly influence the quality of care provided and, ultimately, treatment and patient outcome" (Draper, Felland, Liebhaber, and Melichar, (2008, p. 1). The Institute of Medicine report (IOM) (2004) *Keeping Patients Safe* asserted that "the vigilance function often thrusts nurses into a role that has been described as the 'front line' of patient defense" (p. 35). The IOM's 2011 report on the future of nursing noted: "Leadership from nurses is needed at every level and across all settings. … Nurses must understand that their leadership is as important to providing quality care as is their technical ability to deliver care at the bedside in a safe and effective manner."

Nurses have a particular responsibility and opportunity for assuring safe health care. As nurses we are the largest health care provider, are with patients and their families in the hospital setting around the clock, connect with individuals in a variety of non-acute settings, and frequently are the 'last line of defense' in preventing errors from reaching individuals. Major national nursing organizations are explicitly calling for nurses to exert appropriate leadership in this area. For example, the American Organization of Nurse Executives (2015) has identified leadership as one of its core competencies for nurse executives, calling upon them to develop expertise in foundational thinking skills, a systems orientation, change management, and communication and relationship building, among other areas. More recently, the American Association of Critical-Care Nurses (2016) has published the second edition of its *AACN Standards for Establishing and Sustaining Healthy Work Environments*. In this document, they call upon all nurses to use authentic leadership and "fully embrace the imperative of a healthy work environment, authentically live it, and engage others in its achievement."

One particular challenge for nursing is to have adequate numbers of well-qualified leaders at decision-making tables throughout the organization so that safety and quality issues can be raised and addressed. In a major report on governance in high-performing community health systems, a key recommendation was that "community health system boards and their CEOs should re-examine their current size and composition … [and] consider the appointment of highly-respected and experienced nursing leaders as voting members of the board to complement physician members and strengthen clinical input in board deliberations" (Prybil et al., 2009).

Although there is support for nurses leading the way, Disch and colleagues (2011) found that the specific role of the chief nursing officer (CNO) in promoting quality and safety in organizations was unclear, and that physician leaders and others in the organization were often unaware of the CNO's participation in and impact on quality and safety initiatives. The authors had visited eight medical centers across the country, conducting interviews with senior leaders, physicians and staff to examine the role of leaders in promoting quality and safety, with particular emphasis on the role of the CNO. They found that, in every organization, the CNO was an active and respected member of the senior leadership team, but in no organization did she have a seat on the governance board. Many CNOs were well integrated into the agenda, either giving a routine update or being consulted on a topic. One board chair noted that the "board absolutely listens to the CNO– we are extremely aware of the involvement of nursing in the health care environment."

Unfortunately, little has changed. These findings mirror what Prybil (2016) recently reported. He analyzed the findings from 8 studies that had examined the presence of nurse and physician leaders on boards over the past ten years, and found that the % of nurses ranged each year from 2 to 6%, while that of physicians ranged from 14 to 26%; in a study from 2015, for nurses it was 2% and, for physicians, 19%. His recommendation? "It is my belief that board deliberations are enriched significantly by the presence and contributions of highly qualified nurse leaders, and it is my hope that their presence around boardroom tables will increase markedly in the coming years."

Although organizations such as the Joint Commission and AONE may be targeting chief nurse executives and nurses in formal positions of leadership, nurses within patient care units have many opportunities to exercise leadership in working with and through others to improve something. Depending on the situation, the nurse may work with other staff nurses, physicians, department heads, or other employees. Three examples are provided in Textbox 16.1.

Creating and Sustaining Change

Kotter, author of a well-known model for change, notes that "leaders who successfully transform businesses do eight things right (and they do them in the right order)" (2010). His eight steps are listed in Table 16.1.

Each of the examples noted above reflect aspects of this model, with some steps being more explicit in some examples than in others. Moreover, all nurses– and not just those in traditional leadership roles– can use these principles, and work with and through others to improve something.

Textbox 16.1 Leadership Examples

Nuisance alarms– Sue Sendelbach (2015), a clinical nurse specialist in a large, Midwestern hospital, wanted to reduce the number of duplicative alarms occurring in her intensive care unit. She had researched the issue and found that up to 99% of alarm signals may not need any intervention and can result in patients' deaths. Engaging an interprofessional group of colleagues who were interested in the issue, she spearheaded a quality improvement project that began with collecting data to determine baseline alarm occurrences; and designed and implemented an intervention (which included customizing alarms based on patient need; daily changes of ECG electrodes, standardized skin preparation, and use of disposable ECG monitoring leads). Staff education and buy-in were conducted, and at the end of the study period, they had achieved an 88.5% reduction in ECG alarm signals, from 28.5/day (baseline) to 3.29.

Preventable ulcers– At another large Midwestern Level 1 trauma center, 22 preventable ulcers (PU) were reported for 2011 (Johnson, 2015). The Pressure Ulcer Response Team (PURT), comprised of wound care clinicians and several staff nurses reviewed the data and identified prevention as their top priority. Instituting a multi-pronged approach throughout the organization, they repeated the message of skin safety through multiple means, e.g., rounds, staff meetings, posters in the bathrooms; they invited more staff nurses to attend Root Cause Analysis sessions; they educated all inpatient staff nurses on skin assessment. They conducted daily rounds with health care providers to discontinue unneeded equipment (e.g., c-collars); and they engaged medical residents in simulation training. At the end of 2015, only six PUs were reported. In addition, the team proudly reported a cultural shift in the organization's thinking from "we saved their life" to "we can save their life and protect their skin at the same time."

Early mobility in the ICU– A group of staff nurses in a community hospital were concerned with the associated complications of immobility experienced by ICU patients. Working through a multidisciplinary mobility committee, they launched an intervention that used a baseline assessment to determine which patients were physiologically appropriate for early mobility, and early patient ambulation supported by a consistent group of staff. Results for those engaged in the early mobility included fewer falls, ventilator-associated events, PUs, CAUTIs; fewer days of delirium; and lower hospital costs.

Table 16.1 Kotter's model of change.

---

1) establishing a sense of urgency,
2) forming a powerful guiding coalition,
3) creating a vision,
4) communicating the vision,
5) empowering others to act on the vision,
6) planning for and creating short-term wins,
7) consolidating improvements and producing still more change, and
8) institutionalizing new approaches.

In planning for a change– or something to be improved– leaders should keep five key questions in mind as they create their plan for change. See Figure 16.1 for a view of the model.

1) **What is the impetus for the change?**
   Possible reasons for change can arise from answers to a variety of questions:
   - Has a root cause analysis identified a major safety threat?
   - Has a review of patient satisfaction data indicated an unacceptable level of performance?

Figure 16.1 The 5 Levers for Change: A change model.

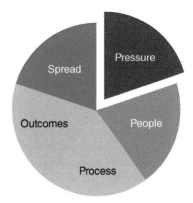

- Are there societal or demographic reasons for the change?
- Is there a competitive reason for the change?
- Is new technology being introduced for which people need to be trained?
- Is there an exciting new approach to patient care that people want to try?

In other words, why is the change necessary? It's obvious that some changes are exciting, eagerly anticipated, and supported, while others may be resisted or rejected, and still other changes will be supported by some people and not others.

The leader or change agent may have to create what could be called the Business, Legal, or Quality (BLQ) case for the change through whatever data would be compelling to those needing to support the change. The Business case covers the financial and resource considerations for the change. The Legal case covers regulatory, statutory, accrediting mandates that the organization must follow, such as The Joint Commission, and state or federal regulations. The Quality case speaks to doing the right thing, or striving for higher quality, or aspiring to become Magnet-recognized or best in the community. Evidence to support aspects of the BLQ case could include data, statistics, compelling stories, appreciative inquiry, benchmarking data, or regulatory mandates.

The needed change should be clearly defined and then linked to the proposed remedy. For example, an unacceptable level of Catheter Associated Urinary Tract Infections (CAUTIs) can be reversed by adopting an evidence-based method for effective and efficient catheter care; or introducing bedside rounding has been implemented to improve communication with patients and prevent unnecessary falls. A compelling, well-stated vision of what you hope to accomplish – and how you intend to go about result in a powerful motivator for change.

2) **Who are the key people who need to be involved?**
Working with and through others requires a careful calculation as to who are all of the individuals or groups that need to be included in some fashion, and what role can they play, for example:

- Who are the people who will want to work with you on this project because they see the need for change, and can become partners and allies?
- Who are the organizational leaders (sometimes called sponsors) who have the power to launch and give approval to the change? These individuals usually have formal authority and the responsibility for holding people accountable. They also usually control the resources. In some instances, one leader can give permission to create the change, while another is the operational leader who provides ongoing support and guidance.
- Who are advocates or champions who will come on board early to support the work? They may be directly or indirectly involved.

- Who are the individuals who will oppose this change? They may feel threatened, or disagree with the plan, or resist change in general. But it's important to identify these people, talk with them and gain their perspectives; often they can provide important insights that need to be considered. At the least, it's important to understand who supports or opposes a proposed change.
- Who is going to be affected in some way by the change? Who will have to change their practices, or routines, or beliefs if the change is adopted? It may be something as simple as a unit secretary who now has to use a different reporting form for supplies. This group of individuals can extend far away from the original change but be affected nonetheless
- Who are the healthy skeptics, those individuals who pose questions about the need for the change, the way in which it's being proposed, or the benefits? While sometimes challenging to deal with, these people can be helpful in identifying potential weaknesses in the need for or plan of change. Asking "under what conditions could this be made to work?" can sometimes elicit helpful suggestions.
- Who needs to be kept updated on progress? This may be the individual who originally gave permission, or your supervisor, or some other organizational leader who is working on a related project. Consideration should especially be given toward keeping nursing staff and relevant physicians updated as pilot projects are being tested.

3) **How will the change be rolled out?**
In his landmark work on the diffusion of innovation, Rogers (2003) identified that certain factors foster the adoption of new ways of doing things, namely the innovation's relative advantage, its compatibility with the current way of doing things, its ease of learning, its testability, among other factors. Several strategies have also helped an innovation gain traction, such as when it is adopted by a highly respected individual who is part of a social network; or providing positive and meaningful feedback to individuals who accept the change in the early stages. Thoughtful planning and gathering of broad input in designing the proposed improvement are key, as are keeping people informed, tracking progress, and making revisions as needed. Use of one of the well-known quality improvement processes is essential in working with and through others to improve something.

It is well known that individuals possess different levels of tolerance for change. Rogers (2003) noted that people range from being active adopters of change to laggards who reluctantly come along when the vast majority of individuals have accepted the change. Bridges (1993) observed that people adapt to change differently, and that many factors enter into a person's ability to change. There are many reasons why people resist change: earlier change attempts that failed, a sense that "this too shall pass," comfort with the status quo, inadequate communication about the benefits of the change, or too many initiatives at once. Given the current dynamic state of the health care industry, the phenomenon of change fatigue is understandable. Change fatigue "refers to impairments in an individual's and organization's abilities to cope with the ever-increasing scope and pace of change" (Valusek, 2007).

In preparing to mount a change initiative, leaders need to assess their organization's change tolerance. What else is occurring at the present time? How could a particular change be connected to something else already going on in the organization? How could it be framed so that it is seen as a helpful adjunct rather than a burdensome interruption? Valusek (2007) advocates implementing a change calendar to manage the timing of changes and using a weekly time line to identify and coordinate the multitude of changes occurring across an organization.

4) **How will success be measured?**
For a change to take hold, tangible results have to be achieved, measured, and communicated – and these have to be tied closely to what you hope to accomplish. As an early step in the process, a desired vision or preferred future should be created and shared, preferably with input by those who will be affected by the change. Kouzes and Posner (2012) describe the importance

of a vision and the leader's role in envisioning the future in a way that inspires others. "Leaders envision the future by imagining exciting and ennobling possibilities. You need to make something happen, to change the way things are, to create something that no one else has ever created before." Leaders also must be able to pragmatically envision better ways of doing immediate tasks, or tackling more mundane challenges. The leader has an idea, and then co-creates it with others to garner their ideas, support, and energy. This can be enjoyable when the change is widely embraced. It can be more difficult when introducing change that is difficult or imposed.

Identifying the specific goal to be achieved, developing concrete, measurable outcomes, and measuring the progress toward the goal are key steps in achieving change. Desired outcomes may be indicators of improved health, decreased use of health resources, prevention of complications, improvement in functional status, cost savings, reduction in lost days from work or school– any reflectors of positive change. It is important to closely match the right outcome measure with the intervention or change being proposed. For example, measuring knowledge when the hoped for outcome is behavioral change is a common example of a mismatch. Similarly, assuming that a certain intervention, such as giving verbal directions for taking a medication, will result in a patient successfully following a medication regimen can also be a mismatch. Nelson, Batalden, and Godfrey (2007) have produced a rich compendium of resources in their book *Quality by Design*. This resource provides useful tools, case studies, references, and recommendations to help formal and informal leaders, students, and educators strengthen their competency in leading change to improve quality and safety.

5) **How can we accelerate the diffusion of health care innovation?**
Parston and colleagues (2015) remind us that there's an acknowledged lag between an invention or innovation and its widespread use across a health system. They attribute this, in part, to a reliance on "*clinical serendipity*, or the belief that one clinician will naturally adopt another's new and improved health care product or process" as potentially being a major factor in this lag. Drawing from case studies from eight countries, they identify factors that can help diffuse innovation whether it be across countries or patient care units. These factors follow:
- Identify the need for a particular change (build the case), provide a clear vision of how things could look and, perhaps most importantly, point out the first practical steps to take.
- Create a specific program or initiative that gives a 'name' to the work, and houses the necessary resources for coordination, implementation, communication…which assumes that those have been secured.
- Select the right leaders to lead the initiative, those with credibility, the capacity to mobilize change, and the necessary skills (technical, communication, project management).
- Establish appropriate systems for monitoring and evaluating the extent and pace of the diffusion process and the innovation's impact over time.
- Design and use an array of communication channels that tap into the various organizational and interpersonal networks of individuals involved.
- Throughout the process, maintain a focus on keeping the vision and strategy visible, sharing data as to progress (and making revisions as warranted), and communicating, communicating, communicating.

A Head, Heart, and Hands Approach to Change

Another way to think about designing an initiative for change is that planning should address the head, heart and hand of a project:

Head: The logic of the analysis and recommendation
Heart: Why the client should change
Hand: How to make the change easy to implement

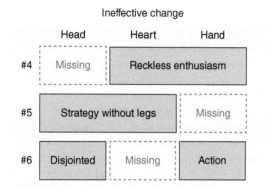

Figure 16.2 Missing elements leading to ineffective change. Source: Change management: You have to appeal to all 3 (head, heart, hands). http://www.consultantsmind.com/2012/09/29/head-heart-hand/ Last accessed July 2016. Reproduced with permission of consultantsmind.com

As was mentioned above, people respond differently to change and that depends on a number of things. Some people are more logical; others rely on persuasion and the emotional side. Skillful planning should pay attention to all three aspects. For example, focusing only on the need for the change (the Head), with the data to vividly describe the reasons why something must change ignores the fear that some individuals may have in changing, or the anticipated loss. Or focusing only on the emotional aspects of the need for change (the Heart), without data or a pragmatic strategy, has been likened to daydreaming. Figure 16.2 provides an example of what happens when any of the components are missing (Consultantsmind, 2012).

Sometimes we learn from failure. Two case studies offer insights and lessons learned from two broad organizational changes that eventually were successful, but experienced setbacks along the way. Barnsteiner and colleagues (2001) describe their journey in establishing a physician discipline policy in a major children's hospital, while Disch and Taranto (2002) describe their experiences in establishing an intraoperative policy for handling emergent situations when there is disagreement over the plan of care.

Implementation Strategies for Education and Practice

In addition to the strategies covered above in structuring change, several specific assignments are offered here to help nurses develop leadership skills for improving quality and safety.

- Select 3 experienced staff nurses to interview on the following questions: What is your definition of leadership? When did you first recognize that you were a leader? What advice would you give to other nurses about being effective in creating change?
- Partner a student nurse with a practicing leader involved in some aspect of operational quality and safety in health care to examine the leader's role.
- Conduct an environmental assessment to identify a threat to quality and safety in the organization or patient care unit, and design a plan for change.
- Participate in a quality/safety committee meeting and analyze the formal and informal leadership roles displayed by members.
- Review issues from the last two years of the *Joint Commission Journal on Quality and Patient Safety*. Which safety issues are most examined? What leadership implications are highlighted?
- Read the *AACN Standards for Creating and Sustaining a Healthy Work Environment*. Which of the six standards do you think are in place in your organization? Which could benefit from some attention?

- Access the AHRQ web site and assess your patient care unit according to questions related to a safety culture: http://www.ahrq.gov/sites/default/files/wysiwyg/professionals/quality-patient-safety/patientsafetyculture/hospital/resources/hospscanform.pdf
- Attend a root cause analysis of a serious reportable event to 1) identify factors contributing to the event stemming from the culture, environment, and educational needs of staff; and 2) develop plans for their improvement
- Watch the video by Helen Haskell on her son's death at (http://qsen.org/faculty-resources/videos/the-lewis-blackman-story/) and reflect on the following questions: 1) Could this happen in your facility? 2) Why or why not? 3) What are leadership implications from this story? 4) What changes would you make for future patient situations such as this?
- Read about high-reliability organizations at (http://www.ahrq.gov/qual/hroadvice/hroadvice.pdf) and reflect on how closely your organization matches the description.
- Attend a staff nurse council meeting, and identify behaviors that you think are effective in engaging people to take a particular course of action.

Conclusion

As the IOM (2011) proclaims in its Key Message #3 in the *Future of Nursing*: "Nurses should be full partners, with physicians and other health care professionals, in redesigning health care in the United States." The tagline for this groundbreaking report is *Leading Change, Advancing Health*. Nursing leaders must be actively involved with others in transforming care delivery, nursing education, and the public's perception of nursing's role if the full impact of the report is to be realized. Nurses have long been known as the frontline of defense in the safety movement. Now nurses at all levels, and in all organizations, are equipped to also be the logical partners in leading this quality and safety journey (IOM, 2011). Nurses as leaders, whether in formal or informal roles, must step forward in identifying the threats to quality and patient safety and in proposing the solutions to make health care safe for all.

References

AHRQ Patient Safety Network (AHRQ PSNet). (2014) *Patient safety primer: Safety culture*. Retrieved March 20, 2016 from https://psnet.ahrq.gov/primers/primer/5.

American Association of Critical-Care Nurses (AACN). (2016) *AACN Standards for establishing and maintaining healthy work environments*. Aliso Viejo CA: AACN.

American Organization of Nurse Executives (AONE). (2015) Nurse executive competencies. Retrieved March 20, 2016 from http://www.aone.org/resources/nec.pdf.

Bagian, J.P. (2005) Patient safety: What really is at issue? *Frontiers of Health Services Management*, 22(1), 3–16.

Barnsteiner, J., Madigan, C., and Spray, T. (2001) Instituting a disruptive conduct policy for medical staff. *AACN Clinical Issues*, 12(3), 378–382.

Bridges, W. (1993) Surviving corporate transition. Mill Valley, CA: William Bridges and Associates.

Consultantsmind. (2012) Change management: You have to appeal to all 3 (head, heart, hands). Retrieved March 20, 2016 from http://www.consultantsmind.com/2012/09/29/head-heart-hand/

Cooper, M. (2000) Towards a model of safety culture. *Safety Science*, 36, 111–136.

Disch, J. (2009) Generative leadership. *Creative Nursing, 15*(4), 172– 177.

Disch, J., Dreher, M., Davidson, P., Sinioris, M., and Wainio, J. (2011) The role of the chief nurse officer in ensuring patient safety and quality. *Journal of Nursing Administration, 41*(4), 179– 185.

Disch, J. and Taranto K (2002) Creating change in the workplace. In D. Mason and J. Leavitt (Eds.). *Policy and politics in nursing and health care.* 4th Ed. St. Louis: Saunders.

Draper, D.A., Felland, L.E., Liebhaber, A., and Melichar, L. (2008) *The role of nurses in hospital quality improvement.* Research Brief #3. Washington, DC: Center for Studying Health System Change.

Geller, E.S. (2000) 10 leadership qualities for a total safety culture. *Professional Safety, 45,* 38– 41.

Hofmann, D.A., and Morgeson, F.P. (2004) The role of leadership in safety. In J. Barling and M. Frone (Eds.), *The psychology of workplace safety* (pp. 159– 180). Washington, DC: American Psychological Association.

Hofmann, D.A., Morgeson, E.P., and Gerras, S.J. (2003) Climate as a moderator of the relationship between LMX and content specific citizenship behavior: Safety climate as an exemplar. *Journal of Applied Psychology, 88,* 17– 178.

Institute of Medicine. (2004) *Keeping patients safe: Transforming the work environment of nurses.* Washington, DC: National Academies Press.

Institute of Medicine. (2011) *The future of nursing: Leading change, advancing health.* Washington, DC: National Academies Press.

Johnson, L. (2016) Personal communication.

Joint Commission. (2009) *Leadership committed to safety.* Sentinel Event #43, Retrieved from http:// www.jointcommission.org/assets/1/18/SEA_43.pdf.

Joint Commission. (2015) Sentinel event data: Root causes by event type. Retrieved March 20, 2016 from http://www.jointcommission.org/assets/1/18/Root_Causes_by_Event_Type_2004-2015.pdf.

Kotter, J.P. (2010) Leading change: Why transformation efforts fail. In *HBR's 10 must reads: The essentials* (pp. 137– 152). Boston: Harvard Business Review Press.

Kouzes, J.M., and Posner, B.Z. (2012) *The leadership challenge.* 5th Ed. San Francisco: Jossey-Bass.

Mullen, J.E., and Kelloway, E.K. (2009) Safety leadership: A longitudinal study of the effects of transformational leadership on safety outcomes. *Journal of Occupational and Organizational Psychology, 82*(2), 253– 272.

National Patient Safety Foundation (NPSF). (2015) *Free from harm: Accelerating patient safety improvement 15 years after To Err is Human.* Boston, MA: NPSF.

Nelson, E.C., Batalden, P.B., and Godfrey, M.M. (2007) *Quality by design: A clinical microsystems approach.* San Francisco: Jossey-Bass.

Northouse, P. (2016) *Leadership: Theory and practice.* 7th Ed. Thousand Oaks, CA: Sage.

Parston, G., McQueen, J., Patel, H., Keown, O.P., Fontana, G., Kuwari, H.A., and Darzi, A. (2015) The science and art of delivery: Accelerating the diffusion of health care innovation. *Health Affairs, 34*(12), 2160– 2166.

Prybil, L., Levey, S., Peterson, R., Heinrich, D., Brezinski, P., Zamba, G., *et al.* (2009) *Governance in high-performing community health systems: A report on trustee and CEO views.* Chicago: Health Research and Educational Trust.

Prybil, L. (2016) Nursing engagement in governing health care organizations. Past, present and future. *Journal of Nursing Care Quality* [in press].

Reason, J. and Hobbs, A. (2003) Safety culture. In J. Reason and A. Hobbs, *Managing maintenance error: A practical guide* (pp. 145– 158). Hampshire, England: Ashgate.

Rogers, E.M. (2003) *Diffusion of innovations.* 5th Ed. New York: Free Press.

Sammer, C.E., Lykens, K., Singh, K.P., Mains, D.A., and Lackan, N.A. (2010) What is patient safety culture: A review of the literature. *Journal of Nursing Scholarship, 42*(2), 156– 165.

Schneider, E.C., Ridgely, M.S., Khodyakov, D., Hunter, L.E., Predmore, Z., and Rudin, R.S. (2014) *Patient safety in the Commonwealth of Massachusetts: Current status and opportunities for improvement.* Santa Monica, CA; The Rand Corporation.

Sendelbach, S., Wahl, S., Anthony, A., and Shotts, P. (2015) Stop the noise: A quality improvement project to decrease electrocardiographic nuisance alarms. *Critical Care Nurse, 35*(4), 15–22.

Valusek, J.R. (2007) The change calendar: A tool to prevent change fatigue. *Joint Commission Journal on Quality and Patient Safety, 33*(6), 355–360.

Zohar, D. (2002a) The effects of leadership dimensions, safety climate and assigned priorities on minor injuries in work groups. *Journal of Organizational Behavior, 23*(1), 75–92.

Zohar, D. (2002b) Modifying supervisory practices to improve sub-unit safety: A leadership-based intervention model. *Journal of Applied Psychology, 87*, 156–163.

Resources

AHRQ (2016). Surveys on patient safety culture. Retrieved from http://www.ahrq.gov/professionals/quality-patient-safety/patientsafetyculture-/index.html.

AHRQ (n.d.) Patient and family engagement. Retrieved from http://www.ahrq.gov/professionals/education/curriculum-tools/cusptoolkit/modules/patfamilyengagement/index.html.

American College of Healthcare Executives (2016) ACHE Healthcare Executive: 2016 Competencies Assessment tool. Retrieved from http://www.ache.org/pdf/nonsecure/careers/competencies_booklet.pdf.

Lucian Leape Institute (2013) *Through the eyes of the workforce: Creating joy, meaning and safer health care.* Boston, MA; National Patient Safety Foundation.

Porter-O'Grady, T., and Malloch K. (2016) Leadership in nursing practice, 2nd ed. Burlington, MA: Jones and Bartlett.

Yoder-Wise, P.S. (2016) Leading and managing in nursing, 6th ed.). St. Louis, MO: Elsevier.

17

Global Perspectives on Quality and Safety

Gwen Sherwood, PhD, RN, FAAN, ANEF

Santos was concerned that patients on the surgical unit where she worked experienced a high rate of hospital-acquired infections (HAI). She began a literature search to investigate possible contributing factors and solutions. She was shocked to see the HAI rates listed for both developed and developing countries. Since she worked in a developing low resource country, she wondered what led health care professionals in developed high resource countries to take short cuts such as failing to wash hands at appropriate times. In her setting clean water could not be taken for granted, nor could adequate resources such as sterile gloves. Still she wanted to follow the evidence-based best practices she read about. Determined, she shared her idea with her unit director to get a group of nurses together to meet with the clinical instructor from the nearby school of nursing who had students on the unit. The instructor had presented a staff development session recently on the need to monitor outcomes of critical data such as HAIs and implement quality improvement projects where needed. Perhaps working together they could collect some data and develop practical solutions for a Plan Do Study Act project to improve quality of care on their unit.

Patient safety and health care quality continue to be significant global health issues. Agencies in nearly every country report quality and safety concerns. With growing awareness of the need to improve outcomes, health care organizations are seeking system improvements and better training for their workers. Sharing evidence, research, and educational approaches across borders can foster broader, even global, solutions. One example is the QSEN project that was initiated in the United States, which is a model framework of the six core competencies for nurses to lead improvements in delivering quality safe care (Cronenwett *et al.*, 2007; Cronenwett *et al.*, 2009; Cronenwett, 2017).

These are the same six competencies identified in 2003 by the IOM for all health professionals if we are to redesign health care to achieve better outcomes: patient-centered care, teamwork and collaboration, evidence-based practice, quality improvement, safety, and informatics (IOM, 2003). The QSEN National Expert Panel developed the definitions along with the KSA objective statements for these six core competencies for prelicensure nursing (Appendix A) and for graduate education (Appendix B), and each competency is further explicated in Chapters 4 through 9 in this book. The integration of these competencies into educational standards and the transformation of nursing curricula and practice are also described in earlier chapters of this book. This chapter will present global challenges in patient quality and safety with exemplar data, examine education as the key to improvement, describe the spread of the US-based QSEN project, explore several dimensions of patient safety such as work

Quality and Safety in Nursing: A Competency Approach to Improving Outcomes, Second Edition.
Edited by Gwen Sherwood and Jane Barnsteiner.
© 2017 John Wiley & Sons, Inc. Published 2017 by John Wiley & Sons, Inc.

force and work environment, and the role of systems thinking, and offer resources available to all. The goal is to consider lessons learned for sharing across borders as we all seek solutions to the global crisis in providing reliable, quality, safe care to all patients. We will also present exemplars of how the QSEN competencies are influencing nursing globally. That the first edition of this book has been translated into three languages (Swedish, Korean, and Chinese) is further evidence of the global significance of improving quality and safety.

Quality and Safety: A Global Perspective

Globalization and increasing mobility of the health care work force has profoundly changed how we address patterns of disease and the supply and availability of health care workers worldwide. It also affects work place environments and culture, which in turn affects health care quality and safety (You *et al.*, 2013). Quality and safety are universal values in health care but are often expressed differently in different locations. We can learn from global cooperation; all countries report the need to improve patient care quality and safety outcomes. Since the US-based IOM released its first quality and safety data in 2000, other startling reports reveal global concerns about quality and safety. Brief examples follow to help understand the depth and breadth of the challenges across the globe.

Global Challenges of Preventable Patient Harm

The World Health Organization (WHO) reports safety issues exist in almost every country with ongoing safety and quality improvement efforts in at least 140 countries (2010). Astounding numbers of preventable deaths are reported worldwide with as many as 254,000 annually in the US (Makary and Daniel, 2016). The *Report of the Mid Staffordshire NHS Foundation Trust Public Inquiry* (2013) indicated patient safety and quality are widespread concerns in the United Kingdom (UK). A European study spanning 11 countries found errors were reported by 11.2% of patients; individual countries ranged from 4 to 17%, mainly due to poor care coordination among providers (Schwappach, 2014).

The WHO reports as many as one in 10 patients in developed countries are harmed by the care they receive due to a range of errors or adverse events (www.who.org). The number is even higher in developing countries, where the risk of health care-associated infection can be as much as 20 times higher. The WHO estimates that at any given time, 1.4 million people worldwide suffer from HAIs. Hand hygiene is the most essential measure for reducing health care-associated infection, yet having a clean, reliable water supply remains a public health problem in low resourced areas. Surgical safety is complex, and problems associated with surgery account for half of the avoidable adverse events that result in death or disability in developing countries.

Comparing health care quality and safety across countries is complicated due to differences in culture, education, language, and roles and responsibilities for nurses. For example, Squires *et al.* (2012) used HCAHPS, a tool developed in the United States and previously translated into English, Spanish, Mandarin, Russian, and Vietnamese to investigate quality in several European countries, which required translation into seven additional languages. This project illustrates the complexity involved in comparing quality across countries that must be addressed with vigorous study approaches.

Challenges in the Workplace

Working to improve quality and safety outcomes addresses both our moral commitment to do no harm and contributes to a healthy work environment that increases worker satisfaction and retention. Workers with the training and opportunities to contribute to improving quality and safety report more satisfaction, which in turn lends to a positive work environment. Nurses help drive quality and safety in all health care delivery settings. The connection of patient safety, satisfaction, and quality of hospital care was investigated in hospitals across Europe and the United States (Aiken *et al.*, 2012). Findings reveal patient care quality varies considerably across countries, and outcomes are significantly affected by the nurse's work environment and nurse-to-patient ratio. A study by You *et al.* (2013) reported nurses in China linked quality of work environment and ratio of nurses to patients with quality of nursing care. In a study of 1117 nurses in South Africa, perceptions of patient safety were not linked to nurse qualifications but did find a link to a positive work culture in which adverse event reporting was encouraged (Blignaut, Coetzee, and Klopper, 2014).

In addressing the problem of patient safety and quality, the Australian Commission on Safety and Quality in Health Care identified the importance of the work environment and ways providers work together in improving quality and safety (2013). The Victoria Commission of Hospital Improvement has developed an accredited leadership program addressing quality and safety challenges through clinical leadership (Commission for Hospital Improvement, 2013). These efforts like those in the United States, England, and elsewhere, demonstrate the impact of organizational leadership and culture in developing work environments conducive to safe quality care.

Sherwood and Shafer (2014) examined quality and safety considerations in the global migration of nurses, noting that nurses have different educational backgrounds depending on their country of origin or different values and attitudes towards health care access and delivery. Safety culture results from the collective values and beliefs of all workers in an organization toward safety, and how that is lived in everyday patient care delivery. How does this affect the responsibilities organizations have to provide adequate training to assure all workers can provide quality safe care? These are questions to be answered as we move forward and share evidence across countries and populations.

Education as the Bridge to Improving Quality and Safety

Transforming health professions education is a primary approach to achieve the quality and safety competencies necessary to implement new roles and responsibilities expected to improve outcomes. In the United States, the IOM (2003) identified the goals for twenty-first century health care delivery: *patient-centered* based on *evidence-based standards,* delivered with *teamwork and collaboration,* within systems focused on continuous *quality improvement* and *safety* science, enhanced by *informatics* (competencies are italicized and reported in Appendices A and B). Earlier chapters in Section 2 of this book explored specific educational approaches and pedagogies to prepare nurses with the necessary KSAs for leading changes in health care delivery systems. Changes to health professions education is a global challenge. We will examine the educational preparation nurses, midwives, and all health professionals must have to develop and implement the competencies to meet expectations for new roles and responsibilities to accomplish the goals for quality and safety.

QSEN: Spreading Beyond the Borders

The unparalleled success of the QSEN project in the United States is now called a social movement as it has permeated nursing education guidelines and professional practice models and invigorated faculty. Offering a robust open access web site (www.QSEN.org) first developed in 2005, nurses from around the world began to access the plethora of free resources made available by the QSEN steering team. Requests for more information and assistance began to come not only from schools and health care organizations in the United States but also from many places around the globe.

Several international conferences applied the QSEN competency framework as the organizing thread for the conference program. In 2007, Macau Polytechnic Institute in Macau held the International Nursing Conference on Quality and Safety of Nursing Practice attended by nurses from 20 countries. The Abu Dhabi Medical Congress first applied the QSEN competencies as the framework for the conference program with modules exploring each competency in turn for application in the local context. The educational collaboration for the annual conference continued for four years. Other international conferences examining the QSEN framework include Taiwan, Hong Kong, Thailand, China, Korea, and Saudi Arabia.

The most intensive application of QSEN has been in Sweden where the Swedish Nursing Society adopted the QSEN framework competencies for nursing education and practice. A more complete description is in Textbox 17.1 from Annette Nygårdh and could be used as a template for other countries.

Textbox 17.1 QSEN: An Integral Part of Nursing in Sweden

By Annette Nygårdh, RN, PhD, Jonkoping University, Sweden

Efforts to integrate the core competencies of nursing started in the US with the project Quality and Safety Education for Nurses (QSEN) (Cronenwett *et al.*, 2007). The QSEN competencies is now included as an integral part of nursing in Sweden (National Association for the nurse in elderly care & Swedish Society of Nursing, 2012) and described as essential to meet the needs of patients and quality of care. In Sweden the quality of care is defined and regulated (Swedish Code of Statutes 2010: 659) to reduce patient suffering and medical injuries. Based on the Institute of Medicine (IOM) report (2003) and in accordance to the Swedish National Board of Health (2011) quality of care is determined by care that is respectful and responsive to individual needs, values and circumstances, and knowledge-based. The waiting times and harmful delays for both the patients and for personnel should be reduced. In addition, the care must be equal regardless of the individual's gender, origin, social and/or economic status and in an appropriate and secure manner.

Donobedian (1966) emphasize that to ensure the quality of care there is a need to study structures (availability, skills, resources), processes (how care is provided, i.e., use of evidence-based practices, person-centered care) and outcomes (i.e., patient satisfaction, mortality, quality of life) within the organization. According to a report from the Institute of Medicine (IOM) (Kohn, Corrigan & Donaldson, 2000), there is a need to critically examine the organization to develop and improve health outcomes and processes.

To improve and assure the quality of care, the care provided needs to be based on relevant data. Data can be used to examine the results of care, and identify areas for improvement. In Sweden there is an ongoing work with collecting patient data and store it in a database, i.e., The Swedish National Quality Register. The Swedish National Quality Register is defined as "an automated and structured set of personal data, set up specifically for the purpose of systematically and continuously developing and securing the quality of care" (Patient Data Act, Chapter 7., §1., 2008: 355). The National Quality Register aims to facilitate the monitoring and evaluation of healthcare performance and quality. This means that the health care organization's own input data can be compared to previous outcomes but also to other health care organizations. The number of quality registers has increased in Sweden and work is ongoing to implement variables that reflect the quality of nursing (SSF 2012).

As a nurse, it is important to know the quality measurements used in the organization (Cronenwett *et al.*, 2009) to evaluate the care given. To mention some of the Swedish national quality registers, the most common register in elderly care is within palliative care, Senior Alert as a register to assess risks of fall, malnutrition, decubitus and unhealthy oral status, and behavioral and psychological symptoms of dementia (BPSD). In accordance to a new law of patient security (SFS 2014:281) there is emphasize on person-centered care and the patients right to participate in health care decisions related to their own care. Based on the law and its emphasis on the patient's perspective of care, an improvement work has started in the context of Coronary diseases. The register (SWEDHEART) have started to implement Patient Reported Outcomes of the care they received (PROM) in the National Quality Register and the next step will be to implement Patient Reported outcomes of the organization of care (PREM). The data collected from PROM and PREM will give the professionals in the organization opportunity to follow-up the care provided and the organization of it to ensure a person-centered care.

The data in the Swedish National Quality Registry is meant to be used in research and to improve and secure quality in health care. According to the specialist nurse's core competence of quality improvement, it is important to ensure that an ethics review is carried out before the start (Cronenwett *et al.*, 2009). The register contains, among other things, information about the individual patient's disease and/or treatment. Therefore, it is important for the nurses to be aware of the legal requirements on patients' right to be informed and secure the process of informed consent before using the data in the register (Patient Data Act).

References

Cronenwett, L., Sherwood, G., Barnsteiner, J., Disch, J., Johnson, J., Mitchell, P., Sullivan, D.T., and Warren, J. (2007). Quality and safety education for nurses. Nursing outlook, 55(3), 122–131.

Cronenwett, L., Sherwood, G., Pohl, J., Barnsteiner, J., Moore, S., Sullivan, D.T., Ward, D., and Warren, J. (2009). Quality and safety education for advanced nursing practice. Nursing Outlook, 57(6), 338–348.

Donabedian, A. (1966). Evaluating the quality of medical care. The Milbank memorial fund quarterly, 44(3), 166–206.

Kohn, L. T., Corrigan, J. M., and Donaldson, M. S. (Eds.). (2000). To err is human: building a Safer Health System (Vol. 6). National Academies Press.

Patient Data Act (SFS, 2008:355). (In Swedish). Stockholm: Socialdepartementet.

Senior Alert. Received from http://plus.rjl.se/infopage.jsf?childId=21157&nodeId=43617

SWEADHEART. Received from http://www.ucr.uu.se/swedeheart/index.php/dokument-sh/arsrapporter

Swedish Society of Nursing (2012). Svensk sjuksköterskeförening (In Swedish). Utveckla och ensa kvalitetsvariabler inom omvårdnadsområden. Received from http://www.swenurse.se/Vi-arbetar-med/Kvalitet/Nationella-Kvalitetsregister/

Swedish Code of Statues, 2010:659. (In Swedish).

The BPSD register. Received from http://www.bpsd.se/other-languages/english/

The National Association of Nurses in Elderly Care & Swedish Society of Nursing. (2012). (In Swedish). Kompetensbeskrivning: Legitimerad sjuksköterska med specialistsjuksköterskeexamen inom vård aväldre. Stockholm: SFF. Received from http://www.swenurse.se/contentassets/4f0b2f399f6c4c649a56a73db77a3340/ssf-aldrekompwebb.pdf

The National Board of Health and Welfare (2011). (In Swedish). Ledningssystem för systematiskt kvalitetsarbete SOSFS 2011:9.

Now, the QSEN Institute is taking the bold step of initiating an International Task Force in recognition of the growing influence of QSEN in multiple countries. Aniko Kukla, chairperson, explains the goals of the task force in Textbox 17.2. Initiated in 2005 as a national project, the consideration of these core competencies in other settings is both exciting and cautioning. What are unique local contexts that impact cultural considerations in providing patient-centered care, or teamwork and collaboration? The Task Force hopes to begin to explore these and other questions. Information is on the QSEN web site, www.QSEN.org.

Textbox 17.2 International QSEN Task Force

By Aniko Kukla, DNP, RN, CPNP
   Veterans Administration Post-Doctoral Quality Scholar
   VA Medical Center, Cleveland, Ohio
   The International QSEN Task Force was established in summer of 2016 with the aim to expand the QSEN community globally. The QSEN community serves as a network of nurses who contribute to the QSEN mission; ensuring that all nurses have the knowledge, skills and attitudes (KSAs) necessary to continuously improve the quality and safety of the healthcare systems within which they work. The aims of the International Task Force are to develop international QSEN initiatives and relationships based upon collaboration and respect.
   The goals of the QSEN International Task Force are:

- Integrate QSEN competencies into academia and practice globally,
- Develop a network of international QSEN scholars and create a Global Listserv,
- Facilitate international initiatives such as teaching strategy submissions, publications, multi-site research projects, conferences, and workshops, and
- Evaluate the global impact.

   The QSEN vision of a global community and a catalyst for change in quality and safety education and competency is a driving force for many networking opportunities. QSEN consultants are collaborating with colleagues in Sweden, Saudi Arabia, Japan, Taiwan, Thailand, and others.
   One of the first initiatives that the International Task Force is involved in is the mapping of the QSEN initiatives globally. A map of the world identifies the initiatives and contacts from the respective countries engaged in the QSEN community. Institutions and healthcare professionals who are active in quality and safety projects and networks are listed at www.QSEN.org. Interested groups may send a brief description of their work in integrating the quality and safety competencies with name and contact information qsen.institute@gmail.com.
   The International QSEN Task force is seeking healthcare professionals who are passionate about global quality and safety initiatives and who are energized to spread the QSEN mission. Members will be connected through virtual meetings with respect to different time zones and needs. The Task Force will meet annually at the QSEN forum. To get involved, contact the leader of the Task Force Dr. Aniko Kukla at axk633@case.edu.

Integrating Quality and Safety in Academic Settings

Few studies compare what students are learning across countries. Tella *et al.* (2015) compared the perceptions of nursing students in two universities in Finland with two universities in Britain about what they learned about patient safety in clinical settings using the Patient Safety in Nursing Education Questionnaire. Students in both settings were motivated to learn about safety and quality in their clinical placements yet experienced some barriers. Patient safety culture and practices in different health care organizations and clinical units vary, posing challenges for nursing students' learning about patient safety during their clinical placements. Students benefitted from a supportive and systems-based approach but rarely had exposure to error reporting systems.

A study from South Korea used the QSEN framework to examine integration and student achievement of quality and safety in four baccalaureate nursing programs (Lee, Jang, and Park, 2015). Results varied across schools although most students reported they had received education about patient safety and quality during their nursing programs. The authors cite the need for curricular standards and attention not only to what is taught but how it is taught.

A three-year cross-sectional survey administered the Health Professional Education in Patient Safety Survey annually to self-assess Canadian baccalaureate nursing students' confidence about patient safety competency (Lukewich *et al.*, 2015). Students reported they were relatively confident in what they were learning about the clinical dimensions of patient safety, but they expressed less confidence about the sociocultural aspects of patient safety although confidence declined as they approached the end of their academic studies. Most students reported they lacked confidence to speak up about patient safety issues.

Few articles explore inclusion of human factors as a specific topic in nursing education and practice yet most safety solutions rely heavily on human factors engineering. A study of 13 schools in England confirmed patient safety was included in the curriculum and allocated more than four hours, but all classes included human factors (Robson *et al.*, 2013).

Two QSEN competencies, patient-centered care and teamwork and collaboration, address patient engagement in their care, also explained in the Foreword (Bataldan, 2017) as co-production. Martin, Navne, and Lipczak (2015) investigated the active involvement of patients with cancer in Denmark. Health professionals in general were found to lack the knowledge and about patient safety, techniques for involving patients in their care, and team communication. These findings are consistent with the emerging emphasis on interprofessional education as a key to improving quality and safety, and the overlay of the QSEN competencies (Dolansky *et al.*, 2017).

Although the QSEN project has described integration of the quality and safety competencies into nursing education in the United States, White *et al.* (2016) describe how safety science was implemented into a large university in the United Kingdom. Yet another study presents findings on visibility of patient safety in nursing curricula in four UK universities as reported from program leaders and students (Steven *et al.*, 2015). Patient safety was not visible as a curricular theme, and faculty struggled to define it. Students felt the emphasis was on what not to do rather than strategies, systems, and procedures to improve patient safety nor was there a focus to place safety within learning about organizational systems and procedures. Students mostly learned by observing staff and felt the pressure of wanting to fit in and to "pass," both of which limited their feelings of emotional safety and willingness to speak up or challenge the process.

Collaborative Health Professions Education: Key to Improvements

To address emerging roles and responsibilities for nurses and other health professionals in quality and safety worldwide, the WHO and the International Council of Nurses (ICN) (www.icn.ch) have each issued position statements, recommendations, and guidelines for improving quality and safety as well as global standards for nursing and midwifery education (WHO, 2009). To improve health care outcomes requires education in the new quality and safety science for all health care providers through changes in academic curricula and clinical education programs to assure a workforce skilled in leading the improvements demanded by regulatory agencies, consumers, and professional organizations (Sherwood, 2012). The United States also issued competencies for all health professionals to improve interprofessional collaboration that is linked to improving quality safe care; the Interprofessional Education Collaborative competency domains are explained in Chapter 14 of this book (Dolansky *et al.*, 2017).

Saleh, Darawad, and Al-Hussami (2105) explored the perceptions of hospital safety culture among 242 registered nurses in five Jordanian hospitals using the Hospital Survey on Patient Safety

Culture. Teamwork within units scored the highest and lowest scores related to nonpunitive response to errors. In South Korea, 459 nurses reported patient safety competency scores ('teamwork,' 'communication,' 'managing safety risks,' 'human and environmental factors,' 'adverse event recognition,' and 'safety culture' dimensions) for 'managing safety risks' as highest and 'teamwork' as lowest (Hwang, 2015). Patient safety competency was higher in older nurses with higher level degrees and longer clinical experience. Hwang and Ahn (2015) further explored teamwork in South Korean hospitals. Of the teamwork subscales, mutual support rated highest, while leadership was lowest. Of the participating nurses, 522 responded that they had experienced at least one clinical error in the last six months, yet only 53.0% responded they report these to their managers and/or the patient safety department. High scores on team communication correlated with higher likelihood of error reporting.

Butterworth and colleagues (2011) describe curriculum revision in England for nurses and physicians in both academia and clinical areas that involve clinical mentors helping with skill development. Working with more than 30 universities, more than 10,000 undergraduate and postgraduate students have completed the curriculum. As in most academic programs, finding time in crowded curricula was a major constraint.

With increasing awareness of the need to improve patient care outcomes, there has been a broad call to improve health professions education. A 20-member international commission examined global concerns about the lag in improving delivery systems and issued recommendations in a seminal report, *Health Professionals for a New Century: Transforming education to strengthen health systems in an interdependent world* (Frenk *et al.*, 2010). The commission noted current health care challenges outstrip traditional educational paradigms. They found evidence of fragmented, outdated, static curricula that focused on competencies that are mismatched for the complex population health needs of the twenty-first century; they further cited weak leadership for initiating change to replace what is now described as tribalism, isolation, and competition among health professionals and their respective education programs with mutual learning, joint solutions, common language, and shared mental models. They called for interactive classrooms led by faculty engaged in creating a dynamic learning environment that learning opportunities among all types of professionals who are involved in the patient's care.

Faculty Development: Modeling Patient Safety

Educator development is important for preparing clinicians, administrators, leaders, and current students across the health professions to model the core quality and safety competencies. Most current educators completed their formal training prior to the emphasis on quality and safety improvements and thus lack the vocabulary, conceptual understanding, and knowledge of the regulations required in clinical settings as well as application to their own educational programs, where evidence-based approaches are equally important. As efforts to integrate patient safety into health professional curricula increase, curricular change is very slow. There is little research that addresses the perspectives of faculty who are on the 'front-lines' of curricular innovation on quality and safety. Tregunno *et al.* (2014) found priorities for the urgency of curricular reform to integrate quality and safety competencies varied among the medical, nursing, and pharmacy faculty who participated in the study. Champions who are also knowledgeable about change can help lead the way for curricular integration and the preparation of safe practitioners. Educators across academic and health care delivery settings and across global regions can develop innovative partnerships to integrate didactic learning with clinical learning opportunities (Sherwood, 2012).

Preparing a Global Work Force to Address Quality and Safety

Numerous systematic reviews and studies from multiple countries report assessment of the KSAs of health care personnel related to patient care quality and safety. Appropriate tools that translate from one language to another yet are sensitive to local culture and context is a major consideration in assessment.

Assessing Quality and Safety Competencies

Tools to assess the preparation of health professionals in both academic and clinical settings are key to accurate findings. A Scandinavian study reported a systematic review of the KSAs among health professionals; findings both indicate the need to change skills and attitudes about patient safety, but also the need for further research (Brasaite, Kaunonen, and Suominen, 2015). A systematic review of assessment tools cited issues in the attempts to develop a comprehensive approach to broad, complex concepts such as quality and safety (Okuyama, Martowirono, and Bijnen, 2011). Most tools assessed teamwork, risk management, and communication and were designed for professionals; two assessed educational outcomes. Mansour's (2012) systematic review of the integration of quality and safety in nursing education found similar results, noting more robust tools will improve accurate assessments of patient safety competencies both in academic and clinical settings.

Reporting Systems and Just Culture

Working in systems that focus on quality and safety can increase awareness of adverse and sentinel events. Health professions education must include preparation in systems for identifying, reporting, and analyzing a near miss or adverse events. In a culture that values quality and safety, there is a process for all workers to disclose near misses and adverse events through a reporting system with systematic analysis and follow up to learn ways to prevent future occurrences (Barnsteiner, 2012).

A long-standing issue, however, is the lack of centralized reporting beyond the single health care setting. Some countries and regions are developing reporting systems to have a more analytic approach to data collection so that aggregated reports can identify gaps in how health care is delivered, identify care interventions for which we need evidence to support, and identify when organizations lack a climate to support quality and safety initiatives. Formal reporting requirements aggregate data on errors, near misses, and poor outcomes from across the industry so that repeated system issues can be detected, analyzed, and changed to establish new evidence-based procedures that may build in a checks and balance to prevent occurrences.

There is increasing interest in sharing data across countries to be able to detect common errors and initiate system improvements. System issues, equipment failures, or high-risk drug packaging may be detected more quickly with aggregate reporting. Medication errors are a universal issue that has been addressed by the International Council of Nurses (www.icn.ch) as a major global patient safety and quality concern. Other high-performance industries such as aviation, nuclear power, and railway have used aggregate reporting to help improve safety outcomes.

Cheng and others (2011) compared incidence-reporting systems for health care risk management in the United Kingdom, United States, Canada, Australia, and Taiwan in developing a health care risk management policy in China. They found many reporting systems have expanded from medication errors and hospital-acquired infections to all patient safety incidents. Management of incidents has become more reliable with increased application of laws, regulations, and reporting standards. The United Kingdom has a government Sentinel Events (Serious Incident Reporting Learning [SIRL] framework) (death or serious injury) database. The United States, the first country to initiate a reporting system, maintains a limited range of incident reporting such as health care-associated infections. Canada and Australia modeled their system after the United States. The Taiwanese system is the most comprehensive.

Research Methods and Priorities in Patient Safety and Quality

The scarcity of research evidence on how to solve the global issue of quality and safety is compounded by a lack of trained researchers in many areas, particularly in developing regions. Andermann and others (2011) developed a research framework for patient safety based on three processes: 1) review existing literature on competencies in patient safety research, 2) consult with end users and international experts, and then 3) conduct a global consensus discussion related to patient safety. WHO (2011) issued three recommendations as *Core Competencies to Carry Out Patient Safety Research* to help strengthen research capacity, particularly useful in locales where there is little data on quality and safety issues. The core competencies document identifies the set of KSAs necessary for patient safety researchers and patient safety officers to effect change through three core competency areas (http://www.who.int/patientsafety/research/methodological_guide/en/index.html):

- Describe the fundamental concepts of the science of patient safety, in their specific social, cultural, and economic context.
- Design and conduct patient safety research.
- Contribute to the process of translating research evidence to improve the safe care of patients.

Resources from a Global Perspective

There are accessible and free resources for organizations in both academic and clinical settings interested in improving quality and safety. Samples are included below.

Institute for Healthcare Improvement (IHI)

The IHI works globally and provides free online patient safety modules for students and can be used by faculty as well (www.IHI.org). There is a global network of student patient safety chapters, and guidelines are available to assist in using new chapters.

Patient Safety Education Project

The Patient Safety Education Project is a core curriculum with practice improvement tool kits to implement patient-centered, systems-based care (Emmanuel *et al.*, 2008). The project uses a train-the-trainer approach and partners with professional organizations in the United States and Australia.

TeamSTEPPS

TeamSTEPPS is now taught around the world and has made adaptions in some settings to adjust to cultural and contextual considerations. This interprofessional, evidence-based curriculum can be downloaded at www.AHRG.gov.

International Society for Quality in Healthcare (ISQUA)

The International Society for Quality in Healthcare (http://www.isqua.org) promotes quality among providers and agencies in more than 70 countries. The society has formal affiliate status with WHO to be able to assist with sharing technical and policy advice based on evidence and best practices.

World Health Organization

WHO offers a variety of guides, curricula, and strategies to improve patient safety and quality with exemplar programs described below. Textbox 17.3 offers examples of the patient safety program areas sponsored by various groups and member states within WHO. More information is available globally on its web site: www.who.int/patientsafety/.

The WHO Patient Safety project convened an international multi-stakeholder working group to identify a set of global priorities for patient safety research using a modified Delphi technique to build consensus. Priorities were based on the severity and frequency of the patient safety issue, magnitude of harm and its distribution, and the impact the issue has on the efficiency of the health system as a whole. The priorities are broad areas that have substantial knowledge gaps for which it is believed that further knowledge will significantly contribute to improving patient safety and reducing harm. Fifty topics have been identified and prioritized according to developing, transitional, and developed countries. Among the top priorities are development and testing of locally effective and affordable solutions, cost-effectiveness of risk-reducing strategies, lack of communication and coordination, and latent organizational failures (www.who.int/patientsafety/research/priority_setting/en/index/html).

Textbox 17.3 Examples of the WHO Patient Safety Program areas (www.who.int/patient/about/programmes/en/index.html) Accessed July 2016. Reproduced with permission of WHO

- Clean Care is Safer Care focuses on health care-associated infection with emphasis on hand hygiene.
- Safe Surgery Saves Lives develops the WHO Safe Surgery Checklist with three phases of safety checks: preanesthesia, before skin incision, and before the patient leaves the operating room; checklists for other hospital areas are now being developed.
- Patients for Patient Safety involves patients and consumers in a global network of patients and patient organizations to champion patient safety.
- Research for Patient Safety established a multifaceted global approach to research in patient safety including education, assessments, and safety measures.
- International Patient Safety Classification defines patient safety concepts with an internationally agreed-upon classlflcatlon system.
- Reporting and Learning generates best practice guidelines for reporting systems.
- Solutions for Patient Safety explores interventions and actions that prevent patient safety problems from occurring and thus reduce patient risk.
- Education for Safer Care developed a model for medical student education in patient safety.

To achieve changes in practice, solutions that redesign care processes can prevent errors that are likely to happen. The World Alliance for Patient Safety issued nine universal patient safety solutions that can help avoid mistakes. These have been translated into Arabic, Chinese, German, and Spanish (WHO, n.d.-b).

- Confusing drug names that sound/look alike
- Confirming patient identification
- Performing correct procedure, correct site
- Controlling concentrated drug solutions
- Assuring medication accuracy during transitions
- Avoiding catheter and tubing misconnections
- Using single-use injection devices
- Improving hand hygiene
- Communicating during patient handovers (handoffs)

The WHO Patient Safety Curriculum Guide now includes a multi-professional edition (www.who.int) jointly developed with the International Confederation of Midwives, International Council of Nurses, International Pharmaceutical Federation, International Pharmaceutical Students Federation, World Dental Federation, and World Medical Association.

The World Alliance for Patient Safety (WHO, 2004), an affiliate of WHO, was formed in response to a World Health Assembly resolution in 2002 that asked WHO member states to focus on patient safety. It has facilitated and promoted patient safety policies and practices around the world in focused areas: safety solutions, global patient safety challenge, patients for patient safety, reporting and learning, taxonomy, research, safety in action, and technology. For example, in 2007–2008, the focus was "Safe Surgery Saves Lives." The cooperative alliance among WHO member states allows faster progress than any one single member can achieve alone.

The International Classification for Patient Safety was developed by the World Alliance for Patient Safety as a conceptual framework to provide a common language and conceptualization around patient safety (www.who.int). Grouping patient safety concepts into an internationally agreed-upon classification enables learning about patient safety across systems throughout the world. The International Classification for Patient Safety is a convergence of international perceptions of the main issues related to patient safety, which facilitates the description, comparison, measurement, monitoring, analysis, and interpretation applicable in regional and national settings. There are subdivisions of concepts for each to allow for regional dialects, different languages and clinical disciplines, and/or provider or patient preferences:

1) Incident type
2) Patient outcomes
3) Patient characteristics
4) Incident characteristics
5) Contributing factors/hazards
6) Organizational outcomes
7) Detection
8) Mitigating factors
9) Ameliorating actions
10) Actions taken to reduce risk

The World Alliance for Patient Safety also works with 40 patient safety champions working to improve safety in health care worldwide, through the Patients for Patient Safety initiative. Consumers consistently rank quality and safety as top concerns in their care and are using their experience to seek system improvements. Patients for Patient Safety (PFPS or P4PS) recognizes the contributions that patients and consumers can have in health care improvement and safety by serving in advisory roles in health care delivery organizations or other agencies. PFPS works with a global network of patients, consumers, caregivers, and consumer organizations that supports patient involvement in patient safety programs, both within countries and globally (WHO, 2004).

Summary

The QSEN project has provided a template to guide nurses in realizing leadership roles for nurses and midwives around the world to help shape the future of health care by helping transform patient care quality and safety outcomes (Sherwood, 2010). The magnitude of the issues in health care quality and safety in all areas of the globe can be addressed through collaboration, partnerships, and sharing to speed progress toward better health for all. The chapter has presented examples of global initiatives, challenges, and partnerships that are promoting quality and safety improvements through programs, core curricula, collaboration, research training, and assessments that are bringing together clinicians, consumers, educators, regulatory agencies, and governmental agencies to focus attention in all locations, both developed and developing or transitional countries. This chapter has presented only a slice of the work ongoing all over the world to honor the commitment of health professionals to first, do no harm. Working together, we continue the transformation of health professions education, train educators, and promote scholarly development to determine evidence-based strategies. Quality and safety are issues of global proportion and require global solutions.

References

Agency for Healthcare Research and Quality. (2009) TeamSTEPPS. Retrieved at www.ahrq.gov.

Aiken, L.H., Clarke, S.P., and Sloane, D.M. (2012) Hospital staffing, organization, and quality of care: Cross-national findings. *International Journal for Quality in Health Care. 14*(1), 5–13.

Andermann, A., Ginsburg, L., Norton, P., Arora, N., Bates, D., Wu, A., Larizgoitia, I., and Patient Safety Research Training and Education Expert Working Group of WHO Patient Safety. (2011) Core competencies for patient safety research: A cornerstone for global capacity strengthening. *British Medical Journal Quality and Safety, 20*(1), 96–101.

Australian Commission on Safety and Quality in Health Care. (2013) Annual Report 2012/2013. Sydney: ACSQHC.

Barnsteiner, J. (2017) Safety. In G. Sherwood and J. Barnsteiner (Eds.), *Quality and safety in nursing: A competency approach to improving outcomes.* 2nd Ed. Hoboken, NJ: Wiley-Blackwell.

Batalden, P. (2017) Foreword. In G. Sherwood and J. Barnsteiner (Eds.), *Quality and safety in nursing: A competency approach to improving outcomes.* 2nd Ed. Hoboken, NJ: Wiley-Blackwell.

Blignaut, A., Coetzee, S., and Klopper, H. (2014) Nurse qualifications and perceptions of patient safety and quality of care in South Africa. *Nursing & Health Sciences, 16*(2): 224–231.

Brasaite, I., Kaunonen, M., and Suominen, T. (2011) Healthcare professionals' knowledge, attitudes and skills regarding patient safety: a systematic literature review. *Scandinavian Journal of Caring Sciences, 29*(1): 30–50.

Butterworth, T., Jones, K., and Jordan, S. (2011) Building capacity and capability in patient safety, innovation and service improvement: An English case study. *Journal of Research in Nursing, 16*(3), 243–251.

Cheng, L., Sun, N., Li, Y., Zhang, Z., Wang, L., Zhou, J., *et al.* (2011) International comparative analyses of incidents reporting systems for healthcare risk management. *Journal of Evidence-Based Medicine.* February 18. doi: 10.1111/j.1756-5391.2011.01119.x. [Epub ahead of print].

Commission for Hospital Improvement. (2013) Clinical Leadership in Quality and Safety http://health.vic.gov.au/chi/cliqs.htm.

Cronenwett, L., and Barnsteiner, J. (2017) A national initiative: Quality and safety education for nurses (QSEN). In G. Sherwood and J. Barnsteiner (Eds.), *Quality and safety in nursing: A competency approach to improving outcomes.* Hoboken, NJ: Wiley-Blackwell.

Cronenwett, L., Sherwood, G., Barnsteiner, J., Disch, J., Johnson, J., Mitchell, P., *et al.* (2007) Quality and safety education for nurses. *Nursing Outlook, 55*(3), 122–131.

Cronenwett, L., Sherwood, G., and Gelmon, S. (2009) Improving quality and safety education: The QSEN Learning Collaborative. *Nursing Outlook, 57*(6), 304–312.

Cronenwett, L., Sherwood, G., Pohl, J., Barnsteiner, J., Moore, S., Taylor Sullivan, D.T., *et al.* (2009) Quality and safety education for advanced practice nursing practice. *Nursing Outlook, 57*(6), 338–348.

Dolansky, M., Singh, M., Luebbers, E., and Moore, S. (2017) Interprofessional approaches to quality and safety education. In G. Sherwood and J. Barnsteiner (Eds.), *Quality and safety in nursing: A competency approach to improving outcomes*. 2nd Ed. Hoboken, NJ: Wiley-Blackwell

Emanuel, L., Walton, M., Hatlie, M., Lau, D., Shaw, T., Shalowitz, J., and Combes, J. (2008) The patient safety education project: An international collaboration. In K. Henriksen, J.B. Battles, M.A. Keyes, and M.L. Grady (Eds.). *Advances in patient safety: New directions and alternative approaches: Vol. 2. Culture and redesign*. Rockville, MD: Agency for Healthcare Research and Quality.

Frenk, J. *et al.* The Lancet Commission. (2010) Health professionals for a new century: transforming education to strengthen health systems in an interdependent world. *The Lancet*. 376(9756):1923–1958.

Hwang, J.I. (2015) What are hospital nurses' strengths and weaknesses in patient safety competence? Findings from three Korean Hospitals. *International Journal of Quality in Health Care*. 27(3):232–238.

Hwang, J.I., Ahn, J.(2015) Teamwork and clinical error reporting among nurses in Korean hospitals. *Asian Nursing Research* (Korean Society of Nursing Science). 9(1):14–20.

Institute of Medicine. (2000) *To err is human: Building a safer health system*. Committee on Quality of Health Care in America, Institute of Medicine. Washington, DC: National Academies Press.

Institute of Medicine. (2003) *Health professions education: A bridge to quality*. Committee on Quality of Health Care in America, Institute of Medicine. Washington, DC: National Academies Press.

International Council of Nurses. (2008) *Positive practice environments for health care professionals: Quality workplaces for quality care*. Retrieved from http://www.ppecampaign.org/content/campaign-toolkit.

Johnson, J. (2017) Quality improvement. In G. Sherwood and J. Barnsteiner (Eds.), *Quality and safety in nursing: A competency approach to improving outcomes*. 2nd Ed. Hoboken, NJ: Wiley-Blackwell.

Lee, N.J., Jang, H., and Park, S.Y. (2016) Patient safety education and baccalaureate nursing students' patient safety competency: A cross-sectional study. *Nursing and Health Sciences*. 18(2):163–171.

Lukewich, J., Edge, D.S., Tranmer, J., Raymond, J., Miron, J., Ginsburg, L., and VanDenKerkhof, E. (2015) Undergraduate baccalaureate nursing students' self-reported confidence in learning about patient safety in the classroom and clinical settings: an annual cross-sectional study (2010–2013). *International Journal of Nursing Studies*. 52(5):930–938.

Makary, M.A. and Daniel, M. (2016) Medical error-the third leading cause of death in the US. *British Medical Journal*. May 3, 2016.353:i2139

Martin, H.M., Navne, L.E., and Lipczak, H. (2013) Involvement of patients with cancer in patient safety: a qualitative study of current practices, potentials and barriers. *British Medical Journal Quality and Safety*, 22(10): 836–842.

Mansour, M. (2012) Current assessment of patient safety education. *British Journal of Nursing*. 21(9): 536–543.

Okuyama, A., Martowirono, K., and Bijnen, B. (2011) Assessing the patient safety competencies of healthcare professionals: a systematic review. *British Medical Journal Quality and Safety*, 20(11): 991–1000.

Robson, W., Clark, D., Pinnock, D., White, N., and Baxendale, B. (2013) Teaching patient safety and human factors in undergraduate nursing curricula in England: A Pilot Survey. *British Journal of Nursing*. 22(17):1001–1005.

Saleh, A.M., Darawad, J.W., and Al-Hussami, M. (2015) The perception of hospital safety culture and selected outcomes among nurses: An exploratory study. *Nursing and Health Science*. 17(3):339–346.

Schwappach, D. (2012) Risk factors for patient-reported medical errors in eleven countries. *Health Expectations*, 17, 321–331.

Sherwood, G. (2010) New views of quality and safety offer new roles for nurses and midwives. *Nursing and Health Sciences*, *12*(3), 281–283.

Sherwood, G. (2017) The imperative to transform education to transform practice. G. Sherwood and J. Barnsteiner (Eds.), *Quality and safety in nursing: A competency approach to improving outcomes.* 2nd Ed. Hoboken, NJ: Wiley-Blackwell.

Sherwood, G., and Shaffer, F. (2014) The role of international educated nurses in a quality safe work force. *Nursing Outlook*, Special Topic Issue. *62*(1): 46–52.

Squires, A., Bruyneel, L., Aiken, L., Van den Heede, K., Brzostek, T., Busse, R., Ensio, A., Schubert, M. Zikos, D., and Sermeus, W. (2012) Cross-cultural evaluation of the relevance of the HCAHPS survey in five European countries. *International Journal for Quality in Health Care 24* (2012): 470–475.

Steven, A., Magnusson, C., Smith, P., and Pearson, P.H. (2014) Patient safety in nursing education: contexts, tensions and feeling safe to learn. *Nurse Education Today. 34*(2):277–284.

Tella, S., Smith, N.J., Partanen, P., Jamookeeah, D., Lamidi, M.L., and Turunen, H. (2015) Learning to ensure patient safety in clinical settings: comparing Finnish and British nursing students' perceptions. *Journal of Clinical Nursing.* 24(19–20): 2954–2964.

The *report of the mid staffordshire NHS foundation trust public inquiry.* (2013) Accessed June 2016 at https://www.gov.uk/government/uploads/system/uploads/attachment_data/file/279124/0947.pdf.

White, N., Clark, D., Lewis, R., and Robson, W. (2016) *International Journal of Nursing Education Scholarship.* 2016 Apr 13;*13*(1). pii:/j/ijnes.2016.13.issue-1/ijnes-2015-0007/ijnes-2015-0007.xml.

World Health Organization. (n.d.–a) *10 Facts on patient safety.* Retrieved July 25, 2011, from http://www.who.int/features/factfiles/patient_safety/en/.

World Health Organization. (n.d.–b) *Patient safety solutions.* Retrieved July 25, 2011, from http://www.who.int/patientsafety/implementation/solutions/patient safety/en/.

World Health Organization. (2004) *World alliance for patient safety.* Retrieved from http://www.who.int/patientsafety/worldalliance/en/.

World Health Organization. (2009) *Global standards for the initial education of nurses and midwives.* Geneva, Switzerland: World Health Organization. Available at http://www.who.int/patientsafety/en/.

World Health Organization. (2011) *Core competencies to carry out patient safety research.* Retrieved from http://www.who.int/patientsafety/research/strengthening_capacity/training_leaders/en/.

World Health Professions Alliance. (2002) *Fact sheet: Patient safety.* Retrieved from http://www.whpa.org/factptsafety.htm.

You, L., Aiken, L., Sloane, D., Liu, K., He, G., Hu, Y., Jianng, S., Li, X., Li, X., Liu, H., and Shang, S. (2013) Hospital nursing, care quality, and patient satisfaction: Cross-sectional surveys of nurses and patients in hospitals in China and Europe. *International Journal of Nursing Studies 50*: 154–161.

Appendix A

Prelicensure Competencies

Table A.1 Patient-centered care.

Knowledge	Skills	Attitudes
Integrate understanding of multiple dimensions of patient-centered care: • patient/family/community preferences, values • coordination and integration of care • information, communication, and education • physical comfort and emotional support • involvement of family and friends • transition and continuity	Elicit patient values, preferences, and expressed needs as part of clinical interview, implementation of care plan, and evaluation of care Communicate patient values, preferences, and expressed needs to other members of health care team Provide patient-centered care with sensitivity and respect for the diversity of human experience	Value seeing health care situations "through patients' eyes" Respect and encourage individual expression of patient values, preferences, and expressed needs Value the patient's expertise with own health and symptoms Seek learning opportunities with patients who represent all aspects of human diversity Recognize personally held attitudes about working with patients from different ethnic, cultural, and social backgrounds Willingly support patient-centered care for individuals and groups whose values differ from own
Describe how diverse cultural, ethnic, and social backgrounds function as sources of patient, family, and community values		
Demonstrate comprehensive understanding of the concepts of pain and suffering, including physiologic models of pain and comfort	Assess presence and extent of pain and suffering Assess levels of physical and emotional comfort Elicit expectations of patient and family for relief of pain, discomfort, or suffering Initiate effective treatments to relieve pain and suffering in light of patient values, preferences, and expressed needs	Recognize personally held values and beliefs about the management of pain or suffering Appreciate the role of the nurse in relief of all types and sources of pain or suffering Recognize that patient expectations influence outcomes in management of pain or suffering

(*Continued*)

Quality and Safety in Nursing: A Competency Approach to Improving Outcomes, Second Edition.
Edited by Gwen Sherwood and Jane Barnsteiner.
© 2017 John Wiley & Sons, Inc. Published 2017 by John Wiley & Sons, Inc.

Table A.1 (Continued)

Knowledge	Skills	Attitudes
Examine how the safety, quality, and cost effectiveness of health care can be improved through the active involvement of patients and families Examine common barriers to active involvement of patients in their own health care processes Describe strategies to empower patients or families in all aspects of the health care process	Remove barriers to presence of families and other designated surrogates based on patient preferences Assess level of patient's decisional conflict and provide access to resources Engage patients or designated surrogates in active partnerships that promote health, safety and well-being, and self-care management	Value active partnership with patients or designated surrogates in planning, implementation, and evaluation of care Respect patient preferences for degree of active engagement in care process Respect patient's right to access to personal health records
Explore ethical and legal implications of patient-centered care Describe the limits and boundaries of therapeutic patient-centered care	Recognize the boundaries of therapeutic relationships Facilitate informed patient consent for care	Acknowledge the tension that may exist between patient rights and the organizational responsibility for professional, ethical care Appreciate shared decision-making with empowered patients and families, even when conflicts occur
Discuss principles of effective communication Describe basic principles of consensus building and conflict resolution	Assess own level of communication skill in encounters with patients and families Participate in building consensus or resolving conflict in the context of patient care	Value continuous improvement of own communication and conflict resolution skills
Examine nursing roles in assuring coordination, integration, and continuity of care	Communicate care provided and needed at each transition in care	

Definition: Recognize the patient or designee as the source of control and full partner in providing compassionate and coordinated care based on respect for patient's preferences, values, and needs.

Table A.2 Teamwork and collaboration.

Knowledge	Skills	Attitudes
Describe own strengths, limitations, and values in functioning as a member of a team	Demonstrate awareness of own strengths and limitations as a team member Initiate plan for self-development as a team member Act with integrity, consistency, and respect for differing views	Acknowledge own potential to contribute to effective team functioning Appreciate importance of intra- and interprofessional collaboration
Describe scopes of practice and roles of health care team members Describe strategies for identifying and managing overlaps in team member roles and accountabilities Recognize contributions of other individuals and groups in helping patient/family achieve health goals	Function competently within own scope of practice as a member of the health care team Assume role of team member or leader based on the situation Initiate requests for help when appropriate to situation Clarify roles and accountabilities under conditions of potential overlap in team member functioning Integrate the contributions of others who play a role in helping patient/family achieve health goals	Value the perspectives and expertise of all health team members Respect the centrality of the patient/family as core members of any health care team Respect the unique attributes that members bring to a team, including variations in professional orientations and accountabilities
Analyze differences in communication style preferences among patients and families, nurses, and other members of the health team Describe impact of own communication style on others Discuss effective strategies for communicating and resolving conflict	Communicate with team members, adapting own style of communicating to needs of the team and situation Demonstrate commitment to team goals Solicit input from other team members to improve individual, as well as team, performance Initiate actions to resolve conflict	Value teamwork and the relationships upon which it is based Value different styles of communication used by patients, families, and health care providers Contribute to resolution of conflict and disagreement
Describe examples of the impact of team functioning on safety and quality of care	Follow communication practices that minimize risks associated with handoffs among providers and across transitions in care	Appreciate the risks associated with handoffs among providers and across transitions in care
Explain how authority gradients influence teamwork and patient safety	Assert own position/perspective in discussions about patient care Choose communication styles that diminish the risks associated with authority gradients among team members	
Identify system barriers and facilitators of effective team functioning Examine strategies for improving systems to support team functioning	Participate in designing systems that support effective teamwork	Value the influence of system solutions in achieving effective team functioning

Definition: Function effectively within nursing and interprofessional teams, fostering open communication, mutual respect, and shared decision-making to achieve quality patient care.

Table A.3 Evidence-based practice (EBP).

Knowledge	Skills	Attitudes
Demonstrate knowledge of basic scientific methods and processes	Participate effectively in appropriate data collection and other research activities	Appreciate strengths and weaknesses of scientific bases for practice
Describe EBP to include the components of research evidence, clinical expertise, and patient/family values	Adhere to Institutional Review Board (IRB) guidelines Base individualized care plan on patient values, clinical expertise, and evidence	Value the need for ethical conduct of research and quality improvement Value the concept of EBP as integral to determining best clinical practice
Differentiate clinical opinion from research and evidence summaries	Read original research and evidence reports related to area of practice	Appreciate the importance of regularly reading relevant professional journals
Describe reliable sources for locating evidence reports and clinical practice guidelines	Locate evidence reports related to clinical practice topics and guidelines	
Explain the role of evidence in determining best clinical practice Describe how the strength and relevance of available evidence influences the choice of interventions in provision of patient-centered care	Participate in structuring the work environment to facilitate integration of new evidence into standards of practice Question rationale for routine approaches to care that result in less than desired outcomes or adverse events	Value the need for continuous improvement in clinical practice based on new knowledge
Discriminate between valid and invalid reasons for modifying evidence-based clinical practice based on clinical expertise or patient/family preferences	Consult with clinical experts before deciding to deviate from evidence-based protocols	Acknowledge own limitations in knowledge and clinical expertise before determining when to deviate from evidence-based best practices

Definition: Integrates best current evidence with clinical expertise and patient/family preferences and values for delivery of optimal health care.

Table A.4 Quality improvement.

Knowledge	Skills	Attitudes
Describe strategies for learning about the outcomes of care in the setting in which one is engaged in clinical practice	Seek information about outcomes of care for populations served in care setting Seek information about quality improvement projects in the care setting	Appreciate that continuous quality improvement is an essential part of the daily work of all health professionals
Recognize that nursing and other health professions students are parts of systems of care and care processes that affect outcomes for patients and families Give examples of the tension between professional autonomy and system functioning	Use tools (such as flow charts, cause-effect diagrams) to make processes of care explicit Participate in a root cause analysis of a sentinel event	Value own and others' contributions to outcomes of care in local care settings
Explain the importance of variation and measurement in assessing quality of care	Use quality measures to understand performance Use tools (such as control charts and run charts) that are helpful for understanding variation Identify gaps between local and best practice	Appreciate how unwanted variation affects care Value measurement and its role in good patient care
Describe approaches for changing processes of care	Design a small test of change in daily work (using an experiential learning method such as Plan-Do-Study-Act)	Value local change (in individual practice or team practice on a unit) and its role in creating joy in work
	Practice aligning the aims, measures, and changes involved in improving care	Appreciate the value of what individuals and teams can to do to improve care
	Use measures to evaluate the effect of change	

Definition: Use data to monitor the outcomes of care processes and use improvement methods to design and test changes to continuously improve the quality and safety of health care systems.

Table A.5 Safety.

Knowledge	Skills	Attitudes
Examine human factors and other basic safety design principles as well as commonly used unsafe practices (such as workarounds and dangerous abbreviations) Describe the benefits and limitations of selected safety-enhancing technologies (such as barcodes, computer provider order entry, medication pumps, and automatic alerts/alarms) Discuss effective strategies to reduce reliance on memory	Demonstrate effective use of technology and standardized practices that support safety and quality Demonstrate effective use of strategies to reduce risk of harm to self or others Use appropriate strategies to reduce reliance on memory (such as forcing functions, checklists)	Value the contributions of standardization/reliability to safety Appreciate the cognitive and physical limits of human performance
Delineate general categories of errors and hazards in care Describe factors that create a culture of safety (such as open communication strategies and organizational error reporting systems)	Communicate observations or concerns related to hazards and errors to patients, families, and the health care team Use organizational error reporting systems for near miss and error reporting	Value own role in preventing errors
Describe processes used in understanding causes of error and allocation of responsibility and accountability (such as root cause analysis and failure mode effects analysis)	Participate appropriately in analyzing errors and designing system improvements Engage in root cause analysis rather than blaming when errors or near misses occur	Value vigilance and monitoring (even of own performance of care activities) by patients, families, and other members of the health care team
Discuss potential and actual impact of national patient safety resources, initiatives, and regulations	Use national patient safety resources for own professional development and to focus attention on safety in care settings	Value relationship between national safety campaigns and implementation in local practices and practice settings

Definition: Minimizes risk of harm to patients and providers through both system effectiveness and individual performance.

Table A.6 Informatics.

Knowledge	Skills	Attitudes
Explain why information and technology skills are essential for safe patient care	Seek education about how information is managed in care settings before providing care Apply technology and information management tools to support safe processes of care	Appreciate the necessity for all health professionals to seek lifelong, continuous learning of information technology skills
Identify essential information that must be available in a common database to support patient care Contrast benefits and limitations of different communication technologies and their impact on safety and quality	Navigate the electronic health record Document and plan patient care in an electronic health record Employ communication technologies to coordinate care for patients	Value technologies that support clinical decision-making, error prevention, and care coordination Protect confidentiality of protected health information in electronic health records
Describe examples of how technology and information management are related to the quality and safety of patient care Recognize the time, effort, and skill required for computers, databases, and other technologies to become reliable and effective tools for patient care	Respond appropriately to clinical decision-making supports and alerts Use information management tools to monitor outcomes of care processes Use high-quality electronic sources of health care information	Value nurses' involvement in design, selection, implementation, and evaluation of information technologies to support patient care

From "Quality and Safety Education for Nurses," by L. Cronenwett *et al.*, 2007, *Nursing Outlook*, 55(3), pp. 122–131. Reprinted with permission from Elsevier Ltd.
Definition: Use information and technology to communicate, manage knowledge, mitigate error, and support decision-making.

Appendix B

Quality and Safety Education for Nurses Graduate/Advanced Practice Nursing Competencies

(Words in bold and italics are different knowledge, skills, and attitudes from the prelicensure competencies.)

Table B.1 Patient-centered care.

Knowledge	Skills	Attitudes
Analyze multiple dimensions of patient-centered care: • Patient/family/community preferences, values • Coordination and integration of care • Information, communication, and education • Physical comfort and emotional support • Involvement of family and friends transition and continuity	Elicit patient values, preferences, and expressed needs as part of clinical interview, *diagnosis*, implementation of care plan, and evaluation of care Communicate patient values, preferences, and expressed needs to other members of health care team Provide patient-centered care with sensitivity, empathy, and respect for the diversity of human experience	Value seeing health care situations "through patients' eyes" Respect and encourage individual expression of patient values, preferences, and expressed needs Value the patient's expertise with own health and symptoms *Honor* learning opportunities with patients who represent all aspects of human diversity
Analyze how diverse cultural, ethnic, spiritual, and social backgrounds function as sources of patient, family, and community values	*Ensure that the systems within which one practices support patient-centered care for individuals and groups whose values differ from the majority or one's own*	*Seek to understand* one's personally held attitudes about working with patients from different ethnic, cultural, and social backgrounds
Analyze social, political, economic, and historical dimensions of patient care processes and the implications for patient-centered care *Integrate knowledge of psychological, spiritual, social, developmental and physiological models* of pain and suffering	*Assess and treat pain and suffering in light of patient values, preferences, and expressed needs* *Respect* the boundaries of therapeutic relationships	Willingly support patient-centered care for individuals and groups whose values differ from own *Value cultural humility*
Analyze ethical and legal implications of patient-centered care Describe the limits and boundaries of therapeutic patient-centered care	*Acknowledge the tension that may exist between patient preferences and organizational and professional responsibilities for ethical care* Facilitate informed patient consent for care	*Seek to understand one's personally held values and beliefs about the management of pain or suffering* *Value* shared decision-making with empowered patients and families, even when conflicts occur

(Continued)

Quality and Safety in Nursing: A Competency Approach to Improving Outcomes, Second Edition.
Edited by Gwen Sherwood and Jane Barnsteiner.
© 2017 John Wiley & Sons, Inc. Published 2017 by John Wiley & Sons, Inc.

Table B.1 (Continued)

Knowledge	Skills	Attitudes
Analyze strategies that empower patients or families in all aspects of the health care process *Analyze features of physical facilities that support or pose barriers to patient-centered care*	Engage patients or designated surrogates in active partnerships *along the health illness continuum* *Create or change organizational cultures so that patient and family preferences are assessed and supported*	Respect patient preferences for degree of active engagement in care process *Honor* active partnerships with patients or designated surrogates in planning, implementation, and evaluation of care
Analyze reasons for common barriers to active involvement of patients and families in their own health care processes	Assess level of patient's decisional conflict and provide access to resources *Eliminate* barriers to presence of families and other designated surrogates based on patient preferences	Respect patient's right to access to personal health records *Value system changes that support patient-centered care*
Integrate principles of effective communication *with knowledge of quality and safety competencies*	*Continuously analyze and improve* own level of communication skill in encounters with patients, families, and teams	Value continuous improvement of own communication and conflict resolution skills
Analyze principles of consensus building and conflict resolution	*Provide leadership in* building consensus or resolving conflict in the context of patient care	*Value consensus*
Analyze advanced practice nursing roles in assuring coordination, integration, and continuity of care *Describe process of reflective practice*	Communicate care provided and needed at each transition in care *Incorporate reflective practices into own repertoire*	*Value the process of reflective practice*

Definition: Recognize the patient or designee as the source of control and a full partner in providing compassionate and coordinated care based on respect for patient's preferences, values, and needs.

Table B.2 Teamwork and collaboration.

Knowledge	Skills	Attitudes
Analyze own strengths, limitations, and values as a member of a team *Analyze impact of own advanced practice role and its contributions to team functioning*	Demonstrate awareness of own strengths and limitations as a team member *Continuously plan for improvement in use of self in effective team development and functioning* Act with integrity, consistency, and respect for differing views	Acknowledge own contributions to effective *or ineffective* team functioning
Describe scopes of practice and roles of all health care team members *Analyze* strategies for identifying and managing overlaps in team member roles and accountabilities	Function competently within own scope of practice as a member of the health care team Assume role of team member or leader based on the situation *Guide the team in managing areas* of overlap in team member functioning *Solicit input from other team members to improve individual, as well as team, performance* *Empower* contributions of others who play a role in helping patients/families achieve health goals	Respect the unique attributes that members bring to a team, including variation in professional orientations, competencies and accountabilities Respect the centrality of the patient/family as core members of any health care team
Analyze strategies that influence the ability to initiate and sustain effective partnerships with members of nursing and inter-professional teams *Analyze impact of cultural diversity on team functioning*	*Initiate and sustain effective health care teams* Communicate with team members, adapting own style of communicating to needs of the team and situation	Appreciate importance of interprofessional collaboration *Value collaboration with nurses and other members of the nursing team*
Analyze differences in communication style preferences among patients and families, *advanced practice* nurses, and other members of the health team *Describe impact of own communication style on others*	*Communicate respect for team member competence in communication* Initiate actions to resolve conflict	Value different styles of communication
Describe examples of the impact of team functioning on safety and quality of care *Analyze* authority gradients and their influence on teamwork and patient safety	Follow communication practices that minimize risks associated with handoffs among providers and across transitions in care Choose communication styles that diminish the risks associated with authority gradients among team members Assert own position/perspective and supporting evidence in discussions about patient care	Appreciate the risks associated with handoffs among providers and across transitions in care *Value the solutions obtained through systematic, interprofessional collaborative efforts*
Identify system barriers and facilitators of effective team functioning Examine strategies for improving systems to support team functioning	*Lead* or participate in the design *and implementation* of systems that support effective teamwork *Engage in state and national policy initiatives aimed at improving teamwork and collaboration*	Value the influence of system solutions in achieving team functioning

Definition: Function effectively within nursing and interprofessional teams, fostering open communication, mutual respect, and shared decision-making to achieve quality patient care.

Table B.3 Evidence-based practice.

Knowledge	Skills	Attitudes
Demonstrate knowledge of *health research* methods and processes	*Use health research methods and processes, alone or in partnership with scientists, to generate new knowledge for practice*	Appreciate strengths and weaknesses of scientific bases for practice Value the need for ethical conduct of research and quality improvement
Describe evidence-based practice to include the components of research evidence, clinical expertise, and patient/family values	Adhere to Institutional Review Board guidelines *Role model clinical decision-making* based on evidence, clinical expertise, and patient/family preferences and values	Value *all components of evidence-based practice*
Identify efficient and effective search strategies to locate reliable sources of evidence	*Employ efficient and effective search strategies to answer focused clinical questions*	*Value development of search skills for locating evidence for best practice*
Identify principles that comprise the critical appraisal of research evidence Summarize current evidence regarding major diagnostic and treatment actions within the practice specialty	*Critically appraise* original research and evidence summaries related to area of practice *Exhibit contemporary knowledge of best evidence related to practice specialty*	*Value knowing the evidence base for practice specialty* *Value public policies that support evidence-based practice*
Determine evidence gaps within the practice specialty	*Promote research agenda for evidence that is needed in practice specialty Initiate changes in approaches to care when new evidence warrants evaluation of other options for improving outcomes or decreasing adverse events*	
Analyze how the strength of available evidence influences the provision of care (assessment, diagnosis, treatment, and evaluation) Evaluate organizational cultures and structures that promote evidence-based practice	*Develop guidelines for clinical decision-making* regarding departure from established protocols/standards of care *Participate in designing systems that support evidence-based practice*	Acknowledge own limitations in knowledge and clinical expertise before determining when to deviate from evidence-based best practices Value the need for continuous improvement in clinical practice based on new knowledge

Definition: Integrate best current evidence with clinical expertise and patient/family preferences and values for delivery of optimal health care.

Table B.4 Quality improvement.

Knowledge	Skills	Attitudes
Describe strategies *for improving* outcomes of care in the setting in which one is engaged in clinical practice *Analyze the impact of context (such as access, cost, or team functioning) on improvement efforts*	*Use a variety of sources of information to review outcomes of care and identify potential areas for improvement* *Propose appropriate aims for quality improvement efforts* *Assert leadership in shaping the dialogue about and providing leadership for the introduction of best practices*	Appreciate that continuous quality improvement is an essential part of the daily work of all health professionals
Analyze ethical issues associated with quality improvement *Describe features of quality improvement projects that overlap sufficiently with research, thereby requiring institutional review board oversight*	*Assure ethical oversight of quality improvement projects* *Maintain confidentiality of any patient information used to determine outcomes of quality improvement efforts*	Value the need for ethical conduct of quality improvement
Describe the benefits and limitations of quality improvement data sources, and measurement and data analysis strategies	*Design and use databases as sources of information for improving patient care* *Select and use relevant benchmarks*	*Appreciate the importance of data that allows one to estimate the quality of local care*
Explain common causes of variation in outcomes of care in the practice specialty	*Select and* use tools (such as control charts and run charts) that are helpful for understanding variation Identify gaps between local and best practice	Appreciate how unwanted variation affects outcomes of care processes
Describe common quality measures in the practice specialty	*Use findings from* root cause analyses to design and implement system improvements *Select and use quality measures to understand performance*	Value measurement and its role in good patient care
Analyze the differences between micro-system and macro-system change *Understand principles of change management* *Analyze the strengths and limitations of common quality improvement methods*	*Use principles of change management to implement and evaluate care processes at the micro-system level* Design, *implement, and evaluate* tests of change in daily work (using an experiential learning method such as Plan-Do-Study-Act) *Align the aims, measures, and changes involved in improving care* Use measures to evaluate the effect of change	Appreciate the value of what individuals and teams can to do to improve care *Value local systems improvement (in individual practice, team practice on a unit, or in the macro-system) and its role in professional job satisfaction* *Appreciate that all improvement is change but not all change is improvement*

Definition: Use data to monitor the outcomes of care processes and use improvement methods to design and test changes to continuously improve the quality and safety of health care systems.

Table B.5 Safety.

Knowledge	Skills	Attitudes
Describe human factors and other basic safety design principles as well as commonly used unsafe practices (such as workarounds and dangerous abbreviations)	*Participate as a team member to design, promote, and model effective use* of technology and standardized practices that support safety and quality	Value the contributions of standardization and reliability to safety *Appreciate the importance of being a safety mentor and role model*
Describe the benefits and limitations of selected safety-enhancing technologies (such as barcodes, computer provider order entry, and electronic prescribing) *Evaluate* effective strategies to reduce reliance on memory	*Participate as a team member to design, promote, and model* effective use of strategies to reduce risk of harm to self and others *Promote a practice culture conducive to highly reliable processes built on human factors research* Use appropriate strategies to reduce reliance on memory (such as forcing functions, checklists)	Appreciate the cognitive and physical limits of human performance
Delineate general categories of errors and hazards in care *Identify best practices for organizational responses to error* Describe factors that create *a just culture* and culture of safety *Describe best practices that promote patient and provider safety in the practice specialty*	Communicate observations or concerns related to hazards and errors to patients, families, and the health care team *Identify and correct system failures and hazards in care* *Design and implement micro-system changes in response to identified hazards and errors* *Engage in a systems focus* rather than blaming individuals when errors or near misses occur *Report errors and support members of the health care team in being forthcoming about errors and near misses*	Value own role in reporting and preventing errors *Value systems approaches to improving patient safety in lieu of blaming individuals* *Value the use of organizational error reporting systems*
Describe processes used to analyze causes of error and allocation of responsibility and accountability (such as root cause analysis and failure mode effects analysis) *Describe methods of identifying and preventing verbal, physical, and psychological harm to patients and staff* *Analyze potential and actual impact* of national patient safety resources, initiatives, and regulations	Participate appropriately in analyzing errors and designing, *implementing, and evaluating* system improvements *Prevent escalation of conflict Respond appropriately to aggressive behavior* Use national patient safety resources: • for own professional development • to focus attention on safety in care settings • *to design and implement improvements in practice*	Value vigilance and monitoring of care, including one's own performance, by patients, families, and other members of the health care team *Value prevention of assaults and loss of dignity for patients, staff, and aggressors* Value relationship between national patient safety campaigns and implementation in local practices and practice settings

Definition: Minimize risk of harm to patients and providers through both system effectiveness and individual performance.

Table B.6 Informatics.

Knowledge	Skills	Attitudes
Contrast benefits and limitations of common information technology strategies used in the delivery of patient care *Evaluate the strengths and weaknesses of information systems used in patient care*	*Participate in the selection, design, implementation, and evaluation of information systems* *Communicate the integral role of information technology in nurses' work* *Model behaviors that support implementation and appropriate use of electronic health records* *Assist team members in adopting information technology by piloting and evaluating proposed technologies*	*Value the use of information and communication technologies in patient care*
Formulate essential information that must be available in a common database to support patient care in the practice specialty	*Promote access to patient care information for all professionals who provide care to patients*	*Appreciate the need for consensus and collaboration in developing systems to manage information for patient care*
Evaluate benefits and limitations of different communication technologies and their impact on safety and quality	*Serve as a resource for how to document nursing care at basic and advanced levels* *Develop safeguards for protected health information* *Champion communication technologies that support clinical decision making, error prevention, care coordination, and protection of patient privacy*	*Value the confidentiality and security of all patient records*
Describe and critique taxonomic and terminology systems used in national efforts to enhance interoperability of information systems and knowledge management systems	*Access and evaluate high quality electronic sources of health care information* *Participate in the design of clinical decision-making supports and alerts* *Search, retrieve, and manage data to make decisions using information and knowledge management systems* *Anticipate unintended consequences of new technology*	*Value the importance of standardized terminologies in conducting searches for patient information* *Appreciate the contribution of technological alert systems* *Appreciate* the time, effort, and skill required for computers, databases, and other technologies to become reliable and effective tools for patient care

From "Quality and Safety Education for Advanced Nursing Practice," by L. Cronenwett *et al.*, 2009, *Nursing Outlook, 57*(6), pp. 122–131. Reprinted with permission from Elsevier Ltd.
Definition: Use information and technology to communicate, manage knowledge, mitigate error, and support decision-making.

Appendix C

Quality and Safety Education for Nurses

Results of a National Delphi Study to Developmentally Level KSAs

Table C.1 Patient-centered care.

Competency	Curricular Introduction			Curricular Emphasis		
Knowledge	Beg	Inter	Adv	Beg	Inter	Adv
Integrate understanding of multiple dimensions of patient-centered care:						
• Patient/family/community preferences, values	X				X	
• Coordination and integration of care	X					X
• Information, communication, and education	X				X	
• Physical comfort and emotional support	X			X		
• Involvement of family and friends	X				X	
• Transition and continuity		X				X
Describe how diverse cultural, ethnic, and social backgrounds function as sources of patient, family, and community values	X				X	
Demonstrate comprehensive understanding of the concepts of pain and suffering, including physiologic models of pain and comfort	X				X	
Examine how the safety, quality, and cost-effectiveness of health care can be improved through the active involvement of patients and families		X				X
Examine common barriers to active involvement of patients in their own health care processes		X			X	
Describe strategies to empower patients or families in all aspects of the health care process		X			X	
Explore ethical and legal implications of patient-centered care	X				X	
Describe the limits and boundaries of therapeutic patient-centered care	X					X
Discuss the principles of effective communication	X			X		

(Continued)

Quality and Safety in Nursing: A Competency Approach to Improving Outcomes, Second Edition.
Edited by Gwen Sherwood and Jane Barnsteiner.
© 2017 John Wiley & Sons, Inc. Published 2017 by John Wiley & Sons, Inc.

Table C.1 (Continued)

Competency	Curricular Introduction			Curricular Emphasis		
Knowledge	Beg	Inter	Adv	Beg	Inter	Adv
Describe basic principles of consensus building and conflict resolution	X					X
Examine nursing roles in assuring coordination, integration, and continuity of care	X					X
Skills						
Elicit patient values, preferences, and expressed needs as part of clinical interview, implementation of care plan, and evaluation of care	X				X	
Communicate patient values, preferences, and expressed needs to other members of health care team	X				X	
Provide patient-centered care with sensitivity and respect for the diversity of human experience	X				X	
Assess presence and extent of pain and suffering	X				X	
Assess levels of physical and emotional comfort	X			X		
Elicit expectations of patient and family for relief of pain, discomfort, or suffering	X				X	
Initiate effective treatments to relieve pain and suffering in light of patient values, preferences, and expressed needs	X				X	
Remove barriers to presence of families and other designated surrogates based on patient preferences	X				**X**	
Assess level of patient's decisional conflict and provide access to resources	X					X
Engage patients or designated surrogates in active partnerships that promote health, safety and well-being, and self-care management	X					X
Recognize the boundaries of therapeutic relationships	X				X	
Facilitate informed patient consent for care	X				X	
Assess own level of communication skill in encounters with patients and families	X				X	
Participate in building consensus or resolving conflict in the context of patient care	X					**X**
Communicate care provided and needed at each transition in care	X				X	
Attitudes						
Value seeing health care situations "through patients' eyes"	X	X				
Respect and encourage individual expression of patient values, preferences, and expressed needs	X				X	
Value the patient's expertise with own health and symptoms	X				X	
Seek learning opportunities with patients who represent all aspects of human diversity	X				X	

Competency	Curricular Introduction			Curricular Emphasis		
Knowledge	Beg	Inter	Adv	Beg	Inter	Adv
Recognize personally held attitudes about working with patients from different ethnic, cultural, and social backgrounds	X			X		
Willingly support patient-centered care for individuals and groups whose values differ from own	X				X	
Recognize personally held values and beliefs about the management of pain or suffering	X				X	
Appreciate the role of the nurse in relief of all types and sources of pain or suffering	X				X	
Recognize that patient expectations influence outcomes in management of pain or suffering	X				X	
Value active partnership with patients or designated surrogates in planning, implementation, and evaluation of care		X			X	
Respect patient preferences for degree of active engagement in care process	X				X	
Respect patient's right to access to personal health records	X				X	
Acknowledge the tension that may exist between patient rights and the organizational responsibility for professional, ethical care	X					X
Appreciate shared decision-making with empowered patients and families, even when conflicts occur		X				X
Value continuous improvement of own communication and conflict resolution skills	X					X

Table C.2 Teamwork and collaboration.

Competency	Curricular Introduction			Curricular Emphasis		
Knowledge	Beg	Inter	Adv	Beg	Inter	Adv
Describe own strengths, limitations, and values in functioning as a member of a team		X				X
Describe scopes of practice and roles of health care team members	X				X	
Describe strategies for identifying and managing overlaps in team member roles and accountabilities		X				X
Recognize contributions of other individuals and groups in helping patient/family achieve health goals		X			X	
Analyze differences in communication style preferences among patients and families, nurses, and other members of the health team		X				X
Describe impact of own communication style on others	X				X	
Discuss effective strategies for communicating and resolving conflict		X				X
Describe examples of the impact of team functioning on safety and quality of care		X				X
Explain how authority gradients influence teamwork and patient safety		X				X
Identify system barriers and facilitators of effective team functioning		X				X
Examine strategies for improving systems to support team functioning				X		X
Skills						
Demonstrate awareness of own strengths and limitations as a team member	X					X
Initiate plan for self-development as a team member			X		X	
Act with integrity, consistency, and respect for differing views	X				X	
Function competently within own scope of practice as a member of the health care team	X					X
Assume role of team member or leader based on the situation			X			X
Initiate requests for help when appropriate to situation	X				X	
Clarify roles and accountabilities under conditions of potential overlap in team-member functioning			X			X
Integrate the contributions of others who play a role in helping patient/family achieve health goals			X			X
Communicate with team members, adapting own style of communicating to needs of the team and situation	X					X
Demonstrate commitment to team goals	X				X	

Competency	Curricular Introduction			Curricular Emphasis		
Knowledge	**Beg**	**Inter**	**Adv**	**Beg**	**Inter**	**Adv**
Solicit input from other team members to improve individual, as well as team, performance			X			X
Initiate actions to resolve conflict			X			X
Follow communication practices that minimize risks associated with handoffs among providers and across transitions in care	X				X	
Assert own position/perspective in discussions about patient care			X			X
Choose communication styles that diminish the risks associated with authority gradients among team members			X			X
Participate in designing systems that support effective teamwork					X	X
Attitudes						
Acknowledge own potential to contribute to effective team functioning	X				X	
Appreciate importance of intra- and interprofessional collaboration	X				X	
Value the perspectives and expertise of all health team members	X				X	
Respect the centrality of the patient/family as core members of any health care team	X				X	
Respect the unique attributes that members bring to a team, including variations in professional orientations and accountabilities			X		X	
Value teamwork and the relationships upon which it is based	X				X	
Value different styles of communication used by patients, families, and health care providers	X				X	
Contribute to resolution of conflict and disagreement			X			X
Appreciate the risks associated with handoffs among providers and across transitions in care	X				X	
Value the influence of system solutions in achieving effective team functioning			X			X

Table C.3 Evidence-based practice (EBP).

Competency	Curricular Introduction			Curricular Emphasis		
Knowledge	Beg	Inter	Adv	Beg	Inter	Adv
Demonstrate knowledge of basic scientific methods and processes	X				X	
Describe EBP to include the components of research evidence, clinical expertise, and patient/family values	X				X	
Differentiate clinical opinion from research and evidence summaries		X				X
Describe reliable sources for locating evidence reports and clinical practice guidelines	X				X	
Explain role of evidence in determining best clinical practice	X				X	
Describe how the strength and relevance of available evidence influences the choice of interventions in provision of patient-centered care		X				X
Discriminate between valid and invalid reasons for modifying evidence-based clinical practice based on clinical expertise or patient/family preferences		X				X
Skills						
Participate effectively in appropriate data collection and other research activities		X				X
Adhere to institutional review board guidelines		X				X
Base individualized care plan on patient values, clinical expertise, and evidence	X				X	
Read original research and evidence reports related to area of practice		X			X	
Locate evidence reports related to clinical practice topics and guidelines		X			X	
Participate in structuring the work environment to facilitate integration of new evidence into standards of practice		X				X
Question rationale for routine approaches to care that result in less than desired outcomes or adverse events		X				X
Consult with clinical experts before deciding to deviate from evidence-based protocols		X				X
Attitudes						
Appreciate strengths and weaknesses of scientific bases for practice		X			X	
Value the need for ethical conduct of research and quality improvement	X				X	
Value the concept of EBP as integral to determining best clinical practice	X				X	
Appreciate the importance of regularly reading relevant professional journals	X					X
Value the need for continuous improvement in clinical practice based on new knowledge	X					X
Acknowledge own limitations in knowledge and clinical expertise before determining when to deviate from evidence-based best practices	X					X

Table C.4 Quality improvement.

Competency	Curricular Introduction			Curricular Emphasis		
Knowledge	Beg	Inter	Adv	Beg	Inter	Adv
Describe strategies for learning about the outcomes of care in the setting in which one is engaged in clinical practice		X				X
Recognize that nursing and other health professions students are parts of systems of care and care processes that affect outcomes for patients and families	X				X	
Give examples of the tension between professional autonomy and system functioning			X			X
Explain the importance of variation and measurement in assessing quality of care			X			X
Describe approaches for changing processes of care			X			X
Skills						
Seek information about outcomes of care for populations served in care setting		X				X
Seek information about quality improvement projects in the care setting		X				X
Use tools (such as flow charts, cause-effect diagrams) to make processes of care explicit		X				X
Participate in root-cause analysis of sentinel event			X			X
Use quality measures to understand performance		X				X
Use tools (such as control charts and run charts) that are helpful for understanding variation		X				X
Identify gaps between local and best practice		X				X
Design a small test of change in daily work (using an experiential learning method such as Plan-Do-Study-Act)		X				X
Practice aligning the aims, measures, and changes involved in improving care			X			X
Use measures to evaluate the effect of change			X			X
Attitudes						
Appreciate that continuous quality improvement is an essential part of the daily work of all health professionals	X				X	
Value own and others' contributions to outcomes of care in local care settings	X				X	
Appreciate how unwanted variation affects care		X				X
Value measurement and its role in good patient care		X			X	
Value local change (in individual practice or team practice on a unit) and its role in creating joy in work		X				X
Appreciate the value of what individuals and teams can do to improve care	X					X

Table C.5 Safety.

Competency	Curricular Introduction			Curricular Emphasis		
Knowledge	Beg	Inter	Adv	Beg	Inter	Adv
Examine human factors and other basic safety design principles as well as commonly used unsafe practices (such as work-arounds and dangerous abbreviations)	X					X
Describe the benefits and limitations of selected safety-enhancing technologies (such as barcodes, computer provider order entry, medication pumps, and automatic alerts/alarms)	X				X	
Discuss effective strategies to reduce reliance on memory	X			X		
Delineate general categories of errors and hazards in care		X			X	
Describe factors that create a culture of safety (such as open communication strategies and organizational error reporting systems)	X				X	
Describe processes used in understanding causes of error and allocation of responsibility and accountability (such as root-cause analysis and failure mode effects analysis)		X				X
Discuss potential and actual impact of national patient safety resources, initiatives, and regulations		X				X
Skills						
Demonstrate effective use of technology and standardized practices that support safety and quality	X				X	
Demonstrate effective use of strategies to reduce risk of harm to self or others	X				X	
Use appropriate strategies to reduce reliance on memory (such as forcing functions, checklists)	X				X	
Communicate observations or concerns related to hazards and errors to patients, families, and the health care team	X				X	
Use organizational error reporting systems for near-miss and error reporting	X				X	
Participate appropriately in analyzing errors and designing system improvements		X				X
Engage in root-cause analysis rather than blaming when errors or near-misses occur			X			X
Use national patient safety resources for own professional development and to focus attention on safety in care settings		X				
Attitudes						
Value the contributions of standardization/reliability to safety	X				X	
Appreciate the cognitive and physical limits of human performance	X			X		
Value own role in preventing errors	X			X		
Value vigilance and monitoring (even of own performance of care activities) by patients, families, and other members of the health care team	X				X	
Value relationship between national safety campaigns and implementation in local practices and practice settings		X				X

Table C.6 Informatics.

Competency	Curricular Introduction			Curricular Emphasis		
Knowledge	Beg	Inter	Adv	Beg	Inter	Adv
Explain why information and technology skills are essential for safe patient care	X			X		
Identify essential information that must be available in a common database to support patient care	X				X	
Contrast benefits and limitations of different communication technologies and their impact on safety and quality		X				X
Describe examples of how technology and information management are related to the quality and safety of patient care		X				X
Recognize the time, effort, and skill required for computers, databases, and other technologies to become reliable and effective tools for patient care		X				X
Skills						
Seek education about how information is managed in care settings before providing care		X				X
Apply technology and information management tools to support safe processes of care	X				X	
Navigate the electronic health record	X				X	
Document and plan patient care in an electronic health record	X				X	
Employ communication technologies to coordinate care for patients		X			X	
Respond appropriately to clinical decision-making supports and alerts		X			X	
Use information management tools to monitor outcomes of care processes		X				X
Use high quality electronic sources of health care information	X				X	
Attitudes						
Appreciate the necessity for all health professionals to seek lifelong, continuous learning of information technology skills	X					X
Value technologies that support clinical decision-making, error prevention, and care coordination	X				X	
Protect confidentiality of protected health information in electronic health records	X			X		
Value nurses' involvement in design, selection, implementation, and evaluation of information technologies to support patient care		X				X

From *Quality and Safety Education for Nurses: Results of a National Delphi Study of Developmentally Level KSAs*, by Barton, Armstrong, and Preheim, 2009. Denver: University of Colorado. Reprinted with permission from the authors.

Glossary

Achieving Competence Today (ACT) an interdisciplinary teaching program that focuses on quality, safety, and health systems improvement.

Adverse event unintentional harm caused by health care management rather than the underlying condition of the patient.

Adverse reaction unexpected harm resulting from a justified action where the correct process was followed for the context in which the event occurred.

Agency for Healthcare Research and Quality (AHRQ) the nation's lead federal agency for research on health care quality, costs, outcomes, and patient safety. AHRQ is the health services research arm of the U.S. Department of Health and Human Services, complementing the biomedical research mission of its sister agency, the National Institutes of Health. The agency is home to research centers that specialize in major areas of health care research, including clinical practice and technology assessment, health care organization and delivery systems, and primary care. AHRQ is a major source of funding and technical assistance for health services research and research training at leading US universities and other institutions. As a science partner, the agency works with the public and private sectors to build the knowledge base for what works and does not work in health and health care and to translate this knowledge into everyday practice and policy making.

American Health Information Community (AHIC) a federally chartered advisory committee that makes recommendations to the secretary of the US Department of Health and Human Services on how to make health records digital and interoperable, encourage market-led adoption, and ensure that the privacy and security of those records are protected at all times. In 2009 AHIC became the National eHealth Collaborative, a new public-private partnership to continue the work of the AHIC (www.nationalehealth.org).

Applicability of study findings whether the effects of the study are appropriate for a particular patient situation.

Background questions questions that need to be answered as a foundation for asking the searchable, answerable foreground question. They are questions that ask for general information about a clinical issue, and they have two components: the starting place of the question (e.g., what, where, when, why, and how), and the outcome of interest (e.g., the clinical diagnosis).

Benchmark (benchmarking) a way for hospitals and doctors to analyze quality data, both internally and against data from other hospitals and doctors, to identify best practices of care and improve quality.

Quality and Safety in Nursing: A Competency Approach to Improving Outcomes, Second Edition.
Edited by Gwen Sherwood and Jane Barnsteiner.
© 2017 John Wiley & Sons, Inc. Published 2017 by John Wiley & Sons, Inc.

Benefits versus risks one way to interpret guideline recommendations. For decisions in which it is clear that benefits far outweigh downsides or downsides far outweigh benefits, the risk/benefit discussion allows the provider to offer a strong recommendation.

Best practices the most up-to-date patient care interventions, which result in the best patient outcomes and minimize patient risk of death or complications.

Bracketing identifying and suspending previously acquired knowledge, beliefs, and opinions about a phenomenon.

Call-out technique for communicating important or critical information by intentionally verbalizing a step in a process.

Care coordination an interdisciplinary approach to the care of a patient.

Care delivery outcomes the outcomes that are influenced by the delivery of clinical care.

Caregiver a person who helps in identifying, preventing, or treating illness or disability.

Carrier an entity that may underwrite or administer a range of health benefit programs; may refer to an insurer or a managed health plan.

Case-control study a type of research that retrospectively compares characteristics of an individual who has a certain condition (e.g., hypertension) with one who does not (e.g., a matched control or similar person without hypertension); often conducted for the purpose of identifying variables that might predict the condition (e.g., stressful lifestyle, sodium intake).

Case series a report on a series of patients with an outcome of interest. No control group is involved.

CCC (Clinical Care Classification) System a standardized, coded nursing terminology that identifies the discrete elements of nursing practice.

Centers for Medicare and Medicaid Services (CMS; formerly Health Care Financing Administration [HCFA]) federal agency that seeks to ensure effective, up-to-date health care coverage and to promote quality care for beneficiaries. Ultimately, CMS is working to transform and modernize the health care system.

Check-back a process that uses closed-loop communication to ensure that information conveyed by the sender is understood by the receiver as intended.

Clinical practice guidelines a set of systematically developed statements, usually based on scientific evidence, that help physicians and their patients make decisions about appropriate health care for specific medical conditions. Clinical practice guidelines briefly identify and evaluate the most current information about prevention, diagnosis, prognosis, therapy, risk/benefit, and cost effectiveness.

Cochrane Collaboration a worldwide association of groups that creates and maintains systematic reviews of the literature for specific topic areas.

Cohort study involves the identification of two groups (cohorts) of patients, one that did receive the exposure of interest and one that did not, and following these cohorts forward for the outcome of interest.

Collaboration process of joint decision making among independent parties involving joint ownership of decisions and collective responsibility for outcomes. The essence of collaboration involves working across professional boundaries.

Commission on Systemic Operability a commission authorized by the Medicare Modernization Act of 2003 and charged with developing strategies to make health care information instantly accessible at all times, by consumers and their health care providers. The group's 12 recommendations and a discussion of the benefits of an interoperable network and the barriers to creating such a network were published in 2005 in a report titled "Ending the Document Game: Connecting and Transforming Your Healthcare Through Information Technology" (http://endingthedocumentgame.gov).

Committee a relatively stable, formally composed group that has an identified purpose as part of an organizational structure.

Communication a process by which information is exchanged between individuals through a common system of symbols, signs, or behavior.

Computerized physician order entry (CPOE) a computerized system that allows a physician's orders for services such as medications, laboratory tests, and other tests to be entered electronically instead of being recorded on order sheets or prescription pads. This allows for the order to be compared against standards for dosing and to be checked for any patient allergies or interactions with other medications, or other potential problems if the order is filled. However, some people prefer to call this **computerized provider order entry system**, thereby recognizing that more than physicians enter orders.

Confidence interval (CI) the range around a study's result within which we would expect the true value to lie. CIs account for the sampling error between the study population and the wider population the study is supposed to represent.

Confounding variable a variable that is not the one in which you are interested but that may affect the results of trial.

Connectivity the physical network and operating rules allowing computerized health information to be stored at one point and retrieved at another by an authorized user. For some people in the health information technology field, connectivity implies having uniform privacy laws protecting individually identifiable medical information from being accessed by unauthorized persons.

Consumer an individual who uses, is affected by, or is entitled or compelled to use a health-related service.

Consumer Assessment of Healthcare Providers and Systems (CAHPS) develops and supports the use of a comprehensive and evolving family of standardized surveys that ask consumers and patients to report on and evaluate their experiences with health care. These surveys cover topics that are important to consumers, such as the communication skills of providers and the accessibility of services. CAHPS originally stood for the Consumer Assessment of Health Plans Study, but as the products have evolved beyond health plans, the name has evolved as well to capture the full range of survey products and tools.

Consumer engagement the situation in which consumers take an active role in their own health care, from understanding their own conditions and available treatments, to seeking out and making decisions based on information about the performance of health care providers.

Consumer-driven (or directed) care a form of health insurance that combines a high-deductible health plan with a tax-favored Health Savings Account, Flexible Spending Account, or Health Reimbursement Account to cover out-of-pocket expenses. These accounts are "consumer driven" in that they give participants greater control over their own health care, allowing individuals to determine on a personal basis how they choose to spend their health care account funds.

Coordination of care comprises mechanisms that ensure patients and clinicians have access to, and take into consideration, all required information on a patient's conditions and treatments to ensure that the patient receives appropriate health care services.

Core measures specific clinical measures that, when viewed together, permit a robust assessment of the quality of care provided in a given focus area, such as acute myocardial infarction.

Critically appraised topic (CAT) a short summary of an article from the literature, created to answer a specific clinical question.

Crew Resource Management (CRM) a training program to improve team functioning in high-stakes industries such as aviation, nuclear power, and health care.

Cultural competence the knowledge, skills, and attitudes necessary for providing quality care to diverse populations.

Culture shared knowledge and behavior of people who interact within distinct social settings and subsystems.

Culture of safety minimizes risk of harm to patients and providers through both system effectiveness and individual performance and recognizes the influence of systems and human factors.

Database of Abstracts of Reviews of Effects (DARE) database that includes abstracts of systematic reviews that have been critically appraised by reviewers at the National Health Service Centre for Reviews and Dissemination at the University of York, England.

Data collection the acquisition of health care information or facts based on patient and consumer race, ethnicity, and language. Data collection provides health care providers with the ability to perform benchmarking measures on health care systems to determine areas where improvement is needed in providing care.

Decision analysis the application of explicit, quantitative methods to analyze decisions under conditions of uncertainty.

Delegation process of transferring authority to a competent individual for completing selected nursing tasks/activities/functions. To assign is to direct an individual to do activities within an authorized scope of practice. Assignment (noun) describes the distribution of work that each staff member is to accomplish in a given work period.

Department of Health and Human Services (HHS) principal federal agency for protecting the health of all Americans and providing essential human services, especially for those who are least able to help themselves.

Design the overall plan for a study that includes strategies for controlling confounding variables, strategies for when the intervention will be delivered (in experimental studies), and how often and when the data will be collected.

Disease management an approach designed to improve the health and quality of life for people with chronic illnesses by working to keep the conditions under control and prevent them from getting worse.

Disease registry a large collection or registry belonging to a health care system that contains information on different chronic health problems affecting patients within the system. A disease registry helps to manage and log data on chronic illnesses and diseases. All data contained within the disease registry are logged by health care providers and are available to providers to perform benchmarking measures on health care systems.

Disparities (in care) differences in the delivery of health care, access to health care services, and medical outcomes based on ethnicity, geography, gender, and other factors that do not include socioeconomic status or insurance coverage. Understanding and eliminating the causes of health care disparities is an ongoing effort of many groups and organizations.

Disruptive behavior behavior that interferes with the ability of everyone on the team to provide safe and effective care, undermines the confidence of any member of the health care team in effectively caring for patients, undermines patients' confidence in the health care team or organization, causes concern for anyone's physical safety, and undermines effective teamwork.

Diversity racial, cultural, or ethnic variation in the demographics of a place, organization, or profession.

Effectiveness a measure of the benefit resulting from an intervention for a given health problem under usual conditions of clinical care for a particular group.

Effective care includes health care services that are of proven value and have no significant trade-offs. The benefits of the services so far outweigh the risks that all patients with specific medical needs should receive them. These services, such as beta-blockers for heart attack patients, are backed by well-articulated medical theory and strong evidence of efficacy, determined by clinical trials or valid cohort studies.

Efficacy a measure of the benefit resulting from an intervention for a given health problem under the ideal conditions of an investigation.

Electronic Health (Medical) Record (EHR or EMR) a computerized medical file that contains the history of a patient's medical care, commonly abbreviated as EHR, in contrast to PHR, which stands for personal health record. An EHR or EMR enables patients to transport their health care information with them at all times.

Emergency department the department within a health care facility that is intended to provide rapid treatment to victims of sudden injury or illness. Emergency departments across the nation struggle with overcrowding, long patient wait periods, and shortages of health care professionals.

Error the failure of a planned action to be completed as intended or the use of an incorrect plan to achieve an aim.

Evidence-based clinical practice guidelines specific practice recommendations that are based on a methodologically rigorous review of the best evidence on a specific topic.

Evidence-based decision making the integration of best research evidence in making decisions about patient care, which should also include the clinician's expertise as well as patient preferences and values.

Evidence-based practice the use of the current, best available scientific research and practices with demonstrated effectiveness in daily medical decision making, including individual clinical practice decisions, by well-trained, experienced clinicians. Evidence is central to developing performance measures for the most common and costly health conditions. The measures allow consumers to compare medical providers and learn which ones routinely offer the highest quality, safest, and most effective care.

Event something that happens to or involves a patient.

Event rate the proportion of patients in a group in whom an event is observed.

Exclusion criteria characteristics possessed by individuals that would exclude them from participating in a study.

Failure Mode Effect Analysis (FMEA) a procedure of analysis of potential failure modes within a system, and classification by severity or determination of the consequences of failures on the system.

Family-centered rounds nursing rounds that include the patient's family with the patient's consent.

Foreground questions those questions that can be answered from scientific evidence regarding diagnosing, treating, or assisting patients with understanding their prognosis, focusing on specific knowledge.

Fully operational electronic health record system system that collects patient information, displays test results, allows providers to enter medical orders and prescriptions, and helps doctors make treatment decisions.

Generalizability the extent to which the findings from a study can be generalized or applied to the larger population (i.e., external validity).

Grading the strength of recommendations:

Level I evidence evidence that is generated from systematic reviews or meta-analyses of all relevant randomized controlled trials or evidence-based clinical practice guidelines based on systematic reviews of randomized controlled trials; the strongest level of evidence to guide clinical practice.

Level II evidence evidence generated from a least one well designed randomized clinical trial (i.e., a true experiment).

Level III evidence evidence obtained from well designed controlled trials without randomization.

Level IV evidence evidence from well designed case-control and cohort studies.

Level V evidence evidence from systematic reviews of descriptive and qualitative studies.

Level VI evidence evidence from a single descriptive or qualitative study.

Level VII evidence evidence from the opinion of authorities and/or reports of expert committees.

Group any collection of interconnected individuals working together for some purpose.

Handoff a time when information is transferred, along with authority and responsibility, during transitions in care across the continuum; provides an opportunity to ask questions, clarify, and confirm responses.

Health care associated harm harm arising from or associated with plans or actions taken during the provision of health care rather than an underlying disease or injury.

Health information exchange (HIE) the mobilization of health care information digitally across organizations within a region or community. HIE provides the capability to move clinical information between separate health care information systems while maintaining the meaning of the information being exchanged.

Health information technology (HIT) a global term, which encompasses electronic health records and personal health records, to indicate the use of computers, software programs, electronic devices and the internet to store, retrieve, update, and transmit information about patients' health.

Health IT Policy Committee a federal advisory committee that makes recommendations to the Office of the National Coordinator for Health Information Technology (ONC) on a policy framework for the development and adoption of a nationwide health information infrastructure, including standards for the exchange of patient medical information (http://healthit.hhs.gov/portal/server.pt/community/healthit_hhs_gov__health_it_policy_committee/1269).

Health IT Standards Committee a federal advisory committee that makes recommendations to ONC on standards, implementation specifications, and certification criteria for the electronic exchange and use of health information (http://healthit.hhs.gov/portal/server.pt/community/healthit_hhs_gov__health_it_standards_committee/1271).

Health literacy the degree to which individuals have the capacity to obtain, process, and understand basic information and services needed to make appropriate decisions regarding their health.

Health Plan Employer Data and Information Set (HEDIS) Measures a set of health care quality measures designed to help purchasers and consumers determine how well health plans follow accepted care standards for prevention and treatment. Formerly known as the Health Plan Employer Data Information Set, health plans can receive accreditation on HEDIS measures from certain organizations, such as the National Committee on Quality Assurance.

Heterogeneity in systematic reviews, the amount of incompatibility between trials included in the review, whether clinical (i.e., the studies are clinically different) or statistical (i.e., the results are different from one another).

High-reliability organization (HRO) organization that maintains culture of safety, fosters a learning environment and evidence-based care, promotes positive working environments, and is committed to improving quality and safety. It incorporates the following: direct involvement of top and middle leadership, safety and quality efforts that are aligned with the organization strategic plan, an established infrastructure for safety and continuous improvement, and active engagement of staff across the organization.

Hierarchy of evidence a mechanism for determining which study designs have the most power to predict cause and effect. The highest level of evidence is systematic reviews of randomized clinical trials, and the lowest level of evidence is expert opinion and consensus statements.

Hospital Consumer Assessment of Healthcare Providers and Systems (H-CAHPS or CAHPS Hospital Survey) a standardized survey instrument and data collection methodology for measuring patients' perspectives of hospital care. Although many hospitals collect information on patient satisfaction, there is no national standard for collecting or publicly reporting this information that would enable valid comparisons to be made across all hospitals. H-CAHPS is a core set of questions that can be combined with customized, hospital-specific items to produce information that complements the data hospitals currently collect to support improvements in internal customer service and quality-related activities.

ICNP (International Classification for Nursing Practice) provides a formal terminology for nursing practice and a framework into which existing vocabularies and classifications can be cross-mapped to enable comparison of nursing data.

Improving Performance in Practice (IPIP) an initiative that is part of a project within the North Carolina Academy of Family Physicians. The program seeks to establish a designated quality improvement consultant (QIC) to work onsite with the practice leadership team to develop a practice-specific redesign plan utilizing the resources of collaborating experts.

Incident characteristics selected attributes of an incident.

Incident type descriptive term for a category made up of incidents of a common nature grouped because of shared, agreed features.

Inclusion criteria essential characteristics of potential participants established by the investigator that must be possessed in order to be considered for a study.

Informed decision-making (IDM) a term used to describe a process designed to help patients understand the nature of the disease or condition being addressed; understand the clinical service being provided including benefits, risks, limitations, alternatives, and uncertainties; consider their own preferences and values; participate in decision making at the level they desire; and make decisions consistent with their own preferences and values, or choose to defer a decision until a later time.

Institute for Healthcare Improvement (IHI) independent nonprofit organization helping to lead the improvement of health care throughout the world. Founded in 1991 and based in Cambridge, Massachusetts, IHI works to accelerate improvement by building the will for change, cultivating promising concepts for improving patient care, and helping health care systems put those ideas into action.

Institute of Medicine (IOM) nonprofit organization and honorific membership organization that works outside the framework of government to ensure scientifically informed analysis and independent guidance on matters of biomedical science, medicine, and health. The institute provides unbiased, evidence-based, and authoritative information and advice concerning health and science policy to policy makers, professionals, leaders in every sector of society, and the public at large. IOM's book on quality and safety, *Crossing the Quality Chasm: A New Health System for the 21st Century*, partially funded by the Robert Wood Johnson Foundation, reported that a huge divide exists between the care we should receive and the care that we get. *Crossing the Quality Chasm* introduces the notion that health care needs to take a page from industry and use its engineering improvement methods to aim for top quality, efficiency, and safety. The report lays out six goals that would become akin to a mantra for the quality improvement movement: care should be "safe, effective, patient-centered, timely, efficient, and equitable." IOM's 2003 landmark report, *Unequal Treatment: Confronting Racial and Ethnic Disparities in Health Care*, demonstrates the reality and effect of health disparities and quality-of-care differences for persons of racial and ethnic minorities.

Integrative reviews systematic summaries of the accumulated state of knowledge about a concept, including highlights of important issues left unresolved.

Interdisciplinary teams individuals from at least two different disciplines who coordinate their expertise to deliver care to patients. More recently, the term used is *interprofessional team.*

Interoperability the ability of different information technology systems and software applications to communicate; to exchange data accurately, effectively, and consistently; and to use the information that has been exchanged.

Interprofessional team a team made up of individuals from at least two distinct professions or disciplines.

Knowledge translation exchange, synthesis, and application of knowledge within a complex system of interactions among researchers and users to improve health, provide more effective health services and products, and strengthen the health care system.

LOINC (Logical Observation Identifiers Names and Codes) a database and universal standard for identifying medical laboratory observations.

Medical error a mistake that harms a patient. Adverse drug events, hospital-acquired infections, and wrong-site surgeries are examples of preventable medical errors.

Medical Subject Headings (MeSH) a thesaurus of medical terms used by many databases and libraries to index and classify medical information.

Meta-analysis a process of using quantitative methods to summarize the results from the multiple studies, obtained and critically reviewed using a rigorous process (to minimize bias) for identifying, appraising, and synthesizing studies to answer a specific clinical question and draw conclusions about the data gathered, to gain a summary statistic (i.e., a measure of a single effect) that represents the effect of the intervention across the multiple studies.

Microsystem small, functional, frontline units that provide most health care to most people. They are the essential building blocks of larger organizations and of the health system. They are the place where patients and providers meet. The quality and value of care produced by a large health system can be no better than the services generated by the small systems of which it is composed.

Misuse occurs when an appropriate process of care has been selected, but a preventable complication arises and the patient does not receive the full potential benefit of the service. Avoidable complications of surgery or medication use are misuse problems. A patient who suffers a rash after receiving penicillin for strep throat, despite having a known allergy to that antibiotic, is an example of misuse. A patient who develops a pneumothorax after an inexperienced operator attempted to insert a subclavian line would represent another example of misuse.

Mitigating factor an action or circumstance that prevents or moderates the progression of an incident toward harming a patient.

Model of care a conceptual object or diagram that provides an outline of how to plan all current and future facility and clinical service. It is important that the model of care be designed and evaluated for its ability to be replicated within the health care system. Models of care can help guide and direct a patient's experience within a health care system.

Multidisciplinary (or interprofessional) teams health care teams made up of health care professionals as well as health educators and/or community leaders.

NANDA-I an organization that catalogues nursing diagnoses to communicate the professional judgments that nurses make every day to patients, colleagues, members of other disciplines, and the public.

National Committee on Vital and Health Statistics a federal committee that makes recommendations to the Secretary of Health and Human Services on health data, statistics, privacy, national health information policy, and the department's strategy to best address those issues (www.ncvhs.hhs.gov).

National Guidelines Clearinghouse a comprehensive database of up-to-date, English-language, evidence-based clinical practice guidelines, developed in partnership with the American Medical Association, the American Association of Health Plans, and the Association for Healthcare Research and Quality.

Nationwide Health Information Network (NHIN) the technologies, standards, laws, policies, programs, and practices that enable health information to be shared among health decision makers, including consumers and patients, to promote improvements in health and health care. The vision for NHIN is said to have begun in 1991 with the publication of an Institute of Medicine report, "The Computer-Based Patient Record." The path to a national network of health care information is through the successful establishment of regional health information organizations. This has been a core component of the work of ONC (Office of the National Coordinator for Health Information Technology) to insure patient information is available at the point of care, regardless of the location of the patient and his or her data.

Near miss an incident that did not cause harm; events, situations, or incidents that could have caused adverse consequences and harmed a patient but did not. Sometimes referred to as a "good catch."

Never event/serious reportable event medical errors with serious consequences for which we have the knowledge to prevent, identified by the National Quality Forum.

NOC (Nursing Outcome Classification) a classification system that describes patient outcomes sensitive to nursing intervention.

Office of the National Coordinator for Health Information Technology (ONC) principal federal entity charged with coordination of nationwide efforts to implement and use the most advanced health information technology and the electronic exchange of health information. The position of National Coordinator was created in 2004, through an executive order, and legislatively mandated in the Health Information Technology for Economic and Clinical Health Act (HITECH Act) of 2009 (healthit.hhs.gov).

Opinion leaders individuals typically highly knowledgeable and well respected in a system; as such, they are often able to influence change.

Outcome the result of a process, including outputs, effects, and impacts.

Outcomes management the use of process and outcomes data to coordinate and influence actions and processes of care that contribute to patient achievement of targeted behaviors or desired effects.

Outcomes measurement a generic term used to describe the collection and reporting of information about an observed effect in relation to some care delivery process or health promotion action.

Outcomes research the use of rigorous scientific methods to measure the effect of some intervention on some outcome(s).

Overuse describes a process of care in circumstances where the potential for harm exceeds the potential for benefit. Prescribing an antibiotic for a viral infection like a cold, for which antibiotics are ineffective, constitutes overuse. The potential for harm includes adverse reactions to the antibiotics and increases in antibiotic resistance among bacteria in the community. Overuse can also apply to diagnostic tests and surgical procedures.

Partnership an explicit relationship with clear roles and responsibilities between two people who share a common goal or vision.

Patient activation the situation in which patients believe they have important roles to play in self-managing care, collaborating with providers, and maintaining their health; they know how to manage their condition and maintain functioning and prevent health declines; and they have the skills and behavioral repertoire to manage their condition, collaborate with their health providers, maintain their health functioning, and access appropriate and high-quality care.

Patient-centered care considers patients' cultural traditions, personal preferences and values, family situations, and lifestyles. Responsibility for important aspects of self-care and monitoring is put in patients' hands, along with the tools and support they need. Patient-centered care also ensures that transitions between different health care providers and care settings are coordinated and efficient. When care is patient-centered, unneeded and unwanted services can be reduced.

Patient-centered environment of care a care setting that is safe and clean, and that guards patient privacy. It also engages all the human senses with color, texture, artwork, music, aromatherapy, views of nature, and comfortable lighting, and considers the experience of the body, mind, and spirit of all who use the facility. Space is provided for loved ones to congregate, as well as for peaceful contemplation, meditation, or prayer; and patients, families, and staff have access to a variety of arts and entertainment that serve as positive diversions. At the heart of the environment of care, however, are the human interactions that occur within the physical structure to calm, comfort, and support those who inhabit it. Together the design, aesthetics, and these interactions can transform an institutional, impersonal, and alien setting into one that is truly healing (Picker Institute).

Patient-centered rounds regular patient visits in which health care professionals are careful to provide medical information to the patient, answer questions, and involve the patient in decisions (IOM).

Patient registry a patient database maintained by a hospital, doctors' practice, or health plan that allows providers to identify their patients according to disease, demographic characteristics, and other factors. Patient registries can help providers better coordinate care for their patients, monitor treatment and progress, and improve overall quality of care.

Patient safety freedom, for a patient, from unnecessary harm or potential harm associated with health care.

Patient safety incident an event or circumstance that could have resulted, or did result, in unnecessary harm to a patient.

Patient satisfaction a measurement designed to obtain reports or ratings from patients about services received from an organization, hospital, physician, or health care provider.

Patient values and preferences values the patient holds; concerns the patient has regarding the clinical decision/treatment/situation, choices the patient has/prefers regarding the clinical decision/treatment/situation.

Pay-for-performance (P4P) a method for paying hospitals and physicians based on their demonstrated achievements in meeting specific health care quality objectives. The idea is to reward providers for the quality, not the quantity, of care they deliver.

Payer the entity that assumes the risk of paying for medical treatments. Examples of payers include uninsured patients, self-insured employers, health plans, or HMOs.

Performance measures sets of established standards against which health care performance is measured. Performance measures are now widely accepted as a method for guiding informed decision making as a strong impetus for improvement.

Personal health record (PHR) a health record that is "owned" and maintained by an individual patient, rather than by payers or providers. Though the term has been around for several decades, it has recently received renewed attention with the adoption of electronic health records. Many health care organizations are offering PHRs to their patients to support their healthy life style and disease management activities.

PICOT format a process in which clinical questions are phrased in a manner that yields the most relevant information; P = patient population; I = intervention of interest; C = Comparison intervention or status; O = outcome; T = time.

Physician Quality Reporting Initiative (PQRI) a measure authorized through the Medicare, Medicaid, and SCHIP Extension Act of 2007. It is a financial incentive for health care professionals to improve the quality of care that they provide.

PNDS (Perioperative Nursing Data Set) a standardized nursing vocabulary that provides perioperative nurses a universal language for similar problems and treatments.

Prevalence the baseline risk of a disorder in the population of interest.

Preventable adverse event an event whose outcome, under the circumstances, was avoidable.

Process Improvement techniques and strategies used to make the processes implemented to solve health care problems better. Process improvement can occur in emergency room or hospital settings as well as in other health-system environments.

Productive pairs individuals who come together and develop a partnership to accomplish a shared goal.

Provider incentives inducements that motivate the regulation of health care. Examples of incentives include monetary rewards for providers who meet specific benchmark standards for their patient care.

p **value** the probability that a particular result would have happened by chance.

Publication or reporting bias a bias in a systematic review caused by incompleteness of the search, such as omitting non-English language sources or unpublished trials (inconclusive trials are less likely to be published than conclusive ones but are not necessarily less valid).

Public reporting information about physician and physician group performance available for consumers to use to compare the performance of local physicians/physician groups. The expectation is that a comparative public report of local physicians' performance in treating people with chronic illnesses will motivate and improve performance.

Purchasers the entity that not only pays the premium for health care costs but also controls the premium dollar before paying it to the provider. Included in the category of purchasers or payers are patients, businesses, and managed care organizations. While patients and businesses function as ultimate purchasers, managed care organizations and insurance companies serve a processing or payer function.

Quality and Safety Education for Nurses (QSEN) project that defined quality and safety competencies (derived from the IOM), including patient-centered care, teamwork and collaboration, evidence-based practice, quality improvement, safety, and informatics (www.QSEN.org).

Quality of care a measure of the ability of a doctor, hospital, or health plan to provide services for individuals and populations that increase the likelihood of desired health outcomes and are consistent with current professional knowledge. Good quality health care means doing the right thing at the right time, in the right way, for the right person, and getting the best possible results. According to the mantra for the quality improvement movement, care should be "safe, effective, patient-centered, timely, efficient, and equitable."

Quality of life the amount of happiness and balance in an individual's life. Attention to good health will create a better quality of life.

Quality improvement (QI) term first coined in the private sector, when corporations began looking at ways to streamline and improve processes and systems. The most well known example of quality improvement methodology is the "Six Sigma" method of change, developed by engineers at Motorola. In the health care context, the goal of quality improvement strategies is for patients to receive the appropriate care at the appropriate time and place with the appropriate mix of information and supporting resources. In many cases, health care systems are designed in such a way as to be overly cumbersome, fragmented, and indifferent to patients' needs. Quality improvement tools range from those that simply make recommendations but leave decision-making largely in the hands of individual physicians (e.g., practice guidelines) to those that prescribe patterns of care (e.g., critical pathways). Typically, quality improvement efforts are strongly rooted in evidence-based procedures and rely extensively on data collected about processes and outcomes.

Quality indicator agreed-upon process or outcome measure that is used to determine the level of quality achieved. It is a measurable variable (or characteristic) that can be used to determine the degree of adherence to a standard or achievement of quality goals.

Quality measures mechanisms used to assign a quantity to quality of care by comparison to a criterion.

Randomized controlled clinical trial a group of patients that is randomized into an experimental group and a control group. These groups are followed up for the variables/outcomes of interest.

Rapid-cycle change a quality improvement method that identifies, implements, and measures changes made to improve a process or a system. At the onset, the team sets an outcome measure based on the system's goals. Improvement occurs through small, rapid PDSA (Plan-Do-Study-Act) cycles to advance practice change. This model requires targeting a specific area to change; planning changes on the basis of sound science, theory, and evidence; piloting several changes with small patient groups; measuring the effects of changes; and acting according to the data. The fundamental concept of rapid-cycle improvement is that health care processes, once defined, in place, and in effect, should be continually improved by instituting a constant cycle of innovations or improvements.

Red rules standards for a particular process without exception.

Regional health information organization (RHIO) a multistakeholder organization, operating in a specific geographical area that enables the exchange and use of health information, in a secure manner, for the purpose of promoting the improvement of health quality, safety, and efficiency. Officials from the U.S. Department of Health and Human Services see RHIOs as the building blocks for the National Health Information Network (NHIN). When complete, the NHIN will provide universal access to electronic health records. As a result of the Health Information Technology for Economic and Clinical Health Act (HITECH Act) of 2009, RHIOs have been replaced with State health information exchange initiatives (http://healthit.hhs.gov/portal/server. pt/community/healthit_hhs_gov_state_health_information_exchange_program/1488).

Report card an assessment of the quality of care delivered by health plans. Report cards provide information on how well a health plan treats its members, keeps them healthy, and provides access to needed care. Report cards can be published by states, private health organizations, consumer groups, or health plans.

Research utilization process by which empirical findings from one or more studies are transformed into nursing interventions and/or tools that support clinical decision making such as guidelines, protocols, or algorithms.

Return on investment (ROI) the amount of improvement in care brought about by a certain investment. ROI can also refer to the theory that if you invest in health care quality now, then the quality of care for patients will improve in the future.

Right care made up of the treatments that, according to evidence-based guidelines, are effective and appropriate for a given condition. Indicators used to define right care are often grouped into two categories: prevention and chronic care.

Root-cause analysis (RCA) set of problem solving methods used to identify the series of actions and circumstances that led to an outcome, usually used to dissect a problem occurrence, although it could also trace the path of success.

Safety safe, effective care requires understanding the complexity of care delivery, the limits of human factors, safety design principles, characteristics of high-reliability organizations, and patient safety resources.

Safety science applies an organizational framework to minimize risk of harm to patients and providers through both system effectiveness and individual performance by applying human factors.

Safe zones designated areas where critical functions requiring concentration, such as medication preparation, are being performed and the clinician is not to be interrupted.

SBAR (situation, background, assessment, recommendation) a structured communication framework that helps health care providers clearly, consistently, and succinctly communicate pertinent information about patient care situations.

Sentinel event any unexpected event in a health care setting that causes death or serious injury to a patient and is not related to the natural course of the patient's illness.

SNOMED-CT (Systematized Nomenclature of Medicine Clinical Terms) a standardized, multilingual vocabulary of clinical terminology that is used by physicians and other health care providers for the electronic exchange of clinical health information.

Standard of care the expected level and type of care provided by the average caregiver under a certain given set of circumstances. These circumstances are supported through findings from expert consensus and based on specific research and/or documentation in scientific literature.

STEEEP Institute of Medicine acronym for six measures of health care quality based on whether care is safe, timely, effective, efficient, equitable, and patient centered.

Systematic review an article in which the authors have systematically searched for, appraised, and summarized all of the medical literature for a specific topic.

Systems a set of interdependent components that interact to achieve a common goal.

Task force a group convened to accomplish a specific objective within a designated period of time.

Team a small number of consistent people committed to a relevant shared purpose.

TeamSTEPPS (Team Strategies and Tools to Enhance Performance and Patient Safety) a training program developed by the Department of Defense and AHRQ that consists of content and exercises on leadership, situation monitoring, mutual support, and communication. It has been widely used outside of health care and, increasingly, within health care settings.

Teamwork a joint action by two or more people, in which each person contributes with different skills and expresses his or her individual interests and opinions to the unity and efficiency of the group in order to achieve common goals.

Throughput the ability of a medical facility, such as an emergency department, to complete a patient input and output cycle (i.e., to provide patients with the full cycle of care).

Translational research activities designed to transform ideas, insights, and discoveries generated through basic science inquiry and from clinical or population studies into effective and widely available clinical applications.

Transparency the process of collecting and reporting health care cost, performance, and quality data in a format that can be accessed by the public and is intended to improve the delivery of services and ultimately improve the health care system as a whole.

Triad for Optimal Patient Safety (TOPS) a multidisciplinary training program.

Underuse the failure to provide a health care service when it would have produced a favorable outcome for a patient. Standard examples include failure to provide appropriate preventive services to eligible patients (e.g., Pap smears, flu shots for elderly patients, screening for hypertension) and proven medications for chronic illnesses (steroid inhalers for asthmatics; aspirin, beta-blockers and lipid-lowering agents for patients who have suffered a recent myocardial infarction).

Validity the extent to which a variable or intervention measures what it is supposed to measure or accomplishes what it is supposed to accomplish. The *internal validity* of a study refers to the integrity of the experimental design. The *external validity* of a study refers to the appropriateness by which its results can be applied to nonstudy patients or populations.

Value purchasing a broad strategy used by some large employers to get more value for their health care dollars by demanding that health care providers meet certain quality objectives or supply data documenting their use of best practices and quality treatment outcomes.

Violation deliberate deviation from an operating procedure, standard, or rules.

Work flow a repeatable pattern of activity enabled by the organization of resources, defined roles, and information into a process that can be documented and learned. Improvements in work flow for health care providers will lessen the burden of providing health care and will lead to greater quality health care overall.

Index

Please note that any suffixes on numbers are as follows: b for boxes; f for figures; t for tables.

Quality and Safety in Nursing: A Competency Approach to Improving Outcomes, Second Edition.
Edited by Gwen Sherwood and Jane Barnsteiner.
© 2017 John Wiley & Sons, Inc. Published 2017 by John Wiley & Sons, Inc.